Low flow anaesthesia

To my wife Hilde
and my children Antje and Jan

Senior Commissioning editor: Melanie Tait
Development editor: Zoë A. Youd
Production controller: Chris Jarvis
Desk editor: Angela Davies
Cover designer: Alan Studholme

Low flow anaesthesia

The theory and practice of low flow, minimal flow and closed system anaesthesia

Second edition

Jan A. Baum Prof Dr med
Department of Anaesthesia and Intensive Care Medicine, Krankenhaus St Elisabeth-Stift, Damme, Germany

English text revised by

Geoffrey Nunn BA(Hons) MB BS FRCA
Consultant Anaesthetist, The General Infirmary at Leeds, Leeds, UK

With a Foreword by **Peter Lawin** Prof Dr med Dr h.c., FCCM
em. Chairman, Klinik and Poliklinik für Anaesthesiologie und operative Intensivmedizin, University of Münster, Germany

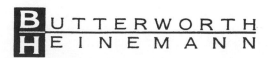

BUTTERWORTH
HEINEMANN

OXFORD   AUCKLAND   BOSTON   JOHANNESBURG   MELBOURNE   NEW DELHI

Butterworth-Heinemann
Linacre House, Jordan Hill, Oxford OX2 8DP
225 Wildwood Avenue, Woburn, MA 01801-2041
A division of Reed Educational and Professional Publishing Ltd

A member of the Reed Elsevier plc group

First German ed. 1988
Second German ed. 1992
Third German ed. 1998
First English ed. 1996
Revised English version 2001
First Chinese ed. 1993
First Italian ed. 1995
First Korean ed. 1999
Second English ed. 2001

British Library Cataloguing in Publication Data
Baum, Jan A.
  Low flow anaesthesia: the theory and practice of low flow,
  minimal flow and closed system anaesthesia. – 2nd ed.
  1 Anesthesiology – Aparatus and instruments   2 Inhalation
  anesthesia
  I. Title
  617.9′6

ISBN 0 7506 4672 1

Library of Congress Cataloguing in Publication Data
A catalogue record for this book is available from the Library of Congress

ISBN 0 7506 4672 1

Typeset by David Gregson Associates, Beccles, Suffolk
Printed and bound in Great Britain by MPG Books, Bodmin, Cornwall

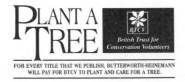

FOR EVERY TITLE THAT WE PUBLISH, BUTTERWORTH-HEINEMANN
WILL PAY FOR BTCV TO PLANT AND CARE FOR A TREE.

Contents

Foreword   xii

Preface to the second English edition   xiv

List of symbols and abbreviations   xix

Conversion table for different physical units of pressure   xxiii

1   Breathing systems – technical concepts and function   **1**
1.1   Classification of breathing systems according to underlying
      technical concepts   1
      1.1.1   Breathing systems without anaesthetic gas reservoir   2
      1.1.2   Non-rebreathing systems   2
              1.1.2.1   Flow-controlled non-rebreathing systems   2
              1.1.2.2   Valve-controlled non-rebreathing systems   7
      1.1.3   Rebreathing systems   7
              1.1.3.1   To-and-fro absorption systems   8
              1.1.3.2   Circle absorption systems   8
      1.1.4   Carbon dioxide absorption   9
      1.1.5   Hybrid breathing systems   10
1.2   Classification of breathing systems in accordance with
      functional criteria   11
      1.2.1   Open breathing systems   11
      1.2.2   Semi-open breathing systems   11
      1.2.3   Semi-closed breathing systems   11
      1.2.4   Closed breathing systems   11
1.3   Breathing systems according to technical and functional
      aspects   12
      1.3.1   Rebreathing systems   12
      1.3.2   Non-rebreathing systems   13
              1.3.2.1   Flow-controlled non-rebreathing systems   13
              1.3.2.2   Valve-controlled non-rebreathing systems   13
      1.3.3   Breathing systems without gas reservoir   14
1.4   Function of breathing systems in relation to the fresh gas
      flow   14

1.5 Advantages and disadvantages of the different breathing systems 15
1.6 References 16

2 Rebreathing systems – the development of a technical concept **18**
2.1 Development of breathing systems – historical perspective 18
    2.1.1 Development of open breathing systems 18
    2.1.2 Development of non-rebreathing systems 19
        2.1.2.1 Valve-controlled non-rebreathing systems 19
        2.1.2.2 Flow-controlled non-rebreathing systems 20
    2.1.3 Development of rebreathing systems 21
2.2 The development of semi-closed use of circle absorption systems – considerations on the current situation 32
2.3 References 35

3 Pharmacokinetics of anaesthetic gases **38**
3.1 Oxygen 38
    3.1.1 Oxygen uptake and consumption 38
    3.1.2 Implications for anaesthetic practice 39
3.2 Nitrous oxide 41
    3.2.1 Nitrous oxide uptake 41
    3.2.2 Implications for anaesthetic practice 42
3.3 Volatile anaesthetics 44
    3.3.1 Uptake of volatile anaesthetics 44
        3.3.1.1 Pharmacokinetics of volatile anaesthetics 44
        3.3.1.2 The Lowe uptake model 46
        3.3.1.3 The Westenskow uptake model 48
        3.3.1.4 The Lin uptake model 48
    3.3.2 Implications for anaesthetic practice 50
3.4 Total gas uptake 51
3.5 References 52

4 Anaesthetic methods with reduced fresh gas flow **54**
4.1 Low flow anaesthesia 57
4.2 Minimal flow anaesthesia 60
4.3 Closed system anaesthesia 61
    4.3.1 Non-quantitative closed system anaesthesia 68
    4.3.2 Quantitative closed system anaesthesia 70
4.4 References 70

5 Control of inhalational anaesthesia **73**
5.1 Computer simulation programs 73
    5.1.1 NARKUP 73
    5.1.2 Gas Man 73
    5.1.3 Clinical relevance of anaesthesia simulation by computer software 74
5.2 Control of inhalational anaesthesia 75
    5.2.1 The induction phase 75
    5.2.2 Maintenance of anaesthesia 79

5.2.2.1   Adapting the fresh gas flow to the uptake   79
5.2.2.2   Influence of the individual uptake   80
5.2.3   The time constant   80
5.2.4   Emergence from anaesthesia   84
5.3   Characteristics of anaesthesia management as a function
of fresh gas flow   85
5.4   Rules on anaesthetic management   86
5.5   References   87

6   **Advantages of the rebreathing techique in anaesthesia**   **88**
6.1   Reduced consumption of anaesthetic gases   88
6.2   Reduced costs   89
6.2.1   Anaesthetic gases   89
6.2.2   Soda lime consumption   94
6.3   Reduced environmental pollution   96
6.3.1   Workplace exposure to anaesthetic gas   96
6.3.2   Reduction of atmospheric pollution   98
6.3.2.1   Nitrous oxide   98
6.3.2.2   Halogenated hydrocarbons   99
6.4   Improved anaesthetic gas climate   100
6.4.1   Breathing gas temperature   101
6.4.2   Breathing gas humidity   103
6.4.3   Body temperature   105
6.4.4   Implications for anaesthetic practice   105
6.5   Extended potentials of patient monitoring and improved
knowledge of machine functions   107
6.6   References   107

7   **Technical requirements for anaesthesia management with reduced
fresh gas flow**   **111**
7.1   Technical regulations and standards   111
7.2   Technical requirements for the anaesthetic equipment with
respect to the extent of fresh gas flow reduction   111
7.2.1   Medical gas supply systems   111
7.2.2   Gas flow control systems   112
7.2.3   Vaporizers   116
7.2.3.1   Precision   117
7.2.3.2   Limitation of vaporizer output   120
7.2.3.3   Specified range of operation   121
7.2.3.4   The Tec 6 desflurane vaporizer   122
7.2.4   Breathing systems   123
7.2.4.1   Gas tightness   123
7.2.4.2   Fresh gas utilization   125
7.2.4.3   Specified range of operation   125
7.2.5   Carbon dioxide absorbers   126
7.2.5.1   Utilization period   126
7.2.5.2   Implications for anaesthetic practice   127
7.2.6   Anaesthesia ventilators   128
7.2.6.1   The gas reservoir   128

7.2.6.1.1   Anaesthetic machines without gas
reservoir   128
7.2.6.1.1.1   Airway pressure and
ventilation characteristics
with fresh gas flow
reduction   130
7.2.6.1.2   Anaesthetic machines with gas
reservoir   133
7.2.6.1.2.1   Bellows-in-box ventilators
with floating bellows   133
7.2.6.1.2.2   Bag-in-bottle ventilators   134
7.2.6.1.2.3   Ventilators with fresh gas
decoupling valve   134
7.2.6.2   Fresh gas flow compensation   135
7.2.6.2.1   Performance of ventilators without
fresh gas flow compensation   135
7.2.6.2.2   Technical possibilities to realize fresh
gas flow compensation   139
7.2.6.2.2.1   Fresh gas decoupling
valve   139
7.2.6.2.2.2   Electronic control of the
ventilator performance   140
7.2.6.2.2.3   Electronic control of
discontinuous fresh gas
supply   140
7.2.6.2.2.4   Electronic control of
discontinuous fresh gas
supply and ventilator
performance   141
7.3   Specific features of different anaesthetic machines   141
7.3.1   Aestiva 3000 (Datex-Ohmeda, Madison, USA)   141
7.3.2   AS/3 ADU Anesthesia Delivery Unit (Datex
Engström, Helsinki, Finland)   142
7.3.3   Cato, and Cicero (Dräger Medizintechnik,   Lübeck,
Germany)   143
7.3.4   Dogma, Access and Narkomat (Heyer, Bad Ems,
Germany)   147
7.3.5   ELSA and EAS 9010 (Gambro–Engström, Bromma,
Sweden)   149
7.3.6   Fabius (Dräger Medizintechnik, Lübeck, Germany)   151
7.3.7   Julian (Dräger Medizintechnik, Lübeck, Germany)   151
7.3.8   Megamed 700 and Mivolan (Megamed, Chain,
Switzerland)   153
7.3.9   Modulus SE and Excel SE (Ohmeda, Madison, USA)   155
7.3.10 Narkomed 4 (North American Dräger, Telford, USA)   156
7.3.11 SA 2 (Dräger Medizintechnik, Lübeck, Germany)   156
7.3.12 Servo Anesthesia System (Siemens–Elema, Solna,
Sweden)   158
7.3.13 Siemens Anesthesia System 711 (Siemens–Elema, Solna,
Sweden)   158

7.3.14 Sulla 909 (Dräger Medizintechnik, Lübeck, Germany) 160
7.3.15 System volumes of different anaesthetic machines 161
7.4 Anaesthetic machines with electronically controlled gas
delivery systems 162
7.4.1 PhysioFlex (Dräger Medizintechnik, Lübeck, Germany) 164
7.5 Implications for anaesthetic practice 166
7.5.1 Closed system anaesthesia 166
7.5.2 Minimal flow anaesthesia 166
7.5.3 Low flow anaesthesia 167
7.6 References 167

8 Monitoring 174
8.1 Technical regulations: safety facilities for inhalation
anaesthetic machines 174
8.2 Main- and side-stream gas analysers 174
8.2.1 Return of sampling gas 176
8.3 Measurement of oxygen concentration 178
8.4 Measurement of volatile anaesthetic concentration 179
8.4.1 Should anaesthetic agent measurement be performed
in the fresh gas or in the breathing system? 180
8.5 Measurement of nitrous oxide concentration 182
8.6 Measurement of carbon dioxide concentration 183
8.6.1 Flow-specific artefacts of the capnogram 183
8.6.2 Zero calibration 185
8.6.3 Implications for anaesthetic practice 187
8.7 Multi-gas analysers 187
8.8 References 189

9 Patient safety aspects of low flow anaesthesia 191
9.1 Specific risks of anaesthetic techniques with reduced fresh
gas flow 191
9.1.1 Risks attributable to inadequate technical equipment 191
9.1.1.1 Hypoxia 191
9.1.1.2 Hypoventilation and alterations in ventilation
patterns 192
9.1.1.3 Carbon dioxide accumulation in the breathing
system 193
9.1.1.4 Accidental increase of the airway pressure 193
9.1.1.5 Accidental overdose of volatile anaesthetics 194
9.1.2 Risks which are directly caused by reduction of the fresh
gas flow 195
9.1.2.1 The long time constant 195
9.1.2.2 Accumulation of foreign gas 196
9.1.2.2.1 Nitrogen 196
9.1.2.2.2 Acetone 197
9.1.2.2.3 Ethanol 198
9.1.2.2.4 Carbon monoxide 198
9.1.2.2.5 Argon 203
9.1.2.2.6 Methane 203

	9.1.2.2.7	Hydrogen	204
	9.1.2.2.8	Haloalkenes	204
	9.1.2.2.9	Implications for anaesthetic practice	206

9.2   Specific safety features of anaesthetic techniques with reduced
      fresh gas flow   207
      9.2.1   Improved equipment maintenance   207
      9.2.2   The long time constant   208
      9.2.3   Improved knowledge of the theory and practice of
              inhalation anaesthesia   210
9.3   Implications for anaesthetic practice   211
9.4   Contraindications for low flow anaesthetic techniques   213
      9.4.1   Relative contraindications   213
      9.4.2   Absolute contraindications   214
9.5   References   214

10   Low flow anaesthesia in clinical practice   220
10.1   Maintenance of the equipment   220
       10.1.1   Are there greater demands on disinfection or
                sterilization of the equipment resulting from fresh gas
                flow reduction?   222
10.2   Practice of low flow anaesthesia with halothane, enflurane and
       isoflurane   225
       10.2.1   Pre-medication and induction   225
       10.2.2   Initial phase of low flow inhalation anaesthesia   225
       10.2.3   The change from high to low fresh gas flow rate   226
                10.2.3.1   Low flow anaesthesia   226
                10.2.3.2   Minimal flow anaesthesia   226
                10.2.3.3   Anaesthetic gas composition   227
                           10.2.3.3.1   Inspired oxygen concentration   227
                           10.2.3.3.2   Metering of inhalation
                                        anaesthetics   231
                                        10.2.3.3.2.1   Isoflurane   231
                                        10.2.3.3.2.2   Enflurane   235
                                        10.2.3.3.2.3   Halothane   235
                           10.2.3.3.3   Control of the concentration of
                                        inhalation anaesthetics   238
       10.2.4   Emergence phase   239
10.3   Practice of low flow anaesthesia with desflurane and
       sevoflurane   241
       10.3.1   Desflurane   241
       10.3.2   Sevoflurane   245
10.4   Gas volume deficiency   247
10.5   Water condensation within the hosing   249
10.6   Economy and efficiency   250
10.7   The laryngeal mask airway   251
10.8   Paediatric anaesthesia   259
10.9   Low flow anaesthesia in cases of short duration (day-case
       surgery)   263
10.10 References   264

11   Low flow anaesthetic techniques without nitrous oxide   **269**
11.1   The routine use of nitrous oxide as carrier gas – pros
       and cons   269
11.2   Inhalation anaesthesia without nitrous oxide – general
       considerations with special respect to low flow anaesthetic
       techniques   271
11.3   Low flow anaesthetic techniques without nitrous oxide –
       clinical practice   272
       11.3.1   Minimal flow anaesthesia without nitrous oxide   272
       11.3.2   Non-quantitative closed system anaesthesia in
                clinical practice   275
11.4   Economics of low flow anaesthetic techniques without nitrous
       oxide   276
11.5   Are there any specific indications for the use of nitrous
       oxide?   278
11.6   References   279

12   Future perspectives   **281**
12.1   Future technical developments   281
12.2   Environmental protection and occupational health and safety   281
12.3   Future inhalational anaesthetics   282
       12.3.1   Xenon   282
       12.3.2   Oxygen as carrier gas   285
12.4   Improvements in patient care   286
12.5   Conclusions   287
12.6   References   287

Index   291

Foreword

The dominant question is no longer whether to use a closed circuit but how to use it safely.

H. J. Lowe and E. A. Ernst, 1981

Methods of anaesthesia with reduced fresh gas flows, up to the technique of 'quantitative anaesthesia' with a completely closed rebreathing system, have gained more and more interest in recent years. The present high standard of medical equipment, the potential for continuous and comprehensive analysis of anaesthetic gas composition, mandatory safety standards for anaesthetic equipment, and increased knowledge of the pharmacokinetics and pharmacodynamics of the inhalational anaesthetics justify the revival of these methods. This calls for a reappraisal of anaesthetic practice since, with a reduction of the fresh gas flow, the gas composition within the breathing system is increasingly determined by the technical and constructional characteristics of the particular breathing system, by the pharmacokinetic properties of the volatile anaesthetics and the individual patient's oxygen consumption, rather than by the composition of the fresh gas itself. Thus, the practical performance of anaesthesia with reduced fresh gas flow requires intense study of technical details, regularities of oxygen and inhalation anaesthetic uptake, and the fundamentals of organ transfer and elimination of anaesthetic gases.

This book, presented by J. Baum, is one of the few monographs on anaesthetic methods with reduced fresh gas flow providing a comprehensive up-to-date overview of the subject. Following discussion of theoretical fundamentals, the author refers in detail to problems and questions arising in the practical performance of these methods. The information on technical details and legal considerations refers to the actual equipment standards and relevant regulations.

Discussion on technical practicality, the potential perspectives of comprehensive non-invasive patient monitoring, and the clinical significance of quantitative anaesthesia is still continuing. However, there can be no doubt that, apart from all known advantages, the concern about anaesthesia with low fresh gas flow intensifies the need for the understanding of equipment function and the pharmacology of inhalational anaesthesia. This is not only an advantage with respect to mastering this anaesthetic method, but is very much also to the benefit of patient safety. Increasing utilization of rebreathing and the reduction of unused excess anaesthetic gas by electronic control of both volume and gas composition in the breathing system will doubtless become the technical concept of future generations of anaesthetic machines.

This book is recommended because of its exceptionally clear didactic concept and its straightforwardly structured, but nevertheless extensive, presentation of this subject. It deserves to be widely read: the interesting and useful methods of anaesthesia with low fresh gas flow will increasingly be applied in daily hospital routine.

Peter Lawin

Preface to the second English edition

As the fundamental books on low flow anaesthetic techniques (H. J. Lowe and E. A. Ernst's *The Quantitative Practice of Anesthesia* and J. A. Aldrete, H. J. Lowe and R. W. Virtue's *Low Flow and Closed System Anesthesia*) at that time were already more than 10 years old, in 1995 it seemed justified to submit a new English textbook, comprehensively describing the different aspects of anaesthesia with reduced fresh gas flow from a current point of view. Due to more stringent regulations on occupational safety and health, an increasing environmental awareness, the development of highly advanced anaesthetic machines and the demand for economical use of anaesthetic gases, there was an increasing interest in this subject. More and more anaesthetists became aware of the absurd anachronism that the majority of anaesthetic machines feature technically advanced rebreathing systems and monitoring devices but are mostly used with fresh gas flows which virtually exclude any rebreathing. A widespread acceptance of low flow anaesthetic techniques was not hindered by insufficient technical equipment but much more by lack of experience and a reluctance to learn new techniques.

The reason for reservations towards anaesthetic techniques with low fresh gas flow was based on the fact that the majority of anaesthetists are unfamiliar with these methods, and there was great uncertainty with respect to dosage of anaesthetic gases and the suitability of available anaesthetic machines for these methods. In addition, there were still concerns about process-inherent hazards such as accidental hypoxia and overdose of volatile anaesthetics.

It was the objective of the first edition of this book to clarify the specific problems of these anaesthetic techniques and available equipment. At the same time, it sought to overcome unjustified reservations by giving practical advice on the performance of these methods.

New technical developments, scientific realizations and professional regulations in recent years now require a comprehensive revision of the first English edition of this book, 4 years after its first publication. In 1999, by submitting a revised draft of the prEN ISO 4135 'Anaesthetic and respiratory equipment – Vocabulary' for statement, the ISO general secretariat took the first steps towards international standardization of the terminology with respect to anaesthetic machines and breathing systems. The new common technical norm EN 740 'Anaesthetic workstations and their modules – Particular requirements' became compulsory in 1998 in all the countries of the European Union. All technical preconditions to safely perform low flow techniques are now met by the standard safety equipment stipulated for all anaesthetic machines. Nearly all new anaesthetic machines are nowadays advertised to be especially suited for low flow anaesthetic techniques, and most of the new anaesthetic ventilators feature fresh gas flow compensation and gas reservoir. An increasing number of scientific publications have focused on the degradation of inhalational anaesthetics by carbon dioxide absorbents. The matter became even more relevant as the first reports on harmful effects of the gaseous degradation products in clinical practice were published. The use of potassium-free soda lime reduces chemical degradation of the anaesthetic agents, the consistent use of calcium hydroxide lime seems to be very promising and may even completely solve this problem. Sevoflurane and desflurane have become the routinely used inhalation anaesthetics in many departments. With respect to economical and ecological aspects, just these anaesthetics, characterized by low solubility and decreasing anaesthetic potency, should only be used with low flow anaesthetic techniques. The routine use of nitrous oxide as a component of the carrier gas has been unanimously called into question in recent surveys. In fact, its use is now recommended in indicated cases only. Although many authors are now ready to dismiss nitrous oxide, there seems to be no consensus yet as to what indications will remain for its use. Omitting the use of nitrous oxide significantly facilitates the performance of low flow techniques. The realization of closed system anaesthesia with conventional anaesthetic machines in routine clinical practice with a fresh gas flow as low as the individual's oxygen uptake becomes possible. Recently the first reports on the advantageous effects of high concentrations of oxygen in the carrier gas were published. This would simplify even more the routine use of extremely low fresh gas flow rates; this matter, however, is still under scientific discussion. New relevant findings on anaesthetic gas climatization by reduction of the fresh gas flow rates were recently released. Xenon will before long be officially approved as a medical gas in the countries of the European Union. All these different topics are comprehensively discussed in the second edition of this book.

As in the preface to the first edition, I wish to thank my esteemed clinical and academic teacher, Prof. Dr med Dr h.c. Peter Lawin, FCCM, em. Chairman and Director of the Klinik und Poliklinik für Anaesthesiologie und operative Intensivmedizin at the University of Münster for his continuous and benevolent support of my clinical and scientific work. The author's own investigations on low flow anaesthetic techniques, which include a vast number of individual measurements, could not have been accomplished without the assistance of my colleagues, Chief Physician Dr G. Sachs and the Senior Anaesthetists Dr Ch. von den Driesch, Dr K. Brauer, Dr B. Sievert and Dr med G. Stanke. I feel greatly obliged for their committed assistance. This also goes for the anaesthetic nursing staff of the author's department, K. Luzak, U. Kramer, Th. Krausse and W. Weitzmann, who took a great interest in the technical details of anaesthetic machines, this being an indispensable requirement for safe performance of this anaesthetic technique. I owe special gratitude to the chief anaesthetic nurse, R. Prior, who made great contributions in preparing the chapter on equipment maintenance.

It would not have been possible to compile all the facts given in this book without any help. Thus, I owe a debt of gratitude to several professional colleagues who supported my scientific work, helped me by benevolent criticism, or made contributions to writing or finalizing of the book's text on different topics: anaesthetic gas climatization: Prof. Dr U. Hölscher, Fachhochschule Münster, Priv. Doz. Dr J. Rathgeber, Albertinen-Krankenhaus, Hamburg and Dr K. Züchner, Universität Göttingen; carbon monoxide, haloalkenes and carbon dioxide absorbents: Dr M. Leier, Städtische Kliniken Nürnberg, Prof. Dr D. Pankow, Universität Halle and Prof. Dr med J. M. Strauß, Medizinische Hochschule Hannover; desflurane and sevoflurane: Dr M. Berghoff, Prof. em. Dr G. Kalff and Dr M. Petermeyer, Rheinisch-Westfälische Technische Hochschule Aachen, and Prof. Dr H. v. Aken, Universität Münster; general and technical aspects of low flow anaesthesia: Prof. Dr A. R. Aitkenhead, University of Nottingham, Dr L. Atzmüller, Linz, Prof. Dr W. Erdmann, University of Rotterdam, Dr Ch. Hönemann, Universität Münster and Prof. Dr G. Rolly, University of Gent; nitrous oxide free inhalational anaesthesia: Prof. Dr J. Coetzee, University of Capetown, Dr G. Fröba, Universität Ulm and Dr J. Mas Marfany, Hospital General de Catalunya, Barcelona; occupational safety and health: Prof. Dr J. Hobbhahn, Universität Regensburg; paediatric anaesthesia: Dr G. Habel, Humboldt-Universität, Klinikum Berlin-Buch; xenon anaesthesia: Prof. Dr C. Lynch III, University of Charlottesville, Priv. Doz. Dr T. Marx, Universität Ulm and Dr R. Tenbrinck, University of Rotterdam. The annual meetings of the Association for Low Flow Anaesthesia are always an occasion for extraordinarily fruitful scientific information and exchange. For continuous benevolent support of and interest in my work I especially want to thank all my friends and colleagues in ALFA. The first English version of my book became the base for editions in other countries. With heartiest gratitude I have to mention the colleagues who took over the tremendous task to translate and publish the work in other languages: in Italian Prof. Dr Francesco Giunta, University of Pisa, in Korean Prof. Dr Suk-Min Yoon, University of Seoul, and in Japanese Prof. Dr Hidenori Toyooka, Tsukuba-University.

Whenever I needed any support or help in understanding or mastering of technical details and problems I always could trustingly turn to Mrs Sandy Brandmeier (USA), Dipl.-Ing. R. Dittmann, Ing. F. Gürtler (Switzerland), Dr M. Graw, Mr M. Holder BSc(Hons) (UK), Dr D.-O. von Karger, Dipl.-Ing. Th. Krießmer, Dr Ciarán Magee (Northern Ireland), Dipl.-Ing. Ch. Manegold, Mr L. Thielen, Dipl.-Ing. Th. Simmerer, Mr J. Vallikari MSc (Finland), Dr-Ing. C. Wallroth, Ing. B. Westerkamp (The Netherlands) and Mr R. Wulf.

The different manufacturers of anaesthetic equipment again generously provided me with all the illustrative material needed to prepare the figures contained in the book.

Last but not least I would like to thank my dear colleague and friend Dr Geoffrey Nunn BA(Hons) MB BS FRCA, The General Infirmary at Leeds, UK, who made a lot of brilliant and essential suggestions to improve the text and its content, and who again will take over the difficult task of transferring my rough 'German English' into a readable and smooth English text. I also owe a debt of gratitude to Dr G. Smaldon, Butterworth-Heinemann, who supported my intention to prepare a second revised edition of this book, and to Mrs Myriam Brearley, Editorial Assistant, and Mrs Melanie Tait, Commissioning Editor, who took care of the manuscript during the publishing process.

Jan Baum
Damme, March 2000

Symbols and abbreviations

$AaDO_2$	Alveolar–arterial oxygen partial pressure difference
AD_{95}	Anaesthetic concentration at which 95% of all patients tolerate skin incision without any motor response
$aeDCO_2$	Arterial–end-expiratory carbon dioxide partial pressure difference
ANSI	American National Standards Institute
APL	Airway pressure limit
APV	Alternating pressure ventilation
bar	Bar
BCDFE	2-Bromo-2-chloro-1,1-difluoroethylene
BMI	Body mass index (kg/m^2): weight (kg) divided by patient's height (m) squared
BW (kg)	Patient's body weight in kilograms
C_A	Alveolar concentration
C_a	Arterial concentration
C_{CO}	Carbon monoxide concentration
CD	Cumulative dose
C_i	Inspiratory concentration
C_f	Fresh gas concentration
CFC	Chlorofluorocarbons
CO	Carbon monoxide
COHb	Carbon monoxide haemoglobin
Compound A	Fluoromethyl-2,2-difluoro-1-trifluoromethyl-vinylether
EN 740	Common European Standard: 'Anaesthetic Workstations and their Modules' Essential Requirements
EU	European Union
$E:I$	Expiratory time to inspiratory time ratio
F_A	Alveolar fraction
FGE valve	Fresh gas decoupling valve (FGE = Frischgasentkoppelung)
FGF	Fresh gas flow
FGU	Fresh gas utilization
F_i	Inspired fraction
F_{iN_2O}	Inspired fraction of nitrous oxide
F_{iO_2}	Inspired fraction of oxygen
h	Hour

HF	High fresh gas flow
HME	Heat and moisture exchanger
$I : E$	Inspiratory time to expiratory time ratio
IPPV	Intermittent positive pressure ventilation
ISO	International Standards Organization
I_{tox}	Toxicity index
kPa	Kilopascal
LMA	Laryngeal mask airway
$\lambda_{B/G}$	Blood–gas partition coefficient
$\lambda_{T/B}$	Tissue–blood partition coefficient
LD_{50}	Lethal dose, 50% of a trial
MAC	Minimum alveolar concentration at which 50% of all patients tolerate skin incision without any motor response
MAC_{N_2O}	Minimum alveolar concentration of nitrous oxide
MAK	Maximale Arbeitsplatzkonzentration (maximum workplace concentration)
mbar	Millibar
MF	Minimal fresh gas flow
MGA	Multi-gas analyser
ms	Millisecond
MV	Ventilatory minute volume
NAD	North American Dräger
NARKUP	Computer simulation program 'NARKUP'
NIOSH	National Institute of Occupational Safety and Health
ORC	Oxygen ratio controller: anti-hypoxic device pneumatically coupling the nitrous oxide to the oxygen flow to guarantee at least 25% oxygen in the fresh gas
$PaCO_2$	Arterial carbon dioxide partial pressure
PaO_2	Arterial oxygen partial pressure
PCV	Pressure-controlled ventilation
PD	Prime dose
PEEP	Positive end-expiratory pressure
$PeCO_2$	End-expiratory carbon dioxide partial pressure
PONV	Postoperative nausea and vomiting
$\dot{Q}$	Cardiac output (dl/min)
$Q_{i/f}$	Inspired concentration/fresh gas concentration quotient
Q_T	Tissue (organ) blood flow
Q_{eff}	Efficiency coefficient
RAM	Random access memory
s	Second
SIMV	Synchronized intermittent mandatory ventilation
T	Time constant
t	Time (min)
TLV list	Table of threshold limit values
TMF	Percentage of time during which minimal flow anaesthesia is performed
TV	Tidal volume
UD	Unit dose
V_A	Alveolar volume
$\dot{V}_A$	Alveolar minute volume

$\dot{V}_{AN}$	Uptake of volatile anaesthetic
$\dot{V}_{CO_2}$	Carbon dioxide production
V_{Del}	Amount of anaesthetic agent (or anaesthetic gas) delivered into the breathing system with the fresh gas flow
$\dot{V}_F$	Fresh gas flow
V_{Fi}	Inspiratory delivered fresh gas volume
$\dot{V}_{FN_2O}$	Nitrous oxide flow (fresh gas)
$\dot{V}_{FO_2}$	Oxygen flow (fresh gas)
$\dot{V}_{ISO}$	Isoflurane uptake
$\dot{V}_{N_2O}$	Nitrous oxide uptake/consumption (ml/min)
$\dot{V}_{O_2}$	Oxygen uptake/consumption (ml/min)
$\dot{V}_{FN_2O}$	Nitrous oxide flow
VIC	Vaporizer inside the circuit
V_L	Lung volume
VOC	Vaporizer outside the circuit
V_S	System volume (gas containing volume of the anaesthetic apparatus)
V_T	Tissue (organ) volume
$\dot{V}_U$	Amount of anaesthetic agent (or anaesthetic gas) taken up by the patient
Xe	Xenon

Conversion table for different physical units of pressure

$1\,\text{mbar} = 100\,\text{Pa} = 1\,\text{hPa}$

$1\,\text{cmH}_2\text{O} = 98.0665\,\text{Pa}$

$1\,\text{kp/cm}^2 = 98066.5\,\text{P} = 98.0665\,\text{kPa}$

$1\,\text{torr} = 133.3\,\text{Pa} = 1.333\,\text{mbar} = 1.333\,\text{hPa}$

$1\,\text{mmHg} = 133.3\,\text{Pa}$

$1\,\text{mbar} \approx 1\,\text{cmH}_2\text{O}$

$1\,\text{cmH}_2\text{O} \approx 0.1\,\text{kPa}$

Breathing systems – technical concepts and function

Breathing systems are the technical elements of anaesthetic machines by means of which anaesthetic gas is administered to the patient. According to the underlying technical concept, the breathing system serves the following purposes:

- making up of the anaesthetic gases from different shares of fresh and expired gas;
- delivery of the anaesthetic gases to the patient;
- elimination of the expired carbon dioxide;
- separation of the anaesthetic gases from the surrounding atmosphere; and
- conditioning of the anaesthetic gases.

All these functions make the breathing system not only the conveyor of the anaesthetic gases but also the interactive technical link between the patient and the apparatus. The breathing system provides and determines the composition and condition of the respired gases.

1.1 Classification of breathing systems according to underlying technical concepts

Up to now there has been no internationally standardized and binding terminology and classification of the breathing systems. In accordance with the recommendations given by E. A. Ernst[1], the ISO norm 4135, being identical to the draft of a common European norm prEN ISO 4135 'Anaesthetic and respiratory equipment – Vocabulary'[2], the classification and terminology should be based on the basic technical concept of the breathing systems. In contrast, the definitions and classifications based on specific individual terminology, for instance: '... a Mapleson A type breathing system [generic terminology] would describe the mode of operation of a Magill breathing system [specific terminology]'[3], significantly contradicts the intention of the above-mentioned technical norms in standardizing the terminology. Great efforts should be made to obtain international agreement on standardizing the classification of breathing systems, which would facilitate scientific and technical exchange.

1.1.1   Breathing systems without anaesthetic gas reservoir (Figure 1.1)

Breathing systems without an anaesthetic gas reservoir cannot ensure the separation of the anaesthetic gases from the surrounding atmosphere. Thus, a precise control of the anaesthetic concentration delivered to the patient is impossible, though accidental uncontrollable admixture of air to the anaesthetic gases remains a real possibility.

These breathing systems are characterized by their extremely simple technical design, and a near-negligible resistance to breathing. The lack of an anaesthetic gas reservoir, however, is responsible for the uncontrolled admission of atmospheric air in the case of a deep inspiration. The term 'breathing system without anaesthetic gas reservoir' covers a wide range of equipment such as anaesthetic drip masks for application of ether or chloroform, including the Schimmelbusch mask, or insufflation systems, like the Boyle–Davies gag.

1.1.2   Non-rebreathing systems (Figure 1.1)

Non-rebreathing systems are intended to be used without rebreathing. They are thus characterized technically by the lack of any means for absorption of the exhaled carbon dioxide. From a technical point of view they are not designed for reusing the anaesthetic gases and vapours contained in the expired gas of an anaesthetized patient during the following inspiration, but rather are designed such that the entire expired gas, or at least the carbon dioxide containing alveolar gas, is removed from the system by venting it as waste into the atmosphere, and replenished by fresh gas.

1.1.2.1   Flow-controlled non-rebreathing systems (Figures 1.1 and 1.2)

In flow-controlled non-rebreathing systems the exhaled air containing carbon dioxide is removed from the breathing system by a sufficiently high fresh gas flow. The fresh gas flow can be uni- or contradirectional to the flow of the expired air. The simplicity of the technical design and the low respiratory resistance are considered to be the particular advantages of these systems.

Flow-controlled non-rebreathing systems are classified according to the scheme devised by Mapleson[11] (Figure 1.3):

Mapleson A: During expiration, the fresh gas flow is counterdirectional to the flow of the expired air, which is vented out of the breathing system via an expiratory valve close to the airway of the patient. Both the Magill and the Lack system in its coaxial and parallel version are variants of the Mapleson A.

Mapleson B and C: The position of the connector for fresh gas delivery and the expiratory valve are both close to the patient connection. The gas reservoir contains a mixture of expired and fresh gas.

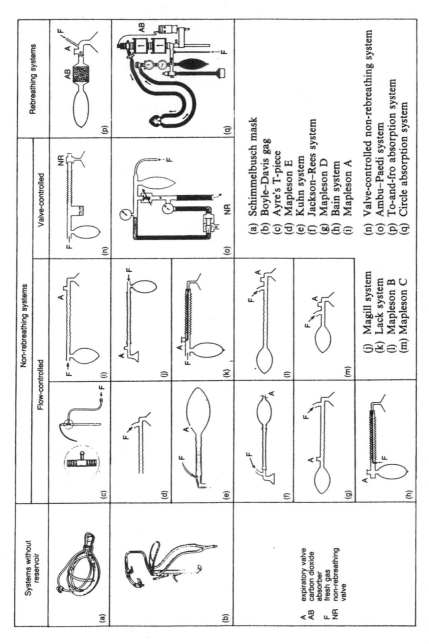

Figure 1.1 Synoptic presentation of breathing systems, classified according to their basic technical concept (from references 4–10)

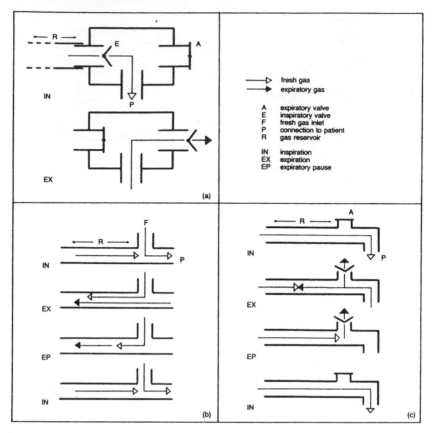

Figure 1.2   Different technical concepts for discharge of exhaled gas: (a) non-rebreathing valve (valve-controlled non-rebreathing system); (b) flow-controlled discharge of the exhaled gas via the reservoir tube (flow-controlled non-rebreathing system, type: Ayre's T-piece); (c) flow-controlled discharge of the exhaled gas via an exhaust port (flow-controlled non-rebreathing system, type: Mapleson A)

Mapleson D: The fresh gas is delivered into the system close to the patient connection, whereas the expired gases are vented out of the system via an expiratory valve at the end of the reservoir hose close to the reservoir bag. During expiration, the fresh gas flow and the flow of the expired gases are unidirectional. The Bain system and the Penlon coaxial system (USA) are both coaxial variants of the Mapleson D.

Mapleson E: From the functional point of view, this is similar to the Mapleson D system, though without a reservoir bag. Since, though, it lacks a reservoir bag, the volume of the hose must at least equal the inspired tidal volume (less the inspiratory phase portion of the fresh gas flow) to avoid admixture of ambient air with the respired gases. The Ayre's T-piece is the most commonly used variant of the Mapleson E system.

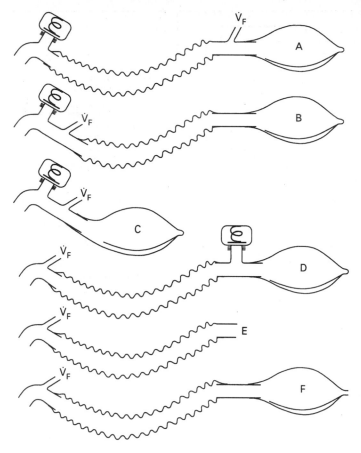

Figure 1.3 Mapleson's classification of the flow-controlled non-rebreathing systems (Mapleson A to F) (from reference 12)

Mapleson F: In 1975 the Jackson–Rees System was added to Mapleson's classification under the term Mapleson F[13]. The Kuhn system, formerly much used in paediatric anaesthesia in Germany, is also a Mapleson F system.

Where Mapleson systems types D, E and F are concerned, the expired gas is washed out of the system during the expiratory phase by a vigorous unidirectional flow of fresh gas (Figure 1.2b). However, with the Mapleson systems types A, B and C, a vigorous fresh gas flow opposes the expiratory flow, increasing the pressure within the system which, in turn, opens an exhaust valve, through which the expiratory volume is discharged out of the system (Figure 1.2c).

Should the fresh gas flow not be sufficiently high, elimination of exhaled gases will be incomplete in all flow-controlled non-rebreathing systems.

Table 1.1   Flow-controlled non-rebreathing systems – recommended fresh gas flow for safe elimination of the carbon dioxide containing exhaled air (12, 14, 17, 18)

	Spontaneous breathing	*Controlled ventilation*
Mapleson A ≡ Magill-System	56–82 ml/kg × min 0.7–1.0 × MV	2–3 × MV
Lack-System	51–85 ml/kg × min 0.6–0.9 × MV	2–3 × MV
Mapleson B	1.5–2 × MV	2–2.5 × MV
Mapleson C	1.5–3 × MV	2–2.5 × MV
Mapleson D	150–300 ml/kg × min 4000–4700 ml/m^2 × min 1.5–3 × MV	0.7–1.5 × MV
Bain-System	200–300 ml/kg × min 2 × MV	70 ml/kg × min 1–1.5 × MV
Mapleson E ≡ Ayre's T-piece	2–4 × MV	2–3 × MV
Mapleson F ≡ Jackson–Rees-System	2–4 × MV	1–2 × MV
Humphrey ADE-System	>50 ml/kg × min	>70 ml/kg × min

Thus, given the basic technical design of all flow-controlled non-rebreathing systems, the rebreathing of exhaled gas is possible in principle. Excessive rebreathing, however, will cause an undesirable carbon dioxide enrichment in the system due to the lack of a carbon dioxide absorber.

Although all these breathing systems comprise similar components, the efficiency of each system is different. They are ranked by the Mapleson classification in order (A to F) of increased requirement of fresh gas flow to safely prevent rebreathing during spontaneous respiration[3]. It is for this reason that specific values are quoted for the fresh gas flow for each of the systems, to prevent excessive rebreathing (Table 1.1). This supports the use of the term 'non-rebreathing' for these types of systems.

The efficiency of the non-rebreathing systems is judged by the lowest fresh gas flow which safely prevents rebreathing of alveolar gas. The wash-out of the expired gas in flow-controlled non-rebreathing systems is governed by:

- the technical design (arrangement of the fresh gas inlet, anaesthetic gas reservoir and exhaust port in relation to the patient connection) and the dimensions of the reservoirs;
- the ventilation mode and pattern (spontaneous or controlled ventilation, tidal volume, breathing frequency, inspiratory–expiratory time relation, duration of the expiratory pause and the dead space of the system); and
- the fresh gas flow.

The efficiency of flow-controlled non-rebreathing systems can be defined by applying the following formula[16]:

$$\text{Efficiency} = \text{Minute Volume/Lowest Fresh}$$
$$\text{Gas Flow}_{\text{(to adequately prevent rebreathing)}}$$

According to Dorsch and Dorsch[14], the efficiency of non-rebreathing systems decreases in the order Mapleson A, D, F, E, C and B in spontaneous breathing, whereas it decreases in the order Mapleson D, F, E, B, C and A in controlled ventilation. Thus, different gas flows are recommended for the different flow-controlled non-rebreathing systems to safely prevent any significant carbon dioxide rebreathing.

Humphrey ADE system: The Humphrey ADE system allows, by means of a lever, a change from the function of a Mapleson A to the function of a Mapleson D or E mode[14,15]. Thus, the breathing system can be adapted to the respective mode of ventilation. During spontaneous breathing the Humphrey ADE system is used as Mapleson A, and during controlled ventilation as a Mapleson D or E system.

1.1.2.2   Valve-controlled non-rebreathing systems (Figures 1.1 and 1.2a)

In valve-controlled non-rebreathing systems, the inspired air is separated completely from the expired gas by a non-rebreathing valve, attached close to the patient's airway. Thus, rebreathing of any exhaled gas is technically impossible, as it is discharged completely into the atmosphere. During inhalation the patient always gets pure fresh gas, the flow of which must equal or exceed the minute volume of the patient. An anaesthetic reservoir bag attached to the inspiratory limb guarantees a sufficient fresh gas volume even if the patient inspires vigorously.

1.1.3   Rebreathing systems (Figure 1.1)

'Rebreathing' describes a technique in which non-consumed gases, contained in the exhaled air, are partially or completely re-routed back to the patient during the following inspiration, purified from carbon dioxide and admixed with a certain amount of fresh gas. This means that devices which eliminate carbon dioxide from the expired gas must be made an indispensable and integral part of such systems. The technical hallmark for rebreathing systems is therefore the carbon dioxide absorber, a container filled with granules of alkali metal and/or alkaline earth metal hydroxides for chemical absorption of the carbon dioxide contained in the exhaled air. It seems more than somewhat absurd to intentionally use the term 'Non-Rebreathing Systems using Carbon Dioxide Absorption'[3] to characterize just these systems which, from a technical point of view, are especially designed for rebreathing. Again, the author refers to the prEN ISO 4135 in which the term 'non-rebreathing system' is defined as 'anaesthesia breathing system from which all the expired mixture is discharged'[2].

1.1.3.1   To-and-fro absorption systems (Figure 1.1)

In the to-and-fro absorption system, the carbon dioxide absorber, via which the patient inhales and exhales the anaesthetic gases, is positioned close to the patient connection port. With prolonged use, due to its preferential exhaustion of the absorbent nearest the patient, the system's dead space increases. Due to its position close to the patient, the handling of a to-and-fro system is cumbersome; its technical design, however, is very simple.

1.1.3.2   Circle absorption systems (Figure 1.1)

Due to the function of the unidirectional inspiratory and expiratory valves, the anaesthetic gas circulates from the expiratory to the inspiratory limb of the circle absorption system, merging at the patient connection. The unidirectional flow of the anaesthetic gases within the circle ensures the separation of the exhaled from the inspired anaesthetic gases. That part of the exhaled air, not discharged out of the system as excess gas, will pass through the carbon dioxide absorber.

In most circle absorption systems the circular flow of the anaesthetic gases derives from the function of the unidirectional valves. In a few other circle systems the flow of the anaesthetic gases is generated by other technical means with the aim of avoiding the use of valves and thus reducing the resistance to gas flow[3,14]. In Revell's circulator, a fan assists the circulation within the circle system, a technique which was realized as early as 1915 in Jackson's rebreathing circle system (Figure 2.8)[19]. This method is in current use in the PhysioFlex anaesthetic machine (Figure 7.34)[20]. In Neff's circulator (Figure 1.4), the propulsion of the gas results from the Venturi effect generated by the fresh gas entering the breathing system.

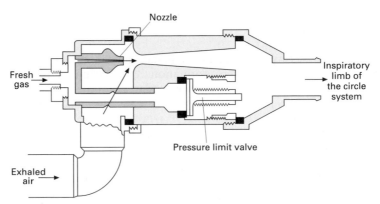

Figure 1.4   Neff's circulator: the anaesthetic gas, driven by a Venturi effect generated by the fresh gas flow, circulates continuously within the circle absorption system (from Davey A, Moyle JTB and Ward CS. Ward's Anaesthetic Equipment, 3rd edn. W.B. Saunders, London, 1992)

1.1.4   Carbon dioxide absorption

The carbon dioxide contained in the exhaled gases is chemically bound by granules of a mixture of alkali metal and alkaline earth metal hydroxides. This absorbent is contained in a canister which is attached to the rebreathing system. Four different absorbents are available. The two classical absorbents are soda lime and barium lime.

Conventional *soda lime* contains 1–4% sodium hydroxide (NaOH), 1–4% potassium hydroxide (KOH), 75–85% calcium hydroxide $(Ca(OH)_2)$ and 14–18% water (H_2O). One hundred grams of soda lime can absorb about 26 litres carbon dioxide according to the following chemical processes:

$$CO_2 + H_2O \rightarrow H_2CO_3$$

$$H_2CO_3 + 2NaOH \rightleftharpoons Na_2CO_3 + 2H_2O$$

$$\text{or}\quad H_2CO_3 + 2KOH \rightleftharpoons K_2CO_3 + 2H_2O$$

$$Na_2CO_3 + Ca(OH)_2 \rightleftharpoons CaCO_3 + 2NaOH$$

$$\text{or}\quad K_2CO_3 + Ca(OH)_2 \rightleftharpoons CaCO_3 + 2KOH$$

During this exothermic reaction 13.7 kcal and 1 mol of water are formed by the absorption of 1 mol of carbon dioxide.

Barium lime contains 20% $Ba(OH)_2 \cdot 8H_2O$ (this corresponds to an additional water content of about 15%), 1–4% KOH and about 65% $Ca(OH)_2$. One hundred grams of barium lime can absorb 27 litres carbon dioxide according to following chemical reactions:

$$CO_2 + H_2O \rightarrow H_2CO_3$$

$$H_2CO_3 + Ba(OH)_2 \rightleftharpoons BaCO_3 + 2H_2O$$

$$BaCO_3 + Ca(OH)_2 \rightleftharpoons CaCO_3 + Ba(OH)_2$$

The alkali metal hydroxides are used to accelerate the absorption of carbon dioxide, KOH in particular speeds up carbon dioxide absorption at lower temperatures. The water is indispensable for starting the chemical reaction between the metal hydroxides and carbon dioxide. Silica, zeolites and kieselguhr, a clay, are used to enhance mechanical stability of the granules and to prevent dust formation[21,22]. Barium lime was used mostly in the USA and, to a lesser extent in some Asian countries, whereas soda lime is generally used world-wide. The absorbents are used as irregular granules or compressed to pellets with a grain size between 2 and 5 mm. The binding capacity of absorbents compressed to pellets was found to be superior to irregular-shaped granules[23,24].

Due to the fact that strong alkali hydroxides are mainly responsible for the degradation of volatile agents, two new kinds of absorbents have recently been introduced into the market omitting or reducing these components, in particular potassium hydroxide (see Sections 6.2.2, 9.1.2.2.4 and 9.1.2.2.8).

The carbon dioxide absorbers of many modern anaesthesia machines, which are referred to as 'Jumbo canisters', mostly contain between 1.5 and

2 litres of absorbent. Formerly, mostly 1 litre canisters were used routinely which, for safety reasons, were used as double absorbers, one on top of the other. The absorption capacity of 1 litre of soda lime is given as 120 litres carbon dioxide under clinical conditions. Assuming the entire exhaled volume passes through the absorber canister, a minute volume of 10 l/min and an expired carbon dioxide concentration of 4.0 vol%, the lifetime of a 1 l canister can be calculated to be 5 h, matching exactly the lifetime measured in laboratory investigations.

Most absorbents contain an indicator dye which changes colour to indicate exhaustion of the absorbent[12,14]:

- ethyl violet: white to purple,
- ethyl orange: orange to yellow,
- cresyl yellow: red to yellow,
- Mimosa Z: red to white.

It has to be emphasized, however, that the colour change of the absorbent is by no means a reliable indicator of soda lime exhaustion[25].

1.1.5   Hybrid breathing systems

Mentell and co-workers[26] were the first in 1994 to introduce a real hybrid breathing system consisting of a Bain system coupled to a circle absorption system (Figure 1.5). Thus, it is a combination of a flow-controlled non-rebreathing and a rebreathing system. Depending on the fresh gas flow rate, the ventilation patterns and the geometry of the coaxial system, the patient inhales back a certain amount of the exhaled air not purged of

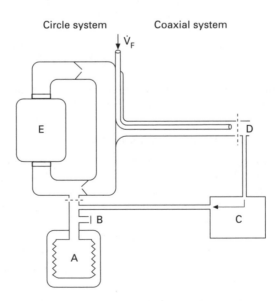

Figure 1.5   Mentell's hybrid system: A: bellows; B: excess gas valve; C: gas analyser, equipped with a hose to return the sampling gas; D: connector to the patient; E: absorber canister (from reference 26)

carbon dioxide beforehand. From a technical point of view, the Mentell system is no more than a circle absorption system with an additive and increased dead space. Only by setting an adequately high fresh gas flow at the controls, adapted to the geometry of the coaxial system, can rebreathing of unpurified exhaled gas be kept within acceptable limits. At high minute ventilation the function of the Mentell system resembles a circle absorption system; if the minute volume is small the system then behaves more like a Bain system. The clinical advantage of the Mentell system, however, remains unproven.

1.2   Classification of breathing systems in accordance with functional criteria

1.2.1   Open breathing systems

Open breathing systems have one characteristic in common: any precise control of the anaesthetic gas composition inhaled by the patient is not possible. The fact that a sufficient fresh gas reservoir is not available may, as a function of the tidal volume, result in uncontrolled entrance of ambient air, or uncontrollable changes in anaesthetic gas concentrations.

1.2.2   Semi-open breathing systems

In the semi-open breathing system, the exhaled gas is completely discharged out of the system, while pure fresh gas is administered to the patient during the following inspiration. This means, depending on the system's design, that the fresh gas flow must be at least equal to the minute volume or be a multiple of it. The amount of oxygen, nitrous oxide and volatile anaesthetic discharged out of the system unused is proportional to the fresh gas flow. The composition of the anaesthetic gas is similar to that of the fresh gas. The inspiratory limb of a semi-open breathing system, thus, is isolated from the atmosphere, whereas the expiratory limb is open to the surrounding air.

1.2.3   Semi-closed breathing systems

In the semi-closed breathing system, the fresh gas flow fed into the breathing system is greater than the uptake, but less than the minute volume. This technique of anaesthetic management is only possible provided the exhaled gas is partially rebreathed, but at the same time, excess gas escapes from the system. The rebreathed gas volume is in inverse proportion to the fresh gas flow and the excess gas volume. As the fresh gas flow is reduced, the difference in composition of the anaesthetic gas and the fresh gas increases as the rebreathing fraction increases.

1.2.4   Closed breathing systems

A breathing system is referred to as being closed if the fresh gas volume that is fed into the system corresponds exactly to the uptake, i.e. the volume of gas which the patient takes up during the respective period of time. Following elimination of carbon dioxide, the entire expiratory gas volume is routed back to the patient in the following inspiratory phase. A sufficient gas volume within the system can only be maintained if the excess gas discharge valve is closed and the system is absolutely gas tight. We refer to 'quantitative anaesthesia with closed breathing system' only if the composition *and* the volume of the fresh gas correspond at any time exactly to those amounts of oxygen, nitrous oxide and volatile anaesthetic which are actually taken up by the patient[27]. However, if only the volume and *not* the composition of the fresh gas corresponds to the uptake of the patient, this is referred to as 'non-quantitative anaesthesia with closed breathing system'.

The classification 'open, semi-open, semi-closed and closed breathing systems' should no longer be used to differentiate breathing systems according to their specific technical properties. These terms are indispensable, however, to describe precisely the function of a breathing system.

1.3   Breathing systems according to technical and functional aspects (Table 1.2)

1.3.1   Rebreathing systems

In terms of the basic technical concept, these breathing systems are especially designed for rebreathing. They are used as *closed breathing systems*

Table 1.2   Alternative possibilities to use the different breathing systems

	Open	semi-open	semi-closed	closed
Rebreathing system	$\varnothing$	+	+	+
Flow-controlled non-rebreathing systems	$(+)^1$	+	$(+)^2$	$\varnothing$
Valve-controlled non-rebreathing systems	$(+)^1$	+	$\varnothing$	$\varnothing$
Systems without reservoir	+	$(+)^3$	$\varnothing$	$\varnothing$

$^+$: Adequate way of use, $(+)$: Unsafe borderline way of use, $\varnothing$: Way of use impossible due to the respective technical concept.

^{1}: Transition to an open system possible in case of inadequate dimension of the reservoir, inadequate low fresh gas flow or high inspiratory volume and resulting entrance of ambient air into the inspiratory limb of the system.

^{2}: The use as semi-closed system is limited, as any rebreathing of carbon dioxide containing exhaled air must be avoided by setting of an adequately high fresh gas flow. Partial rebreathing of the carbon dioxide free exhaled dead space volume, however, is justifiable.

^{3}: Transition to a semi-open system is possible if the inspired volume is small, fresh gas is delivered with continuous flow, and mouth and pharyngeal space or an artificial chimney serve as a gas reservoir. If, under these circumstances, the fresh gas flow is comparatively small, a transition even to a semi-closed system with uncontrolled rebreathing of carbon dioxide containing exhaled air may be possible.

if the fresh gas volume corresponds to the uptake and, following carbon dioxide absorption, the exhaled gas is completely rebreathed by the patient. With respect to function, they are *semi-closed breathing systems* if the fresh gas flow is greater than the uptake, but less than the minute volume, and rebreathing is partial. Inevitably, the rebreathing volume decreases with increasing fresh gas flow, while the excess gas volume increases. Given favourable design of the system – a circle system with the exhaust valve proximal to the expiratory limb and the fresh gas inlet being proximal to the inspiratory limb – plus a fresh gas flow that is greater than the alveolar ventilation volume, the rebreathing proportion is reduced to a negligible minimum[1]. The composition of the inspiratory gas is then virtually identical to the fresh gas, so that the rebreathing system functions as a *semi-open breathing system*. In terms of function, rebreathing systems cannot be *open breathing systems*, since the design renders the free entrance of air impossible.

1.3.2 Non-rebreathing systems

1.3.2.1 Flow-controlled non-rebreathing systems

With respect to the basic technical concept, non-rebreathing systems are not designed for rebreathing, but for elimination of the exhaled gas, and inspiratory supply of fresh gas. Essentially, the efficiency of elimination of the expiratory gas depends on the technical design of the breathing system, the tidal and minute volume and the ventilation patterns[7,28]. Accordingly, precise specifications are given for the different breathing systems, as to the fresh gas flow which has to be selected to reliably prevent rebreathing, for both spontaneous breathing and controlled ventilation (Table 1.1). These recommendations are always made with respect to the minute volume. To obtain the best efficiency of these breathing systems, the fresh gas volume should at least equal the gas volume sufficient to eliminate the entire carbon dioxide containing alveolar gas. Thus, flow-controlled non-rebreathing systems are designed to be used as *semi-open breathing systems*. Should a lower fresh gas flow – as low as 70% of the minute volume – be quoted for a particular system, this results in partial rebreathing without carbon dioxide absorption which can only be acceptable provided that this will not cause a considerable carbon dioxide enrichment. The rebreathed gas should be the dead space volume and not the carbon dioxide containing alveolar ventilation volume[1]. This results in a floating, but rather limited transition to a *semi-closed use* of flow-controlled non-rebreathing systems. If the reservoir volume of the system is comparatively large, increasing reduction of the fresh gas flow causes a drastic rise in carbon dioxide concentration. If, on the other hand, the reservoir volume is comparatively small, air may be drawn into the system during inspiration, which in turn results in a functionally *open breathing system*.

1.3.2.2 Valve-controlled non-rebreathing systems

Where valve-controlled non-rebreathing systems are concerned, rebreathing of the expiratory gas, which necessarily escapes via the non-rebreathing valve, is not possible. These systems cannot be used as closed or semi-closed breathing systems. Since the inspiratory gas reliably consists of pure fresh gas, its flow must equal the minute volume. A further increase of fresh gas flow is unreasonable, since the resultant positive pressure in the inspiratory limb will impair the valve function, causing excess gas to be immediately discharged from the system via the expiratory valve. Thus valve-controlled non-rebreathing systems are used exclusively as *semi-open breathing systems*. Transition to the *open breathing system* may be possible only if the inspiratory limb is open to the atmosphere, while the volume of the gas reservoir is too small or the fresh gas flow too low. Ambient air may thus be drawn into the system during inspiration.

1.3.3   Breathing systems without gas reservoir

In this context, reference is made to the Boyle–Davis gag as an example. If the fresh gas flow is low, ambient air is inhaled in addition to the anaesthetic gas with every inspiration. By definition, this is an *open breathing system*. If however, the fresh gas flow is high and the tidal volume low, the oropharynx, which is filled with fresh gas in the expiratory pause, acts as a fresh gas reservoir, so that the patient inhales fresh gas only. This represents a floating transition from the open to the *semi-open breathing system*.

Generally, it may be possible that all the different breathing systems assume the characteristics of an open system whenever ambient air can enter the system freely, and the entire volume of the fresh gas flow and the reservoir is lower than the inspiratory volume.

1.4   Function of breathing systems in relation to the fresh gas flow (Table 1.3)

In summary, breathing systems must be understood as being the technical elements which, as a function of the fresh gas flow selected, prepare the gas mixture which the patient inhales in a dynamic process from fresh gas, exhaled gas and, perhaps, ambient air. Thus they are not only components which passively administer the fresh gas to the patient prepared by the

Table 1.3   Use of different breathing systems according to the fresh gas flow rate

	Semi-open	*Semi-closed*	*Closed*
Rebreathing systems	$\dot{V}_F \geq MV$	$MV > \dot{V}_F > Uptake$	$\dot{V}_F = Uptake$
Flow-controlled non-rebreathing systems	$\dot{V}_F \gg MV$	$\dot{V}_F \approx MV$	$\emptyset$
Valve-controlled non-rebreathing systems	$\dot{V}_F = MV$	$\emptyset$	$\emptyset$

$\dot{V}_F$: Fresh gas flow, MV: Minute volume, Uptake: Total gas uptake of the patient.

flow control system, the mixer and the vaporizer, but they are the elements by which the composition of the anaesthetic gases finally is determined.

Thus, finally it is the method of anaesthesia management, which itself depends greatly on the selection of the fresh gas flow, that determines the function and dosage characteristics of the respective breathing systems.

1.5   Advantages and disadvantages of the different breathing systems (Table 1.4)

The *advantage of the breathing systems without reservoir* is their extremely simple technical construction. These breathing systems can even be used in the most unfavourable conditions. *Disadvantages* are the lack of any exact control of the anaesthetic gas composition and the possibility of uncontrolled admixture of ambient air. Breathing systems without reservoir are

Table 1.4   Specific characteristics of different breathing systems

	Non-rebreathing systems	**Rebreathing systems**
Technical construction	Simple	Complex
Controllability of the anaesthetic gas composition	Alteration of the fresh gas composition will lead to instant corresponding alteration of the composition of the anaesthetic gas	Alteration of the fresh gas composition will only lead with certain time delay to a corresponding alteration of anaesthetic gas composition
Knowledge about the anaesthetic gas	Anaesthetic gas composition is similar to the composition of the fresh gas	The difference between the anaesthetic gas composition and the composition of the fresh gas is the higher the lower is the fresh gas flow rate
Climatization of the anaesthetic gases	No warming or humidifying effect	The lower the fresh gas flow rate the better the anaesthetic gas climatization
Anaesthetic gas and vapour consumption	High to extremely high	Low in case of judicious use of the rebreathing technique
Pollution with anaesthetic gases and vapours	High to extremely high	Low in case of judicious use of the rebreathing technique
Costs resulting from anaesthetic gas and vapour consumption	The higher the higher is the fresh gas flow rate	The lower the lower is the fresh gas flow rate
Possibilities to alternatively use the breathing system	As semi-open, to a very limited degree as semi-closed system	Depending on the fresh gas flow rate: as semi-open, semi-closed or closed system

not used in developed countries any more but will still play a role if anaesthesia has to be performed under extremely adverse infrastructural conditions.

Similarly, the *advantage of the non-rebreathing systems* lies in their simple technical construction. Furthermore, the anaesthetic gas composition equals that of the fresh gas, which is known to the anaesthetist, and controllability will reach its maximum, as each alteration of the fresh gas composition will instantly lead to a corresponding alteration of the gas composition within the breathing system. The *disadvantages* are the extremely high consumption, poor utilization and correspondingly high costs of anaesthetic gases and vapours, the high workplace and atmospheric pollution, and the lack of any anaesthetic gas climatization.

The *advantages of rebreathing systems* are the potential to significantly reduce consumption and hence costs, the corresponding improved utilization of anaesthetic gases and vapours, the decrease in workplace and atmospheric pollution, and the improved climatization of anaesthetic gases. The lower the fresh gas flow, the higher will be the rebreathing fraction and the more these benefits will be realized. The *disadvantages* are the significantly more sophisticated technical construction of the rebreathing systems, the lack of exact knowledge about the anaesthetic gas composition within the breathing system, and the significant decrease of its controllability.

Whilst, however, the disadvantages of the non-rebreathing systems result from their technical construction and, thus, are fixed, the disadvantages of rebreathing systems can easily be overcome just by varying of the function of these systems. As the specific characteristics of rebreathing systems only become apparent if the fresh gas flow rate is comparatively low, simply increasing the fresh gas flow will change the function of the rebreathing system to that of a non-rebreathing system, eliminating the specific shortcomings of these systems whenever necessary.

The judicious use of rebreathing systems answers the justified public demand for economically and ecologically responsible use of anaesthetic gases and vapours. The improved climatization of the anaesthetic gases together with their flexibility of function are also strong arguments in favour of the rebreathing technique.

1.6   References

1. Ernst EA. Closed circuit anesthesia. In List FW and Schalk HV, eds, *Refresher-Kurs ZAK 85*. Akademische Druck- und Verlagsanstalt, Graz 1985, S127–S137.
2. International Organisation for Standards (ISO). prEN ISO 4135: 1999 – Revision of ISO 4135, second edition: 1995 – Anaesthetic and respiratory equipment – vocabulary. European Committee for Standardisation, Brussels, 1999.
3. Moyle JTB and Davey A, ed. by Ward CS. *Ward's Anaesthetic Equipment*, 4th edn. W. B. Saunders, London, 1998.
4. Barth L and Meyer M. *Moderne Narkose*. Fischer, Stuttgart, 1965.
5. Dick W, Altemeyer KH and Schöch G. Das Paedi-System. Ein neues Narkosesystem für Säuglinge und Kinder. *Anaesthesist* 1977; **26**, 369–371.

6. Dudziak R. *Lehrbuch der Anästhesiologie*. Schattauer, Stuttgart, 1980.
7. Gray TC, Nunn JF and Utting JE. *General Anaesthesia*. Butterworth, London, 1980.
8. Herden HN and Lawin P. *Anästhesie-Fibel*. Thieme, Stuttgart, 1973.
9. Larsen R, Sonntag H and Kettler D. *Anästhesie und Intensivmedizin für Schwestern und Pfleger*. Springer, Berlin, 1984.
10. Lee JA and Atkinson RS. *Synopsis der Anästhesie*. Fischer, Stuttgart, 1978.
11. Mapleson WW. The elimination of rebreathing in various semi-closed anaesthetic systems. *Br J Anaesth* 1954; **26**, 323–332.
12. Ehrenwerth J and Eisenkraft JB. *Anesthesia Equipment: Principles and Applications*. Mosby Year Book, St Louis, 1993.
13. Willis BA, Pender JW and Mapleson WW. Rebreathing in a T-piece: volunteer and theoretical studies of the Jackson–Rees modification of Ayre's T-piece during spontaneous respiration. *Br J Anaesth* 1975; **47**, 1239–1246.
14. Dorsch JA and Dorsch SE. *Understanding Anesthetic Equipment: Construction, Care and Complications*, 3rd edn. Williams & Wilkins, Baltimore, 1994.
15. Humphrey D. A new anaesthetic breathing system combining Mapleson A, D and E principles. *Anaesthesia* 1983; **38**, 361–372.
16. Mushin WW and Jones PL. *Macintosh, Mushin and Epstein: Physics for the Anaesthetist*. Blackwell Scientific Publications, Oxford, 1987.
17. Baum J. Narkosesysteme. *Anaesthesist* 1987; **36**, 393–399.
18. Feiss P. *Sistemi ed Apparecchiature per Anestesia*. Masson, Milan, 1991.
19. Jackson DE. A new method for the production of general analgesia and anaesthesia with a description of the apparatus used. *J Lab Clin Med* 1915; **1**, 1–12.
20. Physio B.V. PhysioFlex, Gesloten Anaesthesie Ventilator. Physio Medical Systems, Hoofddorp, 1990.
21. Baum J. Hinweise zu korrektem Umgang und fachgerechter Nutzung. Stellungnahme der Kommission für Normung und technische Sicherheit der DGAI. *Anästh Intensivmed* 1999; **40**, 507–509.
22. Petty WC. Carbon dioxide absorption. In Petty WC. *The Anesthesia Machine*. Churchill Livingstone, New York, 1987, pp. 67–79. **7
23. Gootjes P and Lagerweij E. Quality comparison of different CO_2 absorbents. *Anaesthesist* 1981; **30**, 261–264.
24. Paravicini D, Henning K and Vietor G. Vergleichende Untersuchungen von verschiedenen Atemkalksorten. *Anästh Intensivther Notfallmed* 1982; **17**, 98–101.
25. Andrews JJ, Johnston RV, Bee DE and Arens JF. Photodeactivation of ethyl violet: a potential hazard of Sodasorb®. *Anesthesiology* 1990; **72**, 59–64.
26. Mentell O, Revenäs B and Jonsson L. A new hybrid anaesthetic circuit for low-flow rebreathing technique. *Acta Anaesth Scand* 1994; **38**, 840–844.
27. Baum J. Clinical applications of low flow and closed circuit anesthesia. *Acta Anaesth Belg* 1990; **41**, 239–247.
28. Nemes C, Niemer M and Noack G. *Datenbuch Anästhesiologie*. Fischer, Stuttgart, 1979.

Rebreathing systems – the development of a technical concept

2.1 Development of breathing systems – historical perspective

The manifold possibilities and variants of inhalational anaesthesia are closely related to the technical development of anaesthetic machines. Competent evaluation of the advantages and disadvantages of rebreathing techniques, as well as of the prejudices with regard to this technique, require such a background knowledge. The following brief, and thus incomplete, description of the development in technology of anaesthetic machines and breathing systems is based essentially on a number of textbooks[1-4] as well as on some review articles and monographs on this topic[5-11].

2.1.1 Development of open breathing systems

The first inhalational anaesthetic was performed by Crawford W. Long (1815–1880) on 3 March 1842 with ether. One of the first chloroform anaesthetics to be published was performed by James Y. Simpson (1811–1870) on 5 November 1847. Both physicians used a cloth soaked with the volatile anaesthetic, held over the mouth and nose of the patient[10,12,13]. The vapours were inhaled by the patient and put him into a narcotic sleep (Figure 2.1). This very simple method of inhalational anaesthesia was soon widely used. In 1862, Skinner developed a mask-like wire frame, into which the cloth was inserted. It was held in front of the patient's face so that skin and mucous tissues were protected from the liquid anaesthetic, while at the same time the narcotizing vapours could be more precisely applied, and the cloth secured in place[10]. This concept was varied and improved in many ways, for example by Esmarch, Kocher and Schimmelbusch. Anaesthesia with these kinds of masks which, in technical terms are systems without gas reservoir, is nowadays rarely performed in developed countries.

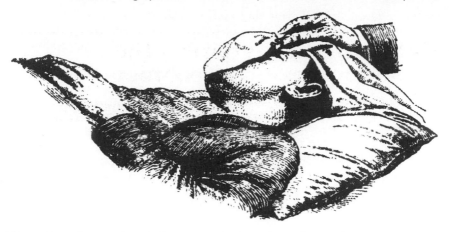

Figure 2.1   Simpson's technique to apply chloroform (from reference 10)

2.1.2   Development of non-rebreathing systems

2.1.2.1   Valve-controlled non-rebreathing systems

The development of valve-controlled non-rebreathing systems is also closely related to the spread of ether anaesthesia. On 16 October 1846, William T. G. Morton (1819–1868) succeeded in demonstrating the first clinical ether anaesthetic at the Massachusetts General Hospital in Boston[13]. He used a special apparatus[10,14], his Morton Ether Inhalator was the very first anaesthetic system (Figure 2.2). The Morton apparatus was a glass ball with two necks, which contained a sponge soaked with ether. One neck was fitted with a mouthpiece through which the patient inhaled the ether vapours. The ambient air which entered the glass ball through the other neck promoted the ether evaporation process. Exhalation took place through the mouthpiece, back into the inhalation system. It was during his first clinical demonstration that Morton realized that the patient's exhalation into the system was disadvantageous. The

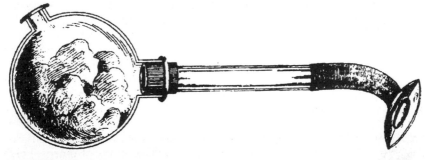

Figure 2.2   Dieffenbach's modification of Morton's apparatus for ether inhalation (from Dieffenbach[14])

system used on the following day and described by H. J. Bigelow[15] was therefore fitted with a valve close to the mouthpiece, allowing exhaled air to escape into the atmosphere. An improvement of this technical concept was the breathing system designed by John Snow (1813–1858). His apparatus was equipped with a generously dimensioned breathing hose, an inspiratory and expiratory valve and a more precisely working ether vaporizer (Figure 2.3). The advantages of this system were a reduced respiratory resistance and the possibility of more accurate dosage of the ether vapour. Further development of this concept in 1941 by Macintosh and Epstein led to the Oxford Vaporizer, the breathing system which was fitted with a non-rebreathing valve in proximity to the patient's airway[10]. Such valve-controlled non-rebreathing systems with precisely operating vaporizers are still manufactured and used nowadays, as is reflected for instance in the AFYA anaesthesia machine of the Dräger company, Lübeck.

2.1.2.2   Flow-controlled non-rebreathing systems

The development of flow-controlled non-rebreathing systems is closely related to the use of nitrous oxide as an anaesthetic gas. Humphry Davy (1778–1829) discussed the possibility of eliminating pain in surgical interventions with the aid of nitrous oxide as early as in 1800: 'As nitrous oxide in its extensive operation appears capable of destroying physical pain, it may probably be used with advantage during surgical operations in which no great effusion of blood takes place'[16]. Following a successful self-test on 11 December 1844, Horace Wells (1815–1848) performed the first clinical demonstration of nitrous oxide as an inhalational anaesthetic at the Massachusetts General Hospital in Boston in January 1845[12,17]. However, this demonstration was not successful and Davy's idea of inhibiting pain by means of nitrous oxide was dismissed by the surgeon Warren as being charlatanry and swindle. Some 18 years later, Gardner Q. Colton (1814–1898) made another attempt to arouse interest in this inhalational anaesthetic[12], but with his method of administration, patients inhaled pure nitrous oxide from a breathing bag up to the state of asphyxia, therefore effect was not obtained reliably and was too brief for longer surgical procedures. In 1868, E. Andrews (1824–1904) was the first to recommend the use of an oxygen–nitrous oxide mixture, for safe anaesthesia even in longer lasting operations[18]. The development of anaesthesia machines (H. Th. Hillischer, 1886; F. W. Hewitt, 1893), by means of which the patient could be supplied with an oxygen–nitrous oxide mixture of defined composition, was a decisive step forward in this direction. In addition, cylinders with pressure regulators were used as oxygen and nitrous oxide reservoirs, which made anaesthetics available at a high continuous flow[10]. M. Neu (1877–1940) introduced an apparatus in 1910 permitting accurate adjustment of nitrous oxide and oxygen flows by means of precision needle valves. The gas flows were measured with the aid of flowmeter tubes[19]. This measurement and dosing principle is still applied in the most advanced present-day machines. From then on it was possible to maintain anaesthesia over lengthy periods without the danger of hypoxia. However, exhaled gas had to be discharged into the atmosphere after each breath via an exhaust valve, since the technique of carbon dioxide absorption was not available in those times. Great volumes of expensive anaesthetic gases, which were very scarce, were inevitably lost.

The construction of the different flow-controlled breathing systems, which are still used today, is based on the development of anaesthetic machines which permit the administration of a defined anaesthetic gas mixture at a high constant flow. These are, for instance, the Ayre's T-piece and the Bain, Kuhn, Lack and Magill systems. A gas mixture consisting of oxygen, nitrous oxide and a volatile anaesthetic agent is administered to the patient. The gas flow must be adjusted to the breathing or ventilation parameters of the patient and to the design of the system in order that rebreathing can be precluded. The technical concept of flow-controlled non-rebreathing systems, thus, requires a constant gas flow at a high rate.

2.1.3   Development of rebreathing systems

As early as 1850 – only 4 years after the first successful clinical perform-ance of ether anaesthesia – John Snow (1813–1858) recognized that ether and chloroform were exhaled unchanged with the expired air[21]. He concluded: 'It follows as a necessary consequence of this mode of excretion of a vapour, that, if its exhalation by the breath could in any way be stopped, its narcotic effects ought to be much prolonged'[22]. To reuse these unchanged vapours in the following inspiration and thereby prolonging the narcotic effect of a given amount of anaesthetic vapour, he converted his ether inhaler (Figure 2.3) into a to-and-fro rebreathing system. The apparatus was equipped with a face mask, without inspiratory or expiratory valves, and a large reservoir bag containing pure oxygen attached to the air inlet; the spiral chamber was filled partially with an aqueous solution of caustic potash which was used as a carbon dioxide absorbent. In several experiments, performed on himself, Snow succeeded in demonstrating that rebreathing of the exhaled vapours was possible following carbon dioxide absorption, and that it resulted in a pronounced prolongation of the narcotic effects of the volatile anaesthetics[21,22]. Furthermore, Snow performed experiments on animals using a closed system (Figure 2.4) for evaluating the carbon dioxide production during anaesthesia[23].

Yet the principle of rebreathing exhaled air via a breathing system after elimination of 'noxious vapours' had long since been known[9]. In 1727, Stephen Hales (1677–1761) described a rebreathing circle system by means of which 'sulphureous steams' could be absorbed, destroying the 'elasticity of the air' and thus rendering impossible free ventilation[24]. His breathing system, which he recommended for rescue purposes, consisted of a gas reservoir made of a bladder into which four diaphragms of flannel were placed, soaked with a solution of highly calcinated tartar, a wide-bore siphon, and unidirectional inspiratory and expiratory valves (Figure 2.5). A mine rescue apparatus from Th. Schwann (1809–1885), which featured a high pressure oxygen reservoir cylinder, reducing and flow control valves

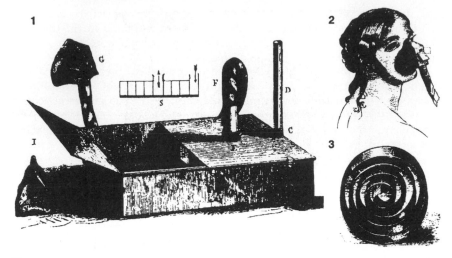

Figure 2.3 Snow's ether inhaler. 1. Overall view of the apparatus (A, metal box serving as a water bath; B, spiral ether chamber; C, opening for filling in ether; D, brass tube by which the air enters which the patient inhales; E, outlet of the ether chamber; F, elastic tube; G, face piece; I, the same face piece compressed, to fit it to a smaller face; S, section of spiral ether chamber). 2. Face piece with inspiratory and expiratory valve. 3. Ether chamber with the bottom removed, showing the volute (from Snow[20])

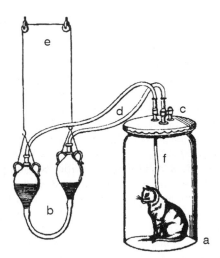

Figure 2.4 Snow's closed system for experimental determination of the amount of carbon dioxide excreted during ether and chloroform anaesthesia. a, Glass jar; b, two glass vessels, filled with an aqueous solution of potash, connected together by an elastic tube; c, airtight lid with an opening for filling in the volatile anaesthetic; d, rubber tubes connecting the jar with the potash apparatus; e, mechanism to move the glass vessels up and down. They alternately filled with the fluid, resulting in a constant circulation of the air within the jar and the vessels and so leading to absorption of the exhaled carbon dioxide by the solution of potash (from Snow[23])

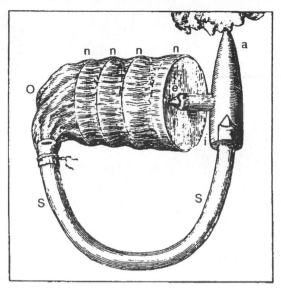

Figure 2.5   Hales' closed rebreathing system of 1727. a, Mouthpiece; e, unidirectional expiratory valve; i, unidirectional inspiratory valve; n, four linen diaphragms clamped into the breathing gas reservoir, soaked with calcinated potassium bitartrate for carbon dioxide absorption; o, flexible breathing gas reservoir; s, inspiratory hose (from Hales[24])

and a circle breathing system with carbon dioxide absorber, was already available in 1856[25].

Alfred Coleman (1828–1902) was the first to use a to-and-fro system with carbon dioxide absorption in clinical practice (Figure 2.6). Nitrous oxide was delivered to a pair of reservoir bags connected together with a unidirectional valve. From the proximal reservoir the patient inhaled the gas, which had to pass a tin box filled with slaked lime, via a wide-bore tubing leading to a face mask. During expiration the air was expired back into the proximal reservoir bag, again passing the metal box where the carbon dioxide was absorbed. By the use of rebreathing technique, Coleman wanted to decrease nitrous oxide consumption, as the usual use of high amounts of this expensive anaesthetic was a serious impediment to the spread of nitrous oxide anaesthesia, and to make it affordable even for his poorer patients[26,27]. As the patients got pure nitrous oxide, this rebreathing technique could only be used in very short surgical procedures. Although Coleman enthusiastically advocated the use of his 'economising apparatus', this technique was not generally adopted[5]. At around the same time, in 1869 in the Berliner Klinische Wochenschrift, Carl Sauer (1835–1892) also described a to-and-fro rebreathing system for the application of nitrous oxide in dentistry[28], which is rarely cited[29].

In 1906, Franz Kuhn (1866–1929) published the constructional details of a concept for a breathing system which incorporated a similar technical component for elimination of carbon dioxide from the exhaled gas (Figure 2.7). Like Coleman and Sauer, Kuhn intended to lead back the unused

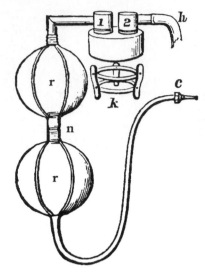

Figure 2.6 Coleman's 'economising apparatus'. c, Adapter to the nitrous oxide cylinder; r, reservoir bags; n, unidirectional valve; 1 and 2, metal box (economizer), filled with small pieces of slaked lime; 1, connector to the reservoir bags; 2, connector to the patient; h, tubing to the face piece; k, frame which supports the economizer on the top of the gas cylinder (from Duncum[5], by permission)

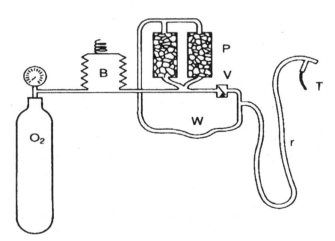

Figure 2.7 Concept of a rebreathing system developed by Franz Kuhn (in 1906). B, bellows; P, carbon dioxide absorber; V, inspiratory valve; W, breathing system; T, airway; r, breathing tube (from Rendell-Baker[9], by permission)

anaesthetic gases, contained in the expired air, to the patient during the following inhalation. The amount of oxygen to be fed into the system then merely had to replenish the volume which had been consumed or lost as a result of leaks. However, this system was never put to clinical use since the flow resistance and the dead space of the breathing system were too great.

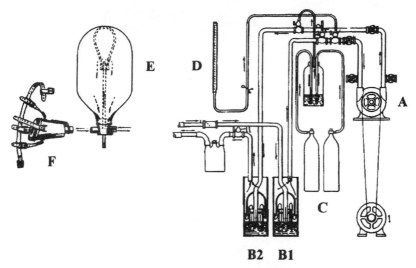

Figure 2.8   Jackson's circle absorption system. The animal inhales gas via a face piece (F) out of a rubber bag which serves as a gas reservoir (E). Anaesthetic gas is continuously sucked out of this reservoir by an air pump (A). The gas passes the wash jar (B1), filled with concentrated sulphuric acid, leaves the pump in the direction of the wash jar (B2), filled with a strong aqueous solution of sodium hydrate and calcium hydrate, passes a Woulff bottle and is then returned back to the gas reservoir. Nitrous oxide and oxygen, obtained from the gas cylinders (C), are fed into the system in just such an amount to keep constant the filling level of the gas reservoir. Fluid ether or chloroform is delivered into the system from the burette (D). (From Jackson[31])

In addition, Kuhn feared that the chemical reaction of chloroform with the absorbing material (caustic soda) might possibly harm the patient[30].

In 1915, Dennis E. Jackson (1879–1980) reported prolonged anaesthesia in animals by means of a closed circle system with carbon dioxide absorption, using a gas mixture of volatile anaesthetics, nitrous oxide and oxygen[31]. The technical concept and details of the circle absorption system designed by Jackson are distinctly forward-looking. Driven by a fan, the anaesthetic gas circulates continuously within the system. Only those amounts of oxygen and nitrous oxide required to maintain adequate filling of the reservoir bag are delivered into the system, ether or chloroform being metered by means of a burette into the circuit in liquid form. The continuous gas flow ensures rapid vaporization and an even distribution of the anaesthetic in the whole gas containing space (Figure 2.8). However, neither the apparatus nor the method met with any interest, although the use of this technology saved considerable amounts of anaesthetic gas and the apparatus itself worked reliably. In 1916, Jackson described a very simple and cheap to-and-fro system for experimental anaesthesia[32], in which a cake pan, partially filled with an aqueous solution of soda lime, was used for absorption of the exhaled carbon dioxide (Figure 2.9).

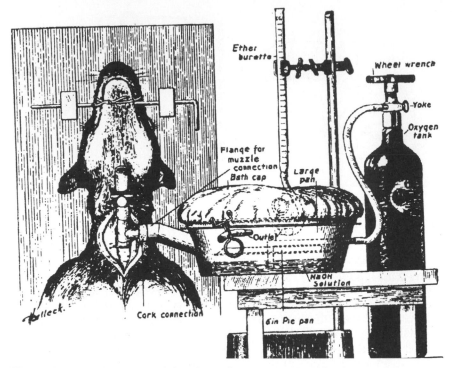

Figure 2.9   Jackson's to-and-fro absorption system. Very simple to-and-fro system built from parts bought in a 10 cent store: the absorber, simultaneously serving as a vaporizer and a gas reservoir, consists of a cake and a pie pan and a bath cap. (From Jackson[32])

It was Ralph M. Waters (1883–1979) who introduced the technique of anaesthesia with closed rebreathing system into medical practice in 1924[33]. In his to-and-fro system, it was a metal canister filled with sodium hydroxide granules which served as a carbon dioxide absorber (Figure 2.10). The patient inhaled anaesthetic gas from a reservoir bag, containing about 10 litres of gas, into which he exhaled again. Adequate oxygenation was achieved by intermittent oxygen supply. Hans Killian (1892–1982) paid a visit to Waters in Madison (USA) in 1928 and was greatly impressed by his work with the to-and-fro system:

... After the patient had been slightly anaesthetised in an anteroom, he [Waters] filled a large 10-litre balloon with an ethylene and oxygen mixture from the Foregger machine, at a ratio of about 80:20%. Then he switched off the machine completely, closed the filling tap of the large rubber bag, attached a soda cartridge to it, and to the other end fitted an anaesthetic mask, which was placed onto the patient's face. The patient inhaled the gas mixture from the rubber bag only and expired back into the balloon. This was in accordance with his to-and-fro system and absorption of carbon dioxide ... He [the patient] remained sleeping, although he did not receive a continuous flow of

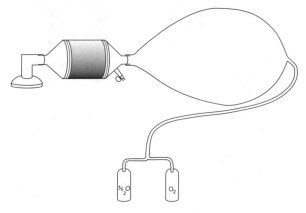

Figure 2.10   The to-and-fro system of R. M. Waters. (From Waters[33])

fresh gas, ethylene–oxygen. This balloon technique did not appear surprising as long as it lasted only 5–10 min for transport from the induction room to the operating theatre. But in this case it lasted much longer, 20–30 min. I noticed that Waters administered oxygen without ethylene into the bag only once, when the patient turned slightly blue. I was somewhat puzzled. Right in front of our eyes, a most remarkable event had taken place, much to my amazement. Though most of the others had not noticed it, Waters had proved that there was something wrong about our pharmacological assumptions that maintenance of the depth of sleep solely depends on the concentration of the inhalational anaesthetic ... One can hardly imagine how this whole story embarrassed me. I lay awake late the following night, thinking and trying with all my might to get behind the secret and to come up with an idea about our anaesthetic methods ... We were really on the verge of an outstanding progress in the field of anaesthesia.[34]

The chemist Hermann D. Wieland (1877–1957) and the gynaecologist Carl J. Gauss (1875–1957), who used purified acetylene (Narcylen) as an anaesthetic gas at the University of Freiburg, were the German protagonists for the use of rebreathing technique in anaesthesia[35,36]. In cooperation with the German engineer Bernhard Dräger (1870–1928), the first anaesthetic apparatus equipped with an anaesthetic circle rebreathing system was developed and put into operation in clinical practice in 1924[36,37]. After carbon dioxide absorption the exhaled gas, still containing unspent anaesthetic gases, was blended with fresh gas and routed back to the patient. This first anaesthetic circle system (Figure 2.11) already featured low resistance inspiratory and expiratory valves, a canister filled with carbon dioxide absorbent and an overflow valve. By introducing the rebreathing technique into anaesthetic practice it was not only possible to reduce the consumption of expensive anaesthetic gases, but also to reduce significantly the discharge of this strange smelling and highly explosive agent.

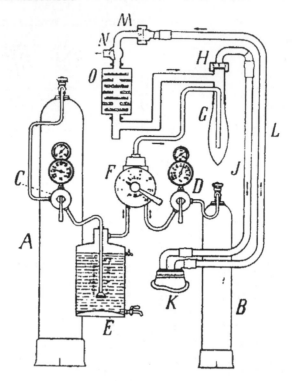

Figure 2.11   The Dräger-Narcylen-Apparat according to Gauss and Wieland (1925). A: Narcylen cylinder, B: oxygen cylinder, C and D: pressure regulator and flow control valve, E: bottle filled with water to purify Narcylen from acetone, F: gas blender, G: reservoir bag, H: inspiratory valve, I: inspiratory limb of the patient hose system, K: face mask, L: expiratory limb of the patient hose system, M: expiratory valve, N: excess gas valve, O: absorber canister (Dräger Kali-Patrone). (From Gauss[36])

Bernhard Dräger applied for a German patent for an anaesthetic circle system (Figure 2.12) on 2 October 1925, which was granted on 26 January 1927[38].

Together with Paul Sudeck (1866–1945) and Helmut Schmidt (1895–1979), University Hospital Hamburg–Eppendorf, Bernhard Dräger developed another anaesthetic apparatus, also equipped with this circle system (Figure 2.13), for the administration of oxygen and nitrous oxide. This became commercially available as the 'Lachgas-Narkose-Apparat Modell A' from 1926 onwards[39–42]. Nitrous oxide and oxygen were obtained from cylinders via pressure regulators, and flowmeters permitted precise dosage of the gas volumes to be fed into the circle system[41].

In the Anglo-American literature the development of the circle absorption system is ascribed to Brian C. Sword (1889–1956)[43]. However, Richard Foregger, the son of the famous engineer Richard von Foregger (1872–1960), recently emphasized that Foregger and Sword constructed

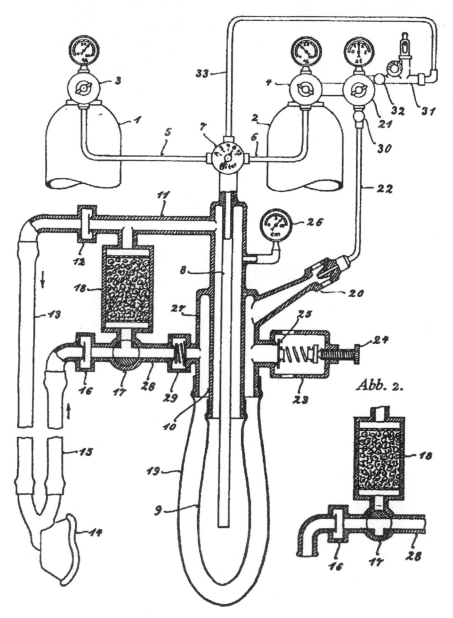

Figure 2.12   Technical sketch of the anaesthesia circle absorber system submitted by Bernhard Dräger for a patent on 2 October 1925. 7: gas blender, 9: reservoir bag, 12: inspiratory valve, 13: inspiratory hose, 14: face mask, 15: expiratory hose, 18: absorber canister, 17: three-way valve (in *Abb. 2* the canister is switched off, the exhaled air is completely is vented out of the system via the excess gas valve: the apparatus works as a non-rebreathing system), 29: excess gas valve. The outer bag (19), the injector nozzle (20) and the airway pressure limit (APL) valve generate a continuous pressure within the breathing system which is displayed at the pressure gauge (26). (From Dräger[38])

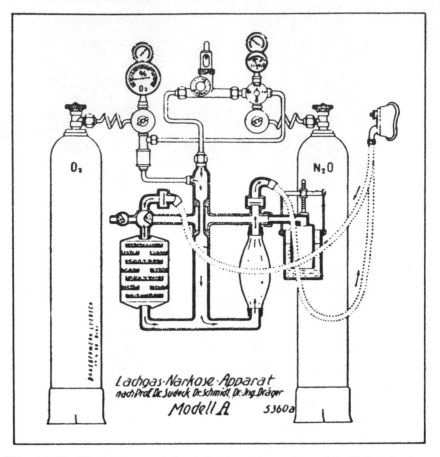

Figure 2.13   Flow diagram of the circle absorption system of the Dräger Lachgas-Narkose-Apparat Modell A of 1925. (From Haupt[6], by permission)

their circle absorption system (Figure 2.14) in the USA between 1928 and 1930, a few years later than the Germans, and that they even followed written recommendations from Hans Killian and Helmut Schmidt[37,44].

In conclusion it should be emphasized that not Waters but Coleman in 1869 was the first to introduce a to-and-fro system into clinical practice, and neither Sudeck and Schmidt nor Sword but Gauss, Wieland and Dräger in 1924 were the first to use a circle absorption system in anaesthesia[45].

Nowadays, the vast majority of anaesthesia machines are equipped with such rebreathing circle absorption systems. The essential advantages of the rebreathing system have already been summarized comprehensively by Ralph Waters[33]:

- considerable savings in anaesthetic gases;
- reduced contamination of the ambient atmosphere;
- reduced danger of explosion when using flammable inhalation anaesthetics;

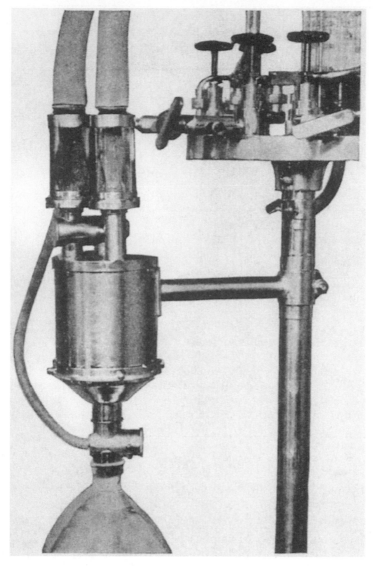

Figure 2.14 The circle absorber system according to B. C. Sword (1930). The photo shows the reservoir bag, the fresh gas delivery hose, the absorber canister and both unidirectional valves. (From Sword[43])

- improved humidification and warming of the anaesthetic gases; and
- reduced loss of heat and moisture.

The following points are regarded as being disadvantageous[3,4]:

- technically involved systems with carbon dioxide absorbers and uni-directional valves;
- increased risk of oxygen deficiency; and

- increased possibility of unnoticed carbon dioxide rebreathing in case of soda lime exhaustion.

However, in evaluating rebreathing systems, Moser[4] comes to the conclusion that the advantages of anaesthesia management with these systems far outweighs the disadvantages.

2.2   The development of semi-closed use of circle absorption systems – considerations on the current situation

Anaesthesia management with closed or virtually closed rebreathing systems had gained increasing popularity since the technical tools for the rebreathing technique had become available[46]. This may also be attributed to the introduction of the flammable and indeed explosive cyclopropane as an anaesthetic agent in 1933[8]. Thanks to the consistent utilization of the rebreathing technique, the discharge of excess gas from the breathing system could be reduced, so that consequently the cyclopropane concentration in the operating theatre could be maintained at the lowest possible level.

With the increasing use of sodium thiopental for rapid induction (1934) and curare (1942) for potent and safe muscle relaxation, the popularity of cyclopropane and, thus, the necessity to extensively reduce the excess gas discharge, declined. Furthermore, the danger of unintended delivery of hypoxic gas mixtures when using rebreathing systems was recognized[8]. A broadsheet against the deliberate application of hypoxic anaesthetic gas mixtures was published by Barach and Rovenstine[47]. They recommended the use of a fixed oxygen nitrous oxide mixture (20% O_2, 80% N_2O), delivered with high flow, from a reservoir tank directly to the patient. This is why in German textbooks the use of fresh gas flows of about 4 l/min or even higher, containing at least 25% oxygen, was urgently recommended as the only way to reliably ensure a sufficient inspired oxygen concentration[1,48].

The introduction of the volatile anaesthetic halothane in 1956 reinforced the tendency for considerable changes in anaesthesia management. From then on, the use of high fresh gas flows, that is, anaesthesia management with a semi-closed rebreathing system, has gained significant prominence. The higher the fresh gas flow, the greater was the volume of excess gas discharged from the system, and the lower the rebreathing volume (Figure 2.15). Thus, the higher the fresh gas flow, the more the composition of the anaesthetic gas corresponded directly to that of the fresh gas. Rebreathing systems were, as a result of this tendency, increasingly used without actually realizing any rebreathing. This development was supported by a number of factors[8,46,49]:

- At that time, the vaporizers available – TEC type or Copper Kettle (Figure 2.16) – did not allow precise metering of halothane at low gas flows[50,51]: patients who were being ventilated suffered from perilous overdosage, on occasions with an even fatal outcome.

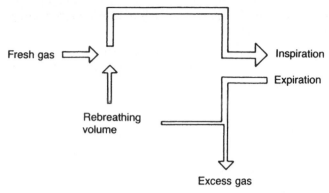

Figure 2.15   Schematic flow diagram of a semi-closed rebreathing circle system.

- There was great uncertainty with respect to the dose and pharmacokinetics of this highly efficient volatile anaesthetic which was characterized by an unusually low therapeutic index.
- Observation of spontaneous breathing as a criterion for evaluation of anaesthetic depth was no longer relevant during controlled ventilation of an anaesthetized and relaxed patient. As an alternative, the depth of anaesthesia was now estimated in accordance with the minimum alveolar concentration (MAC) principle by means of the anaesthetic concentration applied. However, at that time this was only practicable when the composition of anaesthetic gas corresponded approximately to that of the fresh gas.
- The increasing utilization of positive pressure ventilation was accompanied by increasing loss of gas from leaks and this could only be compensated for by an increase in the fresh gas flow.
- The costs involved for oxygen and nitrous oxide could be considerably reduced by using central piping systems for medical gases.
- The practical performance of anaesthesia with a high excess gas volume does not require knowledge of pharmacokinetic characteristics with respect to the uptake and distribution of volatile anaesthetics or a subtle understanding of apparatus functions. The interest in acquiring such knowledge decreased, which may be attributed to the fact that anaesthetists were taking over a great number of new tasks which occupied their attention during anaesthesia.
- The problem of operating theatre contamination by large volumes of excess gas discharged from the systems seemed to be solved by use of activated charcoal filters and the installation of central anaesthetic gas scavenging systems. The unnecessary and possibly ecologically questionable contamination of the atmosphere by anaesthetic gases did not meet with any attention in those days.

Nowadays, preference is given to anaesthesia management with the semi-closed rebreathing system using comparatively high fresh gas flows, presumably for medicolegal reasons. Accordingly, due to lack of education in this field, anaesthetists frequently have not only insufficient knowledge

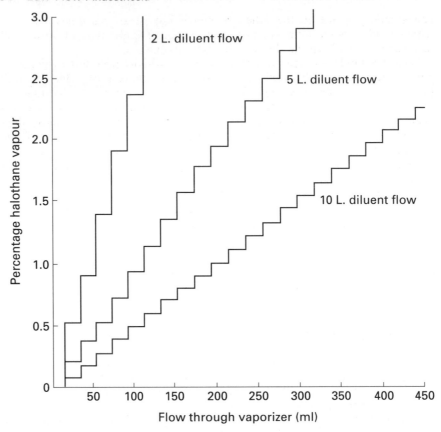

Figure 2.16   Changes in halothane concentration produced by 20 ml increments in flow through the copper kettle at 20°C, with different diluent (fresh gas) flows of 2, 5 and 10 litres per minute. (From Feldman and Morris[50], by permission)

about specific problems, but also about the special advantages of anaesthesia management with low fresh gas flows. Essential knowledge, such as uptake and distribution characteristics of oxygen, nitrous oxide and volatile anaesthetics and the effect of fresh gas flow on the function of breathing systems, is no longer conveyed. The great uncertainty with respect to the nomenclature of breathing systems[46] reflects the generally inadequate knowledge of equipment function. By becoming accustomed to excessive fresh gas flows, less attention is paid to daily equipment maintenance and leak testing. This also applies to technical inspections or the production of anaesthetic machines, since high leakage losses – more than 10 l/min has been quoted at a pressure within the system of 20 cm H_2O – are accepted which, of course, makes flow reduction impossible.

The absolutely incomprehensible contradiction between the high technical specifications placed on equipment that is especially designed for rebreathing – i.e. the new common European Standard on Anaesthetic Work Stations EN 740[53] – on the one hand, and daily anaesthetic practice on the other, in which high fresh gas flows are used which render rebreathing systems with carbon dioxide absorption almost dispensable, has been emphasized by Bergmann[54].

With the circle absorption system, the anaesthetist now has available a perfect, technically advanced and reliable rebreathing tool, which is well proven in daily practice. Mandatory stipulations on safety features of modern anaesthetic machines are entirely focused upon anaesthesia management with rebreathing systems. However, the advantages of this sophisticated equipment cannot be used to their full potential because of the general trend towards the use of high fresh gas flows. This is why Bergmann comes to the conclusion: 'And yet it seems reasonable that in view of today's technical potentials of continuous monitoring of breathing gases, the technical perfection of the system itself, and the importance which is attached to the gas tightness of the systems, and the accuracy of the flow control systems and vaporizers, all further efforts should be focused upon a sure return to the closed system'[54].

2.3   References

1. Barth L and Meyer M. *Moderne Narkose*. Fischer, Stuttgart, 1965.
2. Killian H and Weese H. *Die Narkose*. Thieme, Stuttgart, 1954.
3. Minnitt RJ and Gillies J. *Textbook of Anaesthetics*, 6th edn. E. & S. Livingstone, Edinburgh, 1945.
4. Moser H. Die Praxis der modernen Narkose. In Demel R, ed. *Wiener Beiträge zur Chirurgie*, Vol. VI. Maudrich, Wien, 1951.
5. Duncum BM. *The Development of Inhalation Anaesthesia*. Oxford University Press, London 1947. Reprint edited on behalf of the History of Anaesthesia Society by the Royal Society of Medicine Press, London, 1994.
6. Haupt J. Der *Dräger-Narkoseapparat – historisch gesehen. Sonderdruck MT 105*. Drägerwerk AG, Lübeck, 1983.
7. Just OH, Dresssler P, Böhrer H and Wiedemann K. Zur Geschichte der Anästhesie an der Universität Heidelberg. *Anästh Intensivther Notfallmed* 1986; **21**, 53–59.
8. Onishchuk JL. The early history of low-flow anaesthesia. In Fink BR, Morris LE and Stephen CR, eds. *The History of Anesthesia. Third International Symposium, Proceedings*. Wood Library–Museum of Anesthesiology, Park Ridge, Illinois, 1992, pp. 308–313.
9. Rendell-Baker L. History of thoracic anaesthesia. In Mushin WW, ed. *Thoracic Anaesthesia*. Blackwell Scientific, Oxford, 1963.
10. Thomas KB. *The Development of Anaesthetic Apparatus*. Blackwell Scientific Publications, Oxford, 1980.
11. Wawersik J. Entwicklung der Narkosegeräte. In Zinganell K, ed. *Anaesthesie – historisch gesehen*. Springer, Berlin, 1987.
12. Colton GQ.* *Anaesthesia. Who Made and Developed the Great Discovery?* A. G. Sherwood & Co., New York, 1886.
13. Knight N. *Pain and its Relief*. Smithsonian Institution, Washington, 1988.
14. Dieffenbach JF. Apparate zum Einatmen der Ätherdämpfe. In *Der Äther gegen den Schmerz*. Hirschwald, Berlin, 1847.

15. Bigelow HJ.* Insensibility during surgical operations produced by inhalation. *Boston Medical and Surgical Journal* 1846; **35**, 309–317.

16. Davy H.* *Researches, Chemical and Philosophical; Chiefly Concerning Nitrous Oxide, or Dephlogisticated Nitrous Air, and its Respiration.* Printed for J. Johnson, London by Biggs and Cottle, Bristol, 1800.

17. Wells H.* *A History of the Discovery of the Application of Nitrous Oxide Gas, Ether, and other Vapors to Surgical Operations.* J. G. Wells, Hartford, 1847.

18. Andrews E.* The oxygen mixture, a new anaesthetic combination. *The Chicago Medical Examiner* 1868; **9**, 656–661.

19. Neu M. Ein Verfahren zur Stickoxidulsauerstoffnarkose. *Münch Med Wschr* 1910; **57**, 1873.

20. Snow J. *On the Inhalation of the Vapour of Ether in Surgical Operations.* John Churchill, London, 1847.

21. Baum J. John Snow (1813–1858): Experimentelle Untersuchungen zur Rückatmung der in der Ausatemluft enthaltenen Narkosegase. *Anästhesiol Intensivmed Notfallmed Schmerzther* 1995; **30**, 37–41.

22. Snow J. On narcotism by the inhalation of vapours. Part XV. The effects of chloroform and ether prolonged by causing the exhaled vapour to be reinspired. *London Medical Gazette* 1850; **11**, 749–754.

23. Snow J. On narcotism by the inhalation of vapours. Part XVI. Experiments to determine the amount of carbonic acid gas excreted under the influence of chloroform. *London Medical Gazette* 1851; **12**, 622–627.

24. Hales S. Analysis of the air: experiment CXVI. In Statical Essays: Containing Vegetable Staticks; Or, An Account of some Statical Experiments On The Sap in Vegetables & Also, A Specimen of an Attempt to Analyse the Air, by a great Variety of Chymio-Statical Experiments, which were read at several Meetings before the Royal Society, vol. I, 2nd edn. W. Innys, London 1731, pp. 264–273.

25. Reinhold H. Theodore Schwann and the invention of closed-circuit breathing. In Rupreht J, van Lieburg MJ, Lee JA and Erdmann W, eds, *Anaesthesia – Essays on Its History*, 2nd edn. Springer-Verlag, Berlin, 1998, pp. 169–175.

26. Coleman A. Action of nitrous oxide. *British Medical Journal*, 25 April 1868, 410.

27. Coleman A. Re-inhalation of nitrous oxide. *British Medical Journal*, 1 August 1868, 114–115.

28. Sauer C. Vorläufige Mittheilung der weiteren Versuche, mit Stickstoffoxydul-Gemischen zu anästhesieren. *Berliner Klinische Wochenschrift* 1869; **6**, 366–367.

29. Böhrer H and Goerig M. Kohlendioxid-Absorption. *Anästhesiol Intensivmed Notfallmed Schmerzther* 1996; **31**, 185–186.

30. Kuhn F. Die perorale Intubation mit und ohne Druck. III. Teil. Apparat zur Lieferung des Druckes für die Überdrucknarkose. *Deutsche Zeitschrift für Chirurgie* 1906; **81**, 63–70.

31. Jackson DE.* A new method for the production of general analgesia and anaesthesia with a description of the apparatus used. *J Lab Clin Med* 1915; **1**, 1–12.

32. Jackson DE. The employment of closed ether anesthesia for ordinary laboratory experiments. *J Lab Clin Med* 1916; **2**, 94–102.

33. Waters RM.* Clinical scope and utility of carbon dioxide filtration in inhalation anaesthesia. *Anesth Analg*; **3**, 20–22, 1924.

34. Killian H. 40 *Jahre Narkoseforschung*. Verlag der Deutschen Hochschullehrerzeitung, Tübingen, 1964.

35. Goerig M and Böhrer H. Narcylennarkose. *Anästhesiol Intensivmed Notfallmed Schmerzther* 1994; **29**, 297–299.

36. Gauss CJ. Die Narcylenbetäubung mit dem Kreisatmer. *Zentralblatt für Gynäkologie* 1925; **23**, 1218–1226.
37. Foregger R. A question of priority: who introduced the CO_2 absorption method with the circle breathing into anaesthesia practice? *Anaesthesist* 1995; **44**, 917–918.
38. Dräger AB. Vorrichtung zum Einatmen von Gasen unter Überdruck, insbesondere für Betäubungszwecke. Patentschrift Nr. 439657. Reichsdruckerei, Berlin, 1927.
39. Schmidt H. Über Stickoxidulnarkose. Technische Überlegungen und Erfahrungen. *Bruhns Beiträge Klin Chir* 1926; **137**, 506–518.
40. Sudeck P and Schmidt H. Über Gasnarkosen. *Zentralblatt für Chirurgie* 1926; **20**, 1271–1275.
41. Drägerwerk, ed. Dräger-Stickoxydul-Narkose-Apparat nach Prof. Dr. Sudeck und Dr. Helmut Schmidt. Modell A. Gebrauchsanweisung Nr. 35, Lübeck, 1927.
42. Haupt J. Die Geschichte der Dräger-Narkoseapparate. 1. überarbeitete Version. Drägerwerk AG, Lübeck, 1996, pp. 31–33.
43. Sword BC.* The closed circle method of administration of gas anesthesia. *Current Researches in Anesthesia & Analgesia* 1930; **9**, 198–202.
44. Foregger R. Richard von Foregger, Ph.D., 1872–1960. Manufacturer of anesthesia equipment. *Anesthesiology* 1996; **84**, 190–200.
45. Baum JA. Who introduced the rebreathing system into clinical practice? In Schulte am Esch J. and Goerig, M. eds, *Proceedings of the Fourth International Symposium on the History of Anaesthesia*. Dräger, Lübeck, 1998, pp. 441–450.
46. Lowe HJ and Ernst EA. *The Quantitative Practice of Anesthesia*. Williams & Wilkins, Baltimore, 1979.
47. Barach AL and Rovenstine EA. The hazard of anoxia during nitrous oxide anesthesia. *Anesthesiology* 1945; **6**, 449–461.
48. Herden HN and Lawin P. *Anästhesie-Fibel*. Thieme, Stuttgart, 1973.
49. Buijs BHMJ. Herwaardering van het Gesloten Ademsysteem in de Anesthesiologie (Reevaluation of Closed Circuit Anaesthesia). Diss. der Erasmus-Universitt, Rotterdam, 1988.
50. Feldman SA and Morris LE. Vaporization of halothane and ether in the copper kettle. *Anesthesiology* 1958; **19**, 650–655.
51. Hill DW and Lowe HJ. Comparison of concentration of halothane in closed and semiclosed circuits during controlled ventilation. *Anesthesiology* 1962; **23**, 291–298.
52. Baum J. Narkosesysteme. *Anaesthesist* 1987; **36**, 393–399.
53. CEN – Comité Européen de Normalisation, ed. Anaesthetic Workstations and their modules – Particular requirements. EN 740. Brussels, 1998.
54. Bergmann H. Das Narkosegerät in Gegenwart und Zukunft aus der Sicht des Klinikers. *Anaesthesist* 1986; **35**, 587–594.

* *Source of supply for facsimile prints of these publications: Wood Library–Museum of Anesthesiology, 520 North Northwest Highway, Park Ridge, Illinois 60068-2573, USA.*

Pharmacokinetics of anaesthetic gases

3.1 Oxygen

3.1.1 Oxygen uptake and consumption

According to Brody[1], the oxygen consumption of all homoiotherms can be calculated as an exponential function of the body weight in kilograms (BW (kg)), according to the formula:

$$\dot{V}_{O_2} = 10.15 \times BW(kg)^{0.73} \,(ml/min)$$

Kleiber[2] quoted a simplified formula for calculation of oxygen consumption at resting conditions, which is now generally known as the Brody formula:

$$\dot{V}_{O_2} = 10 \times BW(kg)^{3/4} \,(ml/min)$$

If the shape of the curve calculated by means of the Brody equation is approximated by two straight lines of different gradients, the oxygen consumption of two groups of different weight can be even more easily calculated[3].

For a body weight between 10 and 40 kg:

$$\dot{V}_{O_2} = 3.75 \times BW(kg) + 20 \,(ml/min)$$

For body weight between 40 and 120 kg:

$$\dot{V}_{O_2} = 2.5 \times BW(kg) + 67.5 \,(ml/min)$$

Not only is the oxygen consumption (Figure 3.1) correlated with the body weight raised to the power of 3/4 – $BW(kg)^{3/4}$ – but also the carbon dioxide production, the alveolar ventilation and the cardiac output[2,4-6]. According to H. Lowe, the oxygen consumption decreases during induction of anaesthesia by about 15–30% with respect to the initial preoperative value[6]. Arndt could demonstrate, by his investigations, that during anaesthesia oxygen consumption virtually corresponds to the basal metabolic rate[4]. During anaesthesia, the oxygen consumption may be influenced by a great number of different factors: with a decrease in temperature of 1°C, it falls by about 10%, and in case of acidosis by about 6% per 0.1 pH change. Certain anaesthetic agents such as ether, ketamine and etomidate increase the $\dot{V}_{O_2}$, just as does a respiratory or metabolic

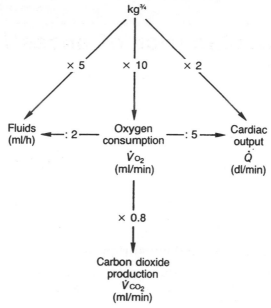

Figure 3.1 Calculation of physiological figures in relation to the body weight $(BW(kg)^{3/4})$. (From Lowe and Ernst[6], by permission)

alkalosis[4]. In addition, the $\dot{V}_{O_2}$ is subject to variations with anaesthetic depth and the degree of relaxation within a range of about 10–25%[7,8]. Changes in cardiac output will also result in alterations of the oxygen uptake. Manawadu *et al.*[9] showed in animal experiments that a blood loss of 30% decreases the oxygen uptake by $30 \pm 10\%$ with respect to the initial value. Furthermore, oxygen consumption is reduced with age, which must be attributed to the reduction of metabolically active muscle mass in favour of fat and connective tissue[6].

In conclusion, the oxygen uptake of a patient undergoing anaesthesia, which represents the oxygen consumption, remains nearly constant in cases of stable circulatory conditions (Figure 3.2). It equals the basic metabolic rate of the patient and, with acceptable accuracy, can be calculated by means of the Brody formula.

3.1.2   Implications for anaesthetic practice

Any general anaesthetic results in a reduction of pulmonary function, irrespective of the anaesthetic method employed, the ventilation pattern and the duration. The alveolar–arterial oxygen partial pressure difference $(AaDO_2)$ and the intrapulmonary shunt will increase, while the functional residual capacity and the compliance of the lung will decrease. These changes are more pronounced in the elderly and obese than in the young and ectomorphic patient[10,11].

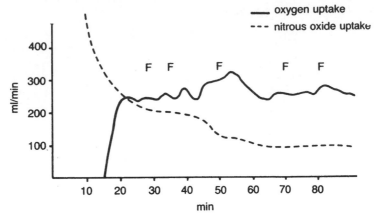

Figure 3.2   Nitrous oxide and oxygen uptake, measured during quantitative closed system anaesthesia with the aid of electronic control of gas dosage by closed-loop feedback. Steady-state conditions are not attained before denitrogenation is completed, approximately 25 min after induction of anaesthesia (F: i.v. administration of 0.05 mg fentanyl). (From Westenskow *et al.*[7], by permission)

In order to reliably prevent hypoxaemia and to ensure continuous and sufficient oxygen supply, the inspired oxygen concentration should be at least 30%[12].

Fresh gas flow and fresh gas composition have a considerable effect on the oxygen concentration of the inspired gas if anaesthesia is performed with a rebreathing circle system. Therefore, the following must be considered if the fresh gas flow is changed:

- Up to a fresh gas flow of 10 l/min the oxygen concentration in the inspiratory limb of a circle system will always be lower than that of the fresh gas[13].
- Given a constant fresh gas composition, the inspired oxygen concentration will certainly drop once the flow is reduced (Figure 3.3).
- Thus, if the fresh gas flow is reduced, its oxygen content must be increased to ensure a sufficient oxygen concentration in the inspired gas (Figure 3.4).

The proportion of exhaled gas contained in the inspired anaesthetic gas increases at low fresh gas flows. An increased oxygen consumption, therefore, by increased alveolar oxygen extraction, results in a reduction of inspired oxygen concentration, as the oxygen concentration of the expired gas declines. Consequently, increased oxygen consumption with low fresh gas flow and a high share of oxygen-depleted rebreathing volume results in a much more marked reduction of the inspired oxygen concentration than with high fresh gas flow and correspondingly low share of oxygen-depleted rebreathing volume (Figure 3.5).

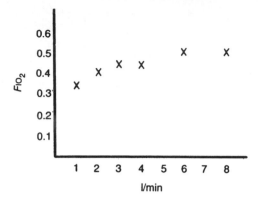

Figure 3.3   With constant fresh gas composition (50% O_2, 50% N_2O), the inspired oxygen concentration (*y*-axis) decreases with reduction of the fresh gas volume (*x*-axis). (From Schilling and Weis[13], by permission)

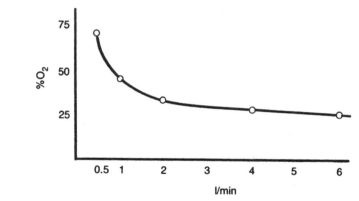

Figure 3.4   To ensure a constant oxygen concentration of 25% by volume, the oxygen content of the fresh gas (*y*-axis) must be increased if the fresh gas volume (*x*-axis) is reduced. (From Schreiber[14], by permission)

3.2   Nitrous oxide

3.2.1   Nitrous oxide uptake

The uptake of nitrous oxide follows an exponential curve: although the nitrous oxide uptake decreases rapidly, it is necessary initially to feed great volumes of nitrous oxide into the breathing system. After this initial period of anaesthesia, lasting about 20–30 min, the further decrease in uptake proceeds very slowly, so that nitrous oxide uptake is virtually constant over lengthy periods. According to Severinghaus[16], and assuming an inspired nitrous oxide concentration of about 80% ($F_{iN_2O} = 0.8$), the nitrous oxide uptake of a normal-weight adult can be approximated by means of the following formula:

$$\dot{V}_{N_2O} = 1000 \times t^{-1/2}(\text{ml/min})$$

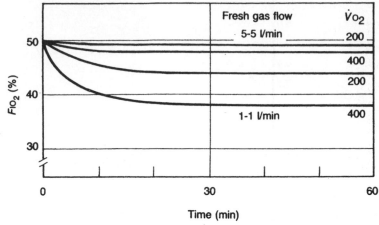

Figure 3.5 If the oxygen consumption ($\dot{V}_{O_2}$) rises to 400 ml/min, a low fresh gas flow (1 l/min O_2 + 1 l/min N_2O) results in a distinctly greater reduction of the inspired oxygen concentration (*y*-axis) than a high flow (5 l/min O_2 + 5 l/min N_2O). (From Westenskow[15], by permission)

where t = time (min). This nitrous oxide uptake characteristic, which corresponds to an exponential function, has been confirmed by Barton and Nunn[17], Spieß[18] and Westenskow *et al.*[7,8] in the range calculated in accordance with the Severinghaus formula.

For calculation of nitrous oxide uptake during the time course of anaesthesia, assuming an inspired nitrous oxide concentration of 75%, Beatty *et al.*[19] quote the following formula:

$$\dot{V}_{N_2O} = 412 \times t^{-0.37}\,(\text{ml/min})$$

The values calculated with this formula are somewhat lower than those calculated using the Severinghaus formula. A significant correlation with body weight or age of the patients could not be established by Beatty *et al.*[19].

3.2.2   Implications for anaesthetic practice

An inspired nitrous oxide concentration of 60–65% permits a satisfactory utilization of the nitrous oxide effect, since the state of amnalgesia with adequate somnolence and distinct analgesia can be attained with this concentration[20]. At the same time, this value corresponds quite well to the recommended inspired oxygen concentration of 30%. The potential to vary these two values, however, is rather limited for safety reasons[17]. A desired oxygen–nitrous oxide mixture can easily be attained using a high fresh gas flow since, with increasing flow, the composition of fresh gas and inspired gas are almost identical. In the case of low fresh gas flows, however, consideration must be given to the following problem: the oxygen uptake is constant within certain limits, while the nitrous oxide

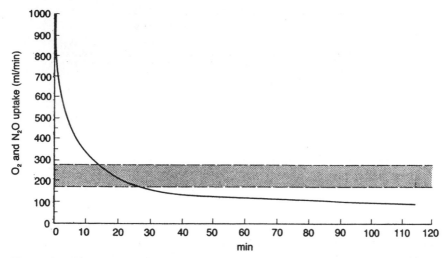

Figure 3.6 While the oxygen uptake during the time course of anaesthesia can be assumed as being constant within certain limits (shaded area), the nitrous oxide uptake decreases exponentially (uptake calculated for a normal-weight adult patient)

uptake decreases continuously, corresponding to an exponential function (Figure 3.6).

Should the fresh gas flow be reduced very early, the volume of nitrous oxide extracted from the system is considerably greater than the volume of oxygen taken up by the patient. The F_{iN_2O} drops while the F_{iO_2} rises. And if, during the initial phase of anaesthesia, the nitrous oxide volume fed into the system with the fresh gas is even lower than the nitrous oxide uptake, this may result in a gas volume deficiency. On the other hand, in the case of long-term anaesthesia, the nitrous oxide uptake drops to comparatively low values. If now the nitrous oxide volume fed into the system becomes greater than the nitrous oxide uptake, in low flow anaesthesia nitrous oxide is liable to accumulate in the breathing system. Correspondingly the F_{iN_2O} increases, and the F_{iO_2} decreases. This is why Lin and Mostert[21] recommend that a 'wash-in phase' with high fresh gas flow should precede the flow reduction. Thereafter, the nitrous oxide uptake remains virtually constant over a long period of time so that a nitrous oxide flow $\dot{V}_{FN_2O}$ calculated in accordance with the following formula:

$$\dot{V}_{FN_2O} = 200 \times \text{desired } F_{iN_2O}(\text{ml/min})$$

and an oxygen flow being equal to the oxygen uptake delivered as the total fresh gas flow will suffice to ensure the desired composition of inspired gas. Smith[22], however, comes to the conclusion that, in the individual case, it will not be possible to make an adequately precise calculation for the composition of inspired gas with any one of these different formulae. The lower the fresh gas flow, the greater are the deviations between calculated and measured concentrations. Given a flow of less than 0.9 l/min, no correlation can be established between the oxygen and nitrous oxide concentrations of the fresh gas and that of the anaesthetic gas.

This makes continuous monitoring of the inspired oxygen concentration an inevitable requirement to ensure an adequate oxygen supply and, thus, the patient's safety, if anaesthesia is performed with reduced fresh gas flows using a nitrous oxide–oxygen mixture.

3.3 Volatile anaesthetics

3.3.1 Uptake of volatile anaesthetics

3.3.1.1 Pharmacokinetics of volatile anaesthetics

Volatile anaesthetics are administered with the objective of attaining an anaesthetic concentration in the central nervous system which affords an adequate pain relief in surgical interventions, and sufficient reduction of consciousness and reflexes at the same time. The amount of anaesthetic required for this purpose must be supplied to the patient's lungs via the breathing system. There the anaesthetic gas or vapour is absorbed by the blood and transported to all organs and tissues, including the brain. The amount of anaesthetic agent entering this tissue compartment brings about anaesthesia. Following a certain period of saturation, it attains the concentration required for sufficient suppression of central nervous tissue functions. Bearing this process in mind, it can clearly be recognized that the uptake of volatile anaesthetics is influenced by a great number of physiological, physicochemical and technical factors.

The transport to the lungs is effected via the whole gas-containing system which consists of the alveolar space, the conducting airways, the breathing system, and possibly a ventilator. The kinetic parameters which influence the uptake in this system are:

- the alveolar minute ventilation volume, $\dot{V}_A$,
- and the anaesthetic alveolar concentration C_A.

Transition into the blood is effected via the alveolar membrane. This stage of the mechanism of anaesthetic uptake is determined by:

- the alveolar–capillary concentration difference
- and the blood/gas partition coefficient $\lambda_{B/G}$ of the anaesthetic selected.

The blood serves as the carrier for the anaesthetic agent. This convective transport is a function of:

- the cardiac output $\dot{Q}$,
- and the anaesthetic arterial concentration C_a.

The transition into the particular tissue compartment, the diffusion transport, is the ultimate stage of anaesthetic uptake and is determined by:

- the organ blood flow, $\dot{Q}_T$;
- the organ's tissue volume, V_T;
- the blood/tissue partial pressure difference of the anaesthetic agent; and
- the tissue and agent specific tissue/blood partition coefficient, $\lambda_{T/B}$.

The total uptake is the sum of the uptakes of all organs, whereby the relevant virtual distribution volume of the individual organ is calculated by multiplying the organ's volume by its specific tissue–blood partition coefficient[23].

Since diffusion transport proceeds rapidly, the concentration of the anaesthetic in the venous limb of the organ's vessel system corresponds to the agent's tissue concentration. This means that the velocity of uptake is mainly determined by the velocity of the convective transport. The anaesthetist, however, is only able to exert an influence on the kinetic parameters determining the agent's transport to the lung. He has no direct influence on the factors influencing the convection and diffusion transport. From the pharmacokinetic point of view, closed and low flow systems are nothing but a special parameter selection with respect to the rebreathing fraction in establishing the desired alveolar concentration of the inhalational anaesthetic[24].

In order to achieve a constant alveolar concentration in non-rebreathing systems, consideration must be given to three different subsets which comprise the BET scheme[24]:

- The amount of anaesthetic agent saturating the alveolar space with the desired concentration (Bolus).
- The substitution of the amount of agent eliminated with the gas exchange caused by the alveolar ventilation (Elimination).
- The substitution of the total anaesthetic uptake, that is, the sum of the uptakes of all individual organs, which can be calculated with the Zuntz equation (Transfer):

$$\dot{V}_A \times C_i = V_A \times C_A + \dot{V}_A \times C_A + C_A \times \lambda_{B/G} \times \Sigma \dot{Q}_T \times e^{-\frac{\dot{Q}_T \times t}{V_T \times \lambda_{B/G}}}$$

where

$\dot{V}_A \times C_I$ = volume of anaesthetic vapour which has to be supplied per time unit (inspiratory supply);

$V_A \times C_A$ = saturation of the alveolar space (bolus);

$\dot{V}_A \times C_A$ = substitution of the anaesthetic volume being eliminated by alveolar ventilation (elimination); and

$C_A \times \lambda_{B/G} \times \Sigma \dot{Q}_T \times e^{-\frac{\dot{Q}_T \times t}{V_T \times \lambda_{B/G}}}$ substitution of the total uptake (transfer).

Pharmacokinetic formulae of this complexity, however, do not provide practical assistance in the dosage of volatile anaesthetics, unless a computer and appropriate software is available at the workplace[25,26].

Since the difference between the anaesthetic concentration of the fresh gas and that of the inspired gas increases with progressive reduction of the fresh gas flow (Figure 3.7) and since a relationship between both figures can no longer be established if the fresh gas flow is less than about 1.5 l/min[17], dosage aids must be provided. This is of particular importance if no monitoring is available for measuring the concentration of volatile anaesthetics within the breathing system.

A poll prompted by Tammisto[28] revealed that even experienced anaesthetists could not estimate the inspired anaesthetic concentration in a

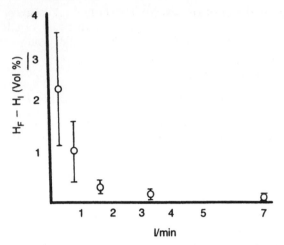

Figure 3.7   The difference between the inspired (H_I) and the fresh gas halothane concentration (H_F) (*y*-axis) increases with decreasing fresh gas flow (*x*-axis). (From Baer[27], by permission)

rebreathing system precisely, although the fresh gas flow and vaporizer settings were known.

3.3.1.2   The Lowe uptake model

Based on the Severinghaus nitrous oxide uptake formula[16], Lowe[6,29] worked out a mathematical concept which approximates the uptake of volatile anaesthetics as a function of the square root of time:

$$\dot{V}_{AN} = C_a \times \dot{Q} \times t^{-1/2} \qquad (1)$$

where $\dot{Q} =$ cardiac output (dl/min), $C_a =$ arterial concentration and $t =$ time (min).

Calculation of the arterial anaesthetic concentration:

$$C_a = C_A \times \lambda_{B/G} \qquad (2)$$

where $C_A =$ alveolar concentration and $\lambda_{B/G} =$ blood/gas partition coefficient.

Calculation of the anaesthetic alveolar concentration as a multiple of MAC:

$$C_A = f \times MAC \qquad (3)$$

where $f =$ calculating factor, which defines the desired alveolar concentration as a fraction of MAC; and MAC = minimum alveolar concentration.

Calculation of the factor f for the AD_{95} concentration (inhalational anaesthetic concentration ensuring sufficient anaesthetic depth for skin incision in 95% of all patients):

$$f = 1.3 - F_{iN_2O} \qquad (4)$$

where $F_{iN_2O} =$ inspired nitrous oxide fraction.

Calculation of the cardiac output according to the Brody formula:

$$\dot{Q} = 2 \times BW(kg)^{3/4} \tag{5}$$

where $BW(kg)$ = patient's body weight in kilograms.

Substitute equations (2)–(5) in (1):

$$\dot{V}_{AN} = (1.3 - F_{iN_2O}) \times MAC \times \lambda_{B/G} \times 2 \times BW(kg)^{3/4} \times t^{-1/2} \tag{6}$$

By integration of this equation the cumulative dose can be calculated (i.e. the total amount of anaesthetic agent delivered to the patient during the time t):

$$KD = 2 \times (1.3 - F_{iN_2O}) \times MAC \times \lambda_{B/G} \times 2 \times BW(kg)^{3/4} \times \sqrt{t} + c \tag{7}$$

where c = arterial prime dose.

At the beginning of anaesthesia, a priming dose (PD) must be fed into the system by means of which the desired concentration of the anaesthetic can be established in the whole gas-carrying space (volume of the lungs, the breathing system and the ventilator), as well as in the blood:

$$PD = C_A \times (V_S + V_L) + C_a \times \dot{Q} \tag{8}$$

where

$$C_A \times (V_S + V_L) = \text{prime dose for the gas-carrying compartments;}$$

$$C_a \times \dot{Q} = \text{prime dose for the blood } (= c: \text{arterial prime dose});$$

$$V_S = \text{system volume (gas containing volume of the}$$

$$\text{anaesthetic apparatus) (dl); and}$$

$$V_L = \text{gas volume of the lungs and the airways (dl).}$$

Substitute (2) and (3) in (8):

$$PD = f \times MAC \times (V_S + V_L) + f \times MAC \times \lambda_{B/G} \times \dot{Q} \tag{9}$$

If the sum of V_S and V_L is assumed to be about 10 litres, equal to 100 dl, the resultant prime dose can be calculated as follows:

$$PD = f \times MAC \times (100 + \lambda_{B/G} \times \dot{Q}) \tag{10}$$

Lowe called the dose to be administered after the first minute the unit dose (UD):

$$UD = 2 \times C_a \times \dot{Q} \text{ (ml anaesthetic vapour)}$$

and recommended the administration of this unit dose in continuously increasing time intervals, that is, after the 1st, 4th, 9th, 16th, etc., minutes. At all these times, the cumulative dose required for maintaining anaesthesia is always a whole-numbered multiple of the unit dose. This results in a dosage scheme for closed system anaesthesia with volatile anaesthetics in which a constant dose of the anaesthetic agent is administered at each time at which the factor $\sqrt{t}$ becomes a whole-numbered figure (Figure 3.8b).

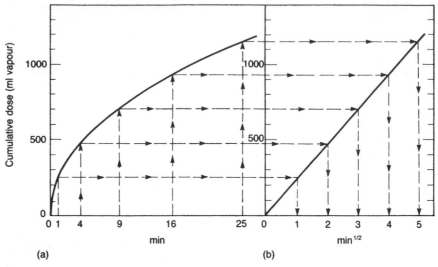

Figure 3.8   Cumulative halothane dose for a patient of 100 kg body weight: in diagram (a) plotted against time t, in diagram (b) against $\sqrt{t}$. The volumes of halothane vapour uptake are identical during whole-numbered intervals. (From Lowe and Ernst[6], by permission)

3.3.1.3   The Westenskow uptake model

Westenskow et al.[30], Thomson et al.[31] and Gorsky et al.[32] pointed out, however, that the doses of inhalational anaesthetic agents calculated according to Lowe's uptake model are too high and that the anaesthetic concentrations are about 25–50% above the desired values (Figure 3.9).

Westenskow summarizes the results of his investigations concerning uptake as follows. The uptake of volatile anaesthetics is neither constant nor does it follow the 'square-root of time' rule of the Lowe model. With semi-logarithmic presentation, the anaesthetic uptake can be described by two straight lines whose intersection point divides anaesthesia into two phases: during the first 10 min, the uptake is high and decreases rapidly, while in the second phase the uptake remains almost constant (Figure 3.10).

This graph results from the calculation of average values of enflurane uptake obtained from 23 patients. Westenskow et al.[30] and Zbinden[33] emphasize, however, that the uptake may differ greatly in individual cases so that at best the graph can be an orientation aid, but in no way provides more than a guideline on dosage.

3.3.1.4   The Lin uptake model

Following mass spectrometric measurements of the uptake of volatile anaesthetics Lin et al.[21,34] came to the conclusion that the rapid initial rise of the quotient F_A/F_I (end-expired (alveolar) to inspired concentration) is based on the wash-in phase. Depending on the fresh gas flow, this

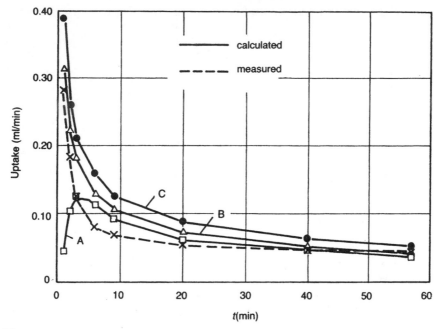

Figure 3.9   Difference in halothane uptake between measured values (– – –) and figures calculated according to the Lowe formula (——). (From Thomson *et al.*[31], by permission)

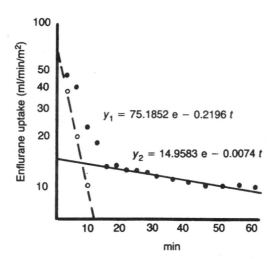

Figure 3.10   In semi-logarithmic presentation, the enflurane uptake during the time course of anaesthesia can be plotted by means of two straight regression lines. The intersection (after 10 min) splits anaesthesia into two phases with different uptake characteristics: the vessel-rich tissues are saturated during the first phase and poorly vascularized tissues in the second phase. (From Westenskow *et al.*[30], by permission)

takes about 3–20 min: during that time the gas concentration is established and brought to equilibrium within the whole gas-containing space. The uptake itself, however, can be assumed to be comparatively constant and is essentially a function of the alveolar–capillary partial pressure difference, provided that the cardiac output and ventilation remain unchanged. Following equilibrium, the uptake of volatile anaesthetics can be approximated for the following period of about 120 min by using the formulae:

$$\dot{V}_{Hal} = 15\text{–}20 \, ml/min \text{ halothane vapour per } \% \text{ desired concentration},$$

$$\dot{V}_{Enf} = 30 \, ml/min \text{ enflurane vapour per } \% \text{ desired concentration}.$$

In addition, the long time constant of the closed system tends to ensure a constant gas concentration.

Referring to a recent investigation on the uptake of isoflurane and desflurane[35], Eger, too, concludes that the individual uptake of volatile anaesthetics changes only slightly during the course of inhalational anaesthesia[36]. The initial high demand for anaesthetic agents could be explained by the need for a sufficient amount of agent to establish the desired agent's concentration within the whole gas containing system, which comprises both the apparatus and the lung volume. Thus, anaesthetists, practising low flow anaesthetic techniques, could renounce the use of any sophisticated mathematical formula to calculate the patient's individual uptake and frequent alterations of the settings of the gas controls, and instead use standardized constant settings of the vaporizers.

Mostert et al.[37] also recommended proceeding as follows. The system should only be closed after an initial phase of anaesthesia with a high fresh gas flow, during which a steady state of gas concentration can be attained. After flow reduction, the loss of volatile anaesthetic resulting from uptake can be replenished by only small amounts of anaesthetic vapour.

3.3.2 Implications for anaesthetic practice

Based on the aforementioned considerations, the following rules may be derived for clinical practice:

- There is no generally accepted dosage pattern for a change from the habitual anaesthetic method with semi-closed system in which gas concentrations are stabilized by the administration of a considerable excess of gas mixture, to the quantitative system of equilibrium using a closed breathing system.
- Each dosage pattern and every pharmacokinetic calculation model will merely offer an aid to orientation. When used in anaesthetic practice, it requires critical verification by careful observation of the individual patient and may have to be adjusted during the course of anaesthesia. This rule is, though, also applicable to anaesthesia management with a high fresh gas flow.
- It should not be overlooked that the goal of such dosage patterns is to establish desired values for anaesthetic concentrations. No statement can be made as to whether in the individual case the resultant depth of

anaesthesia attained with this concentration is adequate for the respective surgical intervention or the individual reaction of the patient.

- The initial phase of anaesthesia is marked by a high demand for nitrous oxide and volatile anaesthetic. In practice, it is of minor significance whether this can be explained by the wash-in process into the gas-carrying space itself or by the high uptake during the induction phase. But at the time when the fresh gas flow is reduced, it must be critically examined whether the selected flow covers the current demand for nitrous oxide and anaesthetic vapour. Otherwise, undesired changes in anaesthetic depth and deficiency of gas volume in the system may result.

3.4 Total gas uptake

The total gas uptake is calculated from the sum of oxygen, nitrous oxide and anaesthetic vapour volumes being taken up at the particular time during anaesthesia. The uptake of nitrous oxide and volatile anaesthetics follows an exponential function, while the uptake of oxygen can be assumed as being constant within certain limits. To this end, the total gas uptake thus decreases with time during the course of anaesthesia (Figure 3.11). The alteration of the uptake during the course of anaesthesia is mainly determined by the nitrous oxide uptake. Thus, consistently

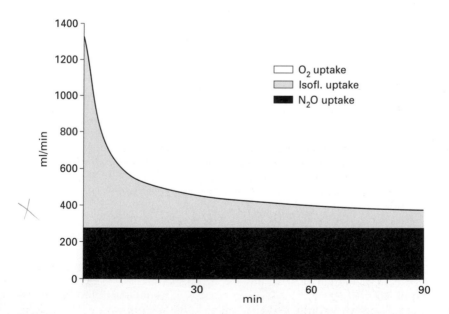

Figure 3.11 The total gas uptake depicted as the sum of oxygen, nitrous oxide and anaesthetic vapour uptake. Calculated for a patient of 75 kg body weight, an inspired nitrous oxide concentration of 65% by volume, and an expiratory isoflurane concentration of 0.75% by volume

omitting the use of any nitrous oxide would exert highly significant implications on the practice of low flow anaesthetic techniques (see Chapter 11).

3.5 References

1. Brody S. *Bioenergetics and Growth.* Reinhold, New York, 1945.
2. Kleiber M. Body size and metabolic rate. *Physiol Rev* 1945; **27**, 511–539.
3. Arndt G and Stock M Ch. Brody's equation: a reinterpretation and its clinical application. *The Circular* 1988; **5**, 5–8.
4. Arndt JO. Inhalationsanästhetika und Stoffwechsel: O_2-Verbrauch wacher, schlafender oder narkotisierter Hunde unter Grundumsatzbedingungen. In Schwilden H and Stoecke H, eds, *Die Inhaltionsnarkose: Steuerung und Überwachung. INA-Schriftenreihe*, vol. 58. Thieme, Stuttgart, 1987, pp. 43–52.
5. Guyton AC, Jones CE and Coleman TC. *Circulatory Physiology: Cardiac Output and Its Regulations.* Saunders, Philadelphia, 1973, pp. 12–14 and 21–24.
6. Lowe HJ and Ernst EA. *The Quantitative Practice of Anesthesia.* Williams & Wilkins, Baltimore, 1981.
7. Westenskow DR, Jordan WS and Gehmlich DS. Electronic feedback control and measurement of oxygen consumption during closed circuit anesthesia. In Aldrete JA, Lowe HJ, Virtue RW, eds, *Low Flow and Closed System Anesthesia.* Grune & Stratton, New York, 1979, pp. 135–146.
8. Westenskow DR and Jordan WS. Automatic control of closed circuit anesthesia and the measurement of enflurane N_2O and oxygen uptake. In *Geschlossenes System für Inhalationsnarkosen*, Internationales Symposium, Düsseldorf, 7–8 May 1982 (abstract).
9. Manawadu BR, Hartwig FE, Sherrill D and Swanson GD. Monitoring oxygen consumption utilizing low flow techniques. In Aldrete JA, Lowe HJ and Virtue RW, eds, *Low Flow and Closed System Anesthesia.* Grune & Stratton, New York, 1979, pp. 147–150.
10. Finsterer U. Lungenfunktion unter Narkose. *Anästh Intensivmed* 1983; **24**, 277–287.
11. Reineke H. Respiratorische Risikofaktoren und Narkosebeatmung. *Anästh Intensivmed* 1983; **24**, 33–36.
12. Don H. Hypoxemia and hypercapnia during and after anesthesia. In Orkin FK and Cooperman LH, eds, *Complications in Anesthesiology.* Lippincott, Philadelphia, 1983, pp. 183–207.
13. Schilling R and Weis KH. Zur Sauerstoffkonzentration im Narkosesystem. *Anaesthesist* 1973; **22**, 198–201.
14. Schreiber P. Anesthesia Systems. In *North American Draeger Safety Guidelines.* Merchants Press, Boston, 1985.
15. Westenskow DR. How much oxygen? *Intl J Clin Monitor Comput* 1986; **2**, 187–189.
16. Severinghaus JW. The rate of uptake of nitrous oxide in man. *J Clin Invest* 1954; **33**, 1183–1189.
17. Barton F and Nunn J F. Totally closed circuit nitrous oxide/oxygen anaesthesia. *Br J Anaesth* 1975; **47**, 350–357.
18. Spieß W. Narkose im geschlossenen System mit kontinuierlicher inspiratorischer Sauerstoffmessung. *Anaesthesist* 1977; **26**, 503–513.
19. Beatty PCW, Kay B and Healy TEJ. Measurement of the rates of nitrous oxide uptake and nitrogen excretion in man. *Br J Anaesth* 1984; **56**, 223–232.
20. Parbrook GD. The levels of nitrous oxide analgesia. *Br J Anaesth* 1967; **39**, 974–982.

21. Lin CY and Mostert JW. Inspired O_2 and N_2O concentrations in essentially closed circuits. *Anaesthesist* 1977; **26**, 514–517.
22. Smith TC. Nitrous oxide and low flow inflow circle systems. *Anesthesiology* 1966; **27**, 266–271.
23. Schwilden H, Stoeckel H, Lauven PM and Schüttler J. Pharmakokinetik und MAC – Praktische Implikationen für die Dosierung volatiler Anästhetika. In Peter K, Brown BR, Martin E and Norlander O, eds, *Inhalationsanästhetika. Anästhesiologie und Intensivmedizin*, vol. 184. Springer, Berlin, 1986, pp. 18–26.
24. Schwilden H, Stoeckel H, Lauven PM and Schüttler J. Pharmakokinetik der Inhalationsansthetika. In *Geschlossenes System für Inhalationsnarkosen, Abstracband*. Internationales Symposium, Düsseldorf, 7–8 May 1982.
25. Schwilden H. *Narkosesimulator*. Deutsche Abbott, Wiesbaden, 1986.
26. Schwilden H. Die rechnergestützte interaktive Dosierung volatiler Anästhetika (AC-Prädiktor). In Schwilden H and Stöckel H, eds, *Die Inhalationsnarkose: Steuerung und Überwachung*. INA Bd. 58. Thieme, Stuttgart, 1987, pp. 167–173.
27. Baer B. Die Abhängigkeit der inspiratorischen Halothankonzentration im Kreisystem von der Höhe der Frischgaszufuhr. *Anaesthesist* 1983; **32**, 6–11.
28. Tammisto T. Monitoring der Konzentration volatiler Anästhetika. In Schwilden H and Stöckel H, eds, *Die Inhalationsnarkose: Steuerung und Überwachung*. INA Bd. 58. Thieme, Stuttgart, 1987, pp. 33–38.
29. Lowe HJ. *Dose-regulated Penthrane Anesthesia*. Abbott Laboratories, Chicago, 1972.
30. Westenskow DR, Jordan WS and Hayes JK. Uptake of enflurane: a study of the variability between patients. *Br J Anaesth* 1983; **55**, 598–610.
31. Thomson D, Zbinden A and Westenskow D. Pharmakokinetik von Inhalationsanästhetika – Untersuchungen mit einem feed-back kontrollierten geschlossenen System. In Peter K, Brown BR, Martin E and Norlander O, eds, *Inhalationsanästhetika. Anästhesiologie und Intensivmedizin*, Bd. 184. Springer, Berlin 1986, pp. 34–42.
32. Gorsky BH, Hall RL and Redford JE. A compromise for closed system anesthesia. *Anesth Analg* 1978; **57**, 18–24.
33. Zbinden AM. *Inhalationsanästhetika: Aufnahme und Verteilung*. Wissenschaftliche Verlagsabteilung, Deutsche Abbott, Wiesbaden, 1987.
34. Lin CY, Mostert JW and Benson DW. Closed circle systems. A new direction in the practice of anesthesia. *Acta Anaesth Scand* 1980; **24**, 354–361.
35. Hendrickx JFA, Soetens M, Van der Donck A, Meeuwis H, Smolders F and De Wolf AM. Uptake of desflurane and isoflurane during closed-circuit anesthesia with spontaneous and controlled mechanical ventilation. *Anesth Analg* 1997; **84**, 413–418.
36. Eger EI, II. Complexities overlooked: things may not be what they seem. *Anesth Analg* 1997; **84**, 239–240.
37. Mostert JW, Goldberg IS, Lanzl EF and Lowe HJ. Das geschlossene System. *Anaesthesist* 1977; **26**, 495–502.

4

Anaesthetic methods with reduced fresh gas flow

Depending on the selection of the fresh gas flow, rebreathing systems may be semi-open, semi-closed or closed. With semi-closed use of a rebreathing system, the fresh gas fed into the system can be arbitrarily set to any value that is less than the minute volume. The fresh gas flow, however, must at least equal that volume, which is lost with the individual uptake by the patient or via leaks from the breathing system at any given time. Only by supplying at least this amount of gas will the appropriate gas volume for ventilation be available. As emphasized beforehand, the lower the fresh gas flow the lower is the amount of gas vented out of the breathing system as waste, and the higher is rebreathing fraction. If a rebreathing system is used with a fresh gas flow equal to the minute volume of the patient, the proportion of gas rebreathed will be negligible. Virtually all the expired gas will be vented out of the system via the excess gas discharge valve and the patient breathes nearly pure fresh gas. If a flow of 4.0 l/min is used, the rebreathing fraction will increase to about 20%. The patient inhales a gas the composition of which still resembles that of the fresh gas. Only once the flow is reduced to 2.0 l/min or lower does the rebreathing fraction reach 50% or more (Figure 4.1). Thus it is only when low fresh gas flows are used that the rebreathing fraction becomes significant, and judicious use is made from the rebreathing technique.

The terminology, by which low flow anaesthetic techniques are catalogued, can be based either on the degree of rebreathing or on the fresh gas flow rate. The fresh gas flow rate mainly determines the rebreathing fraction, as is shown in Figure 4.1; however, in the individual case rebreathing is also significantly influenced by the technical design of the rebreathing system, the ventilation patterns and the individual's total gas uptake. If, for instance, a minimal flow technique using 0.5 l/min fresh gas flow is performed on an adult patient of normal weight, the resulting rebreathing volume will be considerable and the excess gas volume very small. If the same flow, however, is used for a small infant, a considerably higher excess gas and a correspondingly lower rebreathing volume will result. Thus, low flow anaesthetic techniques can only be precisely and unambiguously defined and catalogued by giving exact details about the rebreathing fraction. A precise definition cannot be linked to the fresh gas flow rate in isolation. In the individual case, however, due to the great

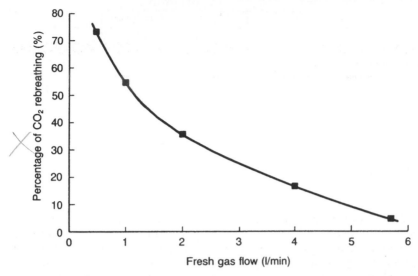

Figure 4.1   Percentage of exhaled carbon dioxide actually reaching the absorber as a function of the fresh gas flow. Measurements at a circle absorption system 8 ISO (Dräger Medizintechnik, Lübeck, Germany), Pat. R.S.: 72 kg, 182 cm, ventilatory minute volume 5.7 l/min

number of variable factors, it will be nearly impossible to calculate exactly or even measure the actual rebreathing fraction.

The term low flow anaesthesia should be restricted to defining inhalational anaesthetic techniques, performed with a semi-closed rebreathing system, in which of rebreathing fraction comes to at least 50%. For most patients, using modern rebreathing systems, this will be achieved only if the fresh gas flow rate is lower than 2.0 l/min[1].

Nevertheless, one has to deal with the fact that a great number of variants of anaesthesia management with different low fresh gas flow rates are described in the literature. It must be accepted that the terminology is still widely linked to a certain fresh gas flow rate. Thus, to avoid extreme confusion in this field, the author suggests the retention of the original terms used by those anaesthetists who introduced the different low flow techniques into clinical practice, such as Waters, Foldes and Virtue[2-4]. From a clinical point of view these terms still serve to distinguish well between the three different low flow anaesthetic techniques: low flow, minimal flow, and closed system anaesthesia (Figure 4.2). The many subsequent attempts to create new terminologies[5-8] are superfluous, since they cannot give any new or more precise information, still relating as they do to the fresh gas flow rates.

According to the literature, four low flow anaesthetic techniques should be distinguished (Figure 4.2): Foldes *et al.*[3,9] were the first to recommend the use of a fresh gas flow rate of 1.0 l/min, as early as in 1952. He called his technique 'Low Flow Anaesthesia'. In 1974 Virtue described a technique called 'Minimal Flow Anaesthesia' in which a fresh gas flow of not more than 0.5 l/min should be used[4,10]. Both low flow anaesthesia

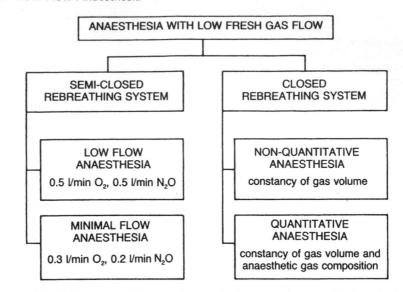

Figure 4.2   Different techniques of anaesthesia management with low fresh gas flows

and minimal flow anaesthesia are extreme variants of the semi-closed use of rebreathing systems. In the latter, the excess gas volume just slightly exceeds the total gas uptake of an adult patient[11]. Low flow anaesthesia and minimal flow anaesthesia are certainly low flow anaesthetic techniques, as the rebreathing fraction can be assumed always to exceed 50%. It must, though, be emphasized, that both terms, low and minimal flow anaesthesia, are defined by the respective fresh gas flow rates. In the individual case these terms do not give any exact information on the respective rebreathing fraction. Both terms allow no more than a rough distinction between a technique realizing good (low flow anaesthesia) or nearly optimal use of rebreathing systems when working with conventional anaesthetic machines. In a considerable number of older type anaesthetic machines, due to their inadequate technical features, a flow reduction to a value as low as 0.5 l/min will be impossible.

In 'Closed System Anaesthesia', by definition, any use of excess gas is avoided, the fresh gas volume delivered into the breathing system just meets the individual's uptake, and the exhaled gas is reused completely after carbon dioxide absorption. Thus, in closed system anaesthesia the flow is reduced to the individual total gas uptake of the patient. If the amount of fresh gas just meets the total uptake, 'Non-quantitative Anaesthesia with Closed System' is realized. However, if not only the gas volume, circulating within the rebreathing system, but also its composition can be kept constant during the whole time course of anaesthesia 'Quantitative Anaesthesia with Closed System' is achieved (Table 4.1).

With all the different low flow anaesthetic techniques the fresh gas flow is more or less adapted to the total gas uptake during the course of anaesthesia (Figure 4.3). Only by proceeding in this way are rebreathing

Table 4.1   Low flow anaesthetic techniques (carrier gas: O_2/N_2O mixture)

Low flow anaesthesia	
Fresh gas flow	constant 1.0 l/min
Fresh gas composition	50% O_2, 50% N_2O
Rebreathing	partial
Use of excess gas	yes
Anaesthetic gas composition	changes with the course of anaesthesia
Technical classification	anaesthetic technique using a semi-closed rebreathing system
Minimal flow anaesthesia	
Fresh gas flow	constant 0.5 l/min
Fresh gas composition	60% O_2, 40% N_2O
Rebreathing	extensive
Use of excess gas	minimal
Anaesthetic gas composition	changes with the course of anaesthesia
Technical classification	anaesthetic technique using a semi-closed rebreathing system
Non-quantitative closed system anaesthesia	
Fresh gas flow	intermittent adaptation of the fresh gas volume to gas loss via uptake or leaks
Fresh gas composition	varies, intermittent alteration according to the anaesthetic gas composition may be necessary
Rebreathing	entire exhaled gas after carbon dioxide elimination
Use of excess gas	no
Anaesthetic gas composition	varies during the course of anaesthesia
Technical classification	anaesthetic technique using a closed rebreathing system
Quantitative closed system anaesthesia	
Fresh gas flow	continuous adaptation of fresh gas flow to the individual total gas uptake
Fresh gas composition	continuous adaptation to individual uptake of anaesthetic gas components
Rebreathing	entire exhaled gas after carbon dioxide elimination
Use of excess gas	no
Anaesthetic gas composition	constant during the whole course of anaesthesia according to preset values
Technical classification	anaesthetic technique using a closed rebreathing system

systems used judiciously and use made of the advantages of the rebreathing technique.

4.1   Low flow anaesthesia

This anaesthetic technique, in which the fresh gas flow is reduced to 1 l/min, was first published by Foldes and co-workers in 1952, after they had used this approach successfully in more than 10 000 patients. As

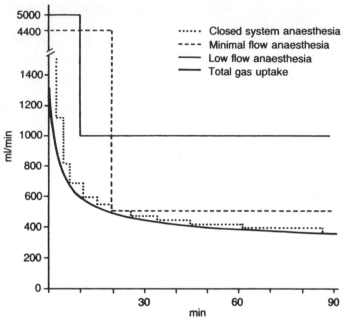

Figure 4.3 Common characteristics of anaesthetic techniques with low fresh gas flow. Following an initial phase using high gas flow, the fresh gas flow rate is reduced and thus adapted to the total gas uptake which continuously decreases during the course of anaesthesia. To achieve the most precise adaptation, frequent adjustments of the flow controls are required

Foldes related, due to the assumption of there being a danger of hypoxia, none of the American anaesthesia journals would accept his paper, so that it finally had to be published in the *Annals of Surgery*[3]. The results of his investigations can be summarized as follows:

The oxygen concentration in the breathing system decreases

- if, with constant fresh gas composition, the total fresh gas flow is reduced;
- if, with constant flow, the fresh gas composition is changed in favour of nitrous oxide; and
- if, with unchanged fresh gas composition and constant flow, the duration of anaesthesia increases.

For calculation of the oxygen and nitrous oxide flows by means of which a desired oxygen concentration can be attained in the system at a pre-selected fresh gas flow, Foldes quoted a simple formula:

$$\dot{V}_{FO_2} = \dot{V}_{O_2} + (\dot{V}_F - \dot{V}_{O_2})/100 \times F_{iO_2}$$

$$\dot{V}_{FN_2O} = \dot{V}_F - \dot{V}_{FO_2}$$

where $\dot{V}_{FO_2}$ = oxygen flow required, $\dot{V}_{FN_2O}$ = nitrous oxide flow required,

$\dot{V}_F$ = fresh gas flow, $\dot{V}_{O_2}$ = oxygen uptake, and F_{iO_2} = desired inspired oxygen concentration.

Foldes and co-workers suggested the following procedure for performance of low flow anaesthesia:

- initial setting of a high fresh gas flow for 3 min (4 l/min N_2O, 1–1.5 l/min O_2);
- thereafter, reduction of the fresh gas flow to 1 l/min, whereby the respective oxygen and nitrous oxide flow should equal the gas volumes calculated from the formulae above;
- should the breathing system be opened to atmosphere for some reason, the first two steps have to be repeated;
- where patients with a high metabolic rate are concerned, a correspondingly higher inspired oxygen concentration must be given.

With a standardized setting of the fresh gas composition (0.5 l/min O_2, 0.5 l/min N_2O), an average inspired oxygen concentration of $30 \pm 5\%$ was attained, and in no case did this value drop below 20%.

In 1985, Foldes and Duncalf presented a somewhat modified concept[9]. The flow reduction is preceded by an initial phase of 10 min with high fresh gas flow (2 l/min O_2, 3 l/min N_2O), to ensure adequate denitrogenation. Thereafter, a standard fresh gas flow of 1 l/min (0.5 l/min O_2, 0.5 l/min N_2O) should be set. Since nitrous oxide uptake decreases continuously during the course of anaesthesia, Foldes recommended modifying the fresh gas composition after another 10 min to 0.7 l/min O_2, 0.3 l/min N_2O. Should rapid changes in concentrations be necessary, the fresh gas flow should be increased.

Foldes preferred low flow anaesthesia to methods with an even lower fresh gas volume, proposing the following arguments:

- the technique of low flow anaesthesia can easily be learned;
- the monitoring demands, oxygen and carbon dioxide measurement as specified by Foldes, are low;
- the demands placed on gas tightness of the system can easily be satisfied with routine maintenance of the machines;
- the dosage of volatile anaesthetics is easy and simple;
- with a flow less than 1 l/min, even minor inaccuracies of the flow control of oxygen and nitrous oxide may result in grave alterations of oxygen concentration within the breathing system;
- with an even lower flow, special water traps, inserted in the patient's hose system, will be required; and
- the advantages of a further fresh gas flow reduction, and thus further improved utilization of rebreathing, are rather insignificant, whereas anaesthesia management will become considerably more difficult.

The low flow technique was somewhat modified by Grote et al. in 1982[12]. Following an initial phase with high flow (2 l/min O_2, 4 l/min N_2O) over 5 min they also recommended fresh gas flow reduction to 1 l/min (0.5 l/min O_2, 0.5 l/min N_2O). According to Grote, the inspiratory oxygen concentration never dropped below 30% with these standardized settings, so that they even considered continuous oxygen measurement unnecessary. They did, however, recommend changing the fresh gas composition to 0.6 l/min O_2 and 0.4 l/min N_2O after 1–2 h.

Grote and co-workers also judge low flow anaesthesia as being advantageous since it is easily understood and simple in performance. However, they emphasize that closed system anaesthesia should be preferred if adequate monitoring devices are available for measuring the concentrations of oxygen and volatile anaesthetics in the anaesthetic gas.

4.2   Minimal flow anaesthesia

In 1974, Virtue[4] introduced an anaesthetic method, termed 'minimal flow anaesthesia', in which the fresh gas flow is reduced to 0.5 l/min. This method could be performed without risk of hypoxia, since in those days, devices for continuous monitoring of the inspiratory oxygen concentration were already available.

Following induction in the usual manner, muscle relaxation, intubation and controlled ventilation, anaesthesia is initially performed with a high fresh gas flow (1.5 l/min O_2 and 3.5 l/min N_2O) for 15–20 min. During this phase, nitrogen is washed out of the body and the breathing system. Adequate volumes of nitrous oxide and anaesthetic vapour corresponding to the initial high uptakes are fed into the system so that the desired concentrations can be established and homogenized in the entire gas-containing space. After this initial phase using high flow, the fresh gas volume is reduced to a standardized setting of 0.5 l/min and simultaneously its composition changed to 60% O_2 (0.3 l/min O_2) and 40% N_2O (0.2 l/min N_2O). For a patient of 80 kg body weight, the oxygen consumption can be calculated according to the Brody formula (see Section 3.1.1) at 267 ml/min, and the nitrous oxide uptake is calculated after 20 min according to the Severinghaus formula (see Section 3.2.1) at 223 ml/min. Thus, after flow reduction, oxygen is administered in excess, while the amount of nitrous oxide fed into the system is somewhat less than the actual uptake. It must be considered, though, that the nitrous oxide uptake decreases exponentially, so that after another 10 min it amounts to only 183 ml/min. That in turn means that, at this time, nitrous oxide is also being fed into the breathing system in excess. With patients of lower weight, the excess gas volume is accordingly higher. Thus, minimal flow anaesthesia is an extreme variant of semi-closed system anaesthesia, using the lowest practicable excess gas volume and virtually complete rebreathing.

It goes without saying that, with such low fresh gas volumes of standardized composition, the question of the course of the inspiratory oxygen concentration had to be answered by Virtue. On average, the F_{iO_2} drops within a period of 120 min, from an initial value of 0.42 to 0.33, and after 3 h to a value of 0.29. The lowest value measured in an individual case was 0.22 after 3 h[4]. The decrease in the inspired oxygen concentration, depending on the duration of the anaesthetic procedure, can be attributed to the fact that with the continuing reduction in nitrous oxide uptake this gas accumulates in the breathing system. This is why Virtue recommends that, where patients of more than 80 kg body weight are concerned, the inspiratory oxygen concentration should be monitored continuously. Whenever the oxygen concentration drops to the lower limit, the oxygen flow should be increased. Alternatively, a higher fresh gas flow with higher oxygen portion, about 0.4 l/min O_2, 0.2 l/min N_2O, could be used right from the beginning. Compared with low flow anaesthesia, there is no essential difference with respect to the inspiratory oxygen concentration, within 3 h the F_{iO_2} drops from an initial 0.37 to 0.30.

Virtue summarizes that an adequate oxygen supply can be ensured over a period of almost 3 h with the recommended fresh gas composition and the use of a flow of 500 ml/min. According to him, the advantages of minimal flow anaesthesia can be attributed to

- An extensive utilization of the advantages inherent in rebreathing.
- Bridging the initial phase of anaesthesia, during which the patient takes up large volumes of nitrous oxide and anaesthetic vapour, by the use of a high fresh gas flow; during this initial phase, furthermore, nitrogen is washed out completely and the desired gas concentrations are evenly flushed into the system.
- The fact that, although the fresh gas flow is considerably reduced, there remains an excess gas volume, which can compensate for leakage losses.

Spieß[13–15] has continuously emphasized the exceptional practicability of this anaesthetic method in routine practice. The disadvantages with respect to closed system anaesthesia are, according to Spieß, the decrease in F_{iO_2} resulting from the standardized and fixed setting of the fresh gas composition. Furthermore, this method does not enable the anaesthetist to measure precisely oxygen consumption as well as nitrous oxide and volatile anaesthetic uptake[13]. Minimal flow anaesthesia, however, can be performed all the more readily without serious problems if new and advanced anaesthetic machines are used[16].

4.3 Closed system anaesthesia

If the composition of the fresh gas and its volume are precisely adapted to the patient's individual uptake of nitrous oxide, oxygen and volatile anaesthetic, maximal reduction of fresh gas flow will be achieved. Since the fresh gas volume which is fed into the breathing system corresponds quantitatively to the gas volume extracted from the system, the excess gas discharge valve will remain closed. The entire exhaled volume is rebreathed after carbon dioxide absorption. While low flow and minimal flow anaesthesia are performed at constant fresh gas flows, closed system anaesthesia requires continuous adaptation of the fresh gas volume to match the current uptake. This is awkward, especially during the initial phase of anaesthesia, when the uptake of nitrous oxide and volatile anaesthetic, and to a certain extent even oxygen, are still subject to rapid changes. Although the management of anaesthesia may be greatly facilitated by a time-limited use of high fresh gas flows, the objective is an early closing of the system, so that advantages of this anaesthetic method may be fully exploited.

The problems, involved in an early transition to closed system anaesthesia, were summarized by Nunn[17] as follows:

- Denitrogenation must be completed prior to closing the breathing system, otherwise the nitrogen concentration in the system will increase.
- During the first minutes, the nitrous oxide flow has to be virtually continuously readjusted in accordance with the rapid initial decrease of its uptake.
- During the initial phase the oxygen consumption may differ considerably from the calculated basic consumption.
- If the anaesthetic machines used are equipped with vaporizers of limited output mounted in the fresh gas supply (VOC – vaporizer outside the circuit), then with early fresh gas flow reduction it will not be possible to administer that amount of vapour required to meet the initial high uptake of volatile anaesthetic. Thus, the alveolar anaesthetic concentration cannot be kept at the desired constant level.

This can be explained by a brief calculation: Given the maximum setting of the Vapor halothane vaporizer (Dräger Medizintechnik, Lübeck) of 4%, no more than 20 ml/min of vaporized halothane can be delivered into the system at a fresh gas flow of 0.5 l/min. In accordance with Lowe's uptake formula, a patient of 100 kg, however, requires as much as 148 ml halothane vapour during the first minute to attain an alveolar concentration of 0.65 × MAC, and then 50 ml/min during the following 3 min. It is not until 16 min later that the uptake declines to about 20 ml/min, thus matching the vaporizer's maximum output at a flow of 0.5 l/min. This means that the vaporizer would have to have a maximum output of 20–30% to cover the high initial demand.

The problems discussed could be solved as follows:

- Denitrogenation can be achieved prior to induction of anaesthesia, if, for a period of at least 5 min, the patient inhales pure oxygen which is fed into the system at a high flow rate.
- With the objective of feeding an adequate nitrous oxide volume rapidly into the system to meet the initially high nitrous oxide uptake, Barton and Nunn[18] recommended proceeding as follows. After rapid denitrogenation as described above, anaesthesia is induced with barbiturate in the usual manner, and the intubated patient is connected to a breathing system previously filled with pure nitrous oxide. Assuming the volume of the system to be 4 litres and the functional residual capacity of the patient's lung as being 2 litres, after a few ventilation cycles the gas of the two compartments is mixed and the resulting alveolar nitrous oxide concentration amounts to about 65%. Thus, the nitrous oxide flow can be immediately set to 0.25 l/min and the oxygen flow to the calculated oxygen demand.
- Ernst[19] recommends that, following denitrogenation and induction of anaesthesia, a high nitrous oxide flow of 6–9 l/min and an oxygen flow

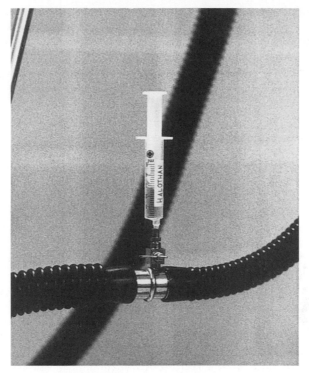

Figure 4.4   Injection port for administration of liquid volatile anaesthetic directly into the expiratory limb of the breathing system

of about 0.25–0.3 l/min, which corresponds to the calculated consumption, should be set at the gas flow controls. With hyperventilation, it should be possible to achieve a rapid and homogeneous wash-in of the desired gas concentrations of 65% N_2O and 35% O_2 in the entire system. The nitrous oxide flow should be reduced to 0.6 l/min as soon as the F_{iO_2} has dropped to a value of 0.35. Further corrections of the fresh gas flow and its composition should ensure constancy of the gas volume circulating in the system and the desired inspiratory oxygen concentration.

- The greatest problem involved in an extremely early reduction of the fresh gas flow, however, is the supply of a sufficient amount of anaesthetic vapour to meet the initial high uptake.
- Weingarten[20] and Lowe and Ernst[21] recommend the injection of liquid volatile anaesthetic directly into the breathing system (Figure 4.4). By separating delivery and metering of the anaesthetic agent from the fresh gas supply, it is possible to feed adequate amounts of volatile anaesthetic into the system, independently of the fresh gas flow. White[22], however, points out that consideration must be given to possible great fluctuations of anaesthetic concentration with such a technique, and that an even and rapid evaporation of volatile anaesthetic cannot be guaranteed without auxiliary equipment such as

vaporizing sieves and circle system blowers. Finally, there is the danger of inadvertent intravenous injection of the volatile anaesthetic drawn up in a syringe.

- Droh[23] suggested the use of vaporizers with a higher output which, however, were not available for use in human medicine at that time. According to an agreement of the manufacturers, up to now, the maximum output of vaporizers was limited to about 3–5 × the MAC of the respective inhalational anaesthetic (see Section 7.2.3.2). This was the reason why the recommendations for an initial vaporizer setting (enflurane 7.0%), given by Ernst[19] for the TEC vaporizer, could not be realized. Only recently, with the Vapor 2000 series (Dräger Medizintechnik, Lübeck, Germany), the first vaporizers with a somewhat increased maximum output became available: 8% instead of 5% for enflurane, 6% instead of 5% for isoflurane, and 6% instead of 4% for halothane. Penlon actually is offering halothane vaporizers with a maximum output at 4, 5 or 8% and enflurane vaporizers at 5 or 7%.
- Another alternative could be the use of vaporizers which are mounted in the breathing system (VIC – vaporizer inside the circuit), by means of which the volatile anaesthetic could be administered independently of the fresh gas flow. In recent years there has been a marked resurgence of interest in this technique, which has been advocated by some authors[24–27].

These vaporizers are technically very simple. A certain part of the anaesthetic gas circulating within the breathing system is passed through the vaporizing chamber (Figure 4.5). These devices are neither flow- nor temperature-compensated, the dial is not calibrated and only roughly graduated. The amount of vaporized agent delivered into the system is

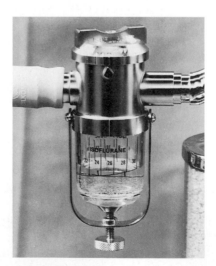

Figure 4.5 Komesaroff vaporizer within a circle absorption system, VIC. (Medical Developments Australia, Melbourne)

mainly dependent on the minute volume, the ventilation patterns, the ambient temperature, the agent in use, and any other odd factors such as supernatant water. The agent concentration achieved in the breathing system predominantly depends on the fresh gas flow rate. The performance characteristics of a vaporizer mounted in the circle can be described as follows:

- A constant setting of the vaporizer dial assumed, the higher the minute volume, the greater is the amount of vaporized agent delivered into the breathing system. An increase of the minute volume will result in an almost immediate increase of the anaesthetic concentration. This effect is the more pronounced the lower is the fresh gas flow (Figure 4.6a). An alteration of the ventilatory pattern – frequency or volume – will lead directly to parallel alterations of the agent's concentration within the breathing system.
- The higher the fresh gas flow rate, the greater the amount of excess gas vented out of the system and so the greater will be the amount of anaesthetic vapour leaving the system at a given time. Therefore, assuming a constant setting of the vaporizer dial, the agent concentration of the anaesthetic gas will be lower, at higher fresh gas flow rates (Figure 4.6b). Conversely, a reduction of the fresh gas flow rate will directly lead to a significant increase of the anaesthetic concentration within the breathing system.
- Due to the rough graduation of these vaporizers, alterations of the anaesthetic concentration can be achieved by controlled alteration of the dial's setting only when using high fresh gas flows. With low fresh gas flow rates, even minor alterations of the dial setting may cause significant changes in the anaesthetic concentration (Figure 4.6c).

Since the anaesthetic concentration developing within the rebreathing system is thus influenced by several factors other than just the vaporizer dial setting, the use of a VIC can only be justified if reliable continuous measurement of the agent concentration within the breathing system can be provided. It has to be considered, however, that in this case the agent monitor itself should be regarded as an integral part of the metering system. According to current technical regulations, a second supervising gas monitoring device would thus be required to safeguard against hazardous misdosage in the event of single fault condition. During more prolonged use of a VIC, the temperature within the vaporizing chamber decreases significantly. Because of this, water condenses, forming a mixture with the liquid anaesthetic agent. This mixture poses a waste disposal problem since it cannot be returned to the agent bottle. Although the use of a vaporizer in the circuit technically seems to be a very simple and fascinating alternative, due to the high risk of misdosage of anaesthetic agents it should be regarded as being an obsolete method, particularly if the fresh gas flow rate is very low[22,28–30].

All the different methods mentioned above have been used to try to achieve closed system anaesthesia in spite of grave inadequacies in terms of anaesthetic machinery. The procedure is difficult to perform if conventional anaesthetic machines are used[31]. The use of the existing simple VIC

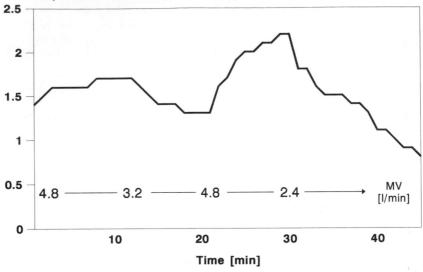

(a)

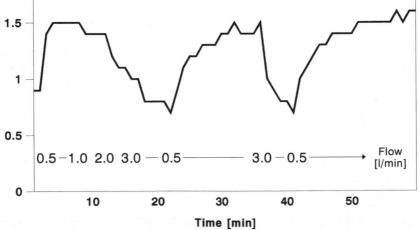

(b)

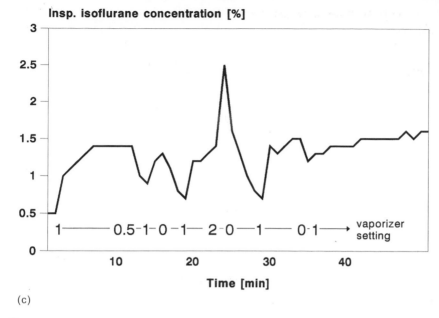

(c)

Figure 4.6 (a) VIC: Inspiratory isoflurane concentration depending on the expired minute volume at a given setting of the vaporizer dial and a fresh gas flow of 0.5 l/min (Komesaroff vaporizer, dial setting position 1). (b) VIC: Inspiratory isoflurane concentration depending on the fresh gas flow rate at a given setting of the vaporizer dial and unchanged ventilation (Komesaroff vaporizer, dial setting position 1). (c) VIC: Inspiratory isoflurane concentration depending on the setting of the vaporizer dial at a given fresh gas flow of 0.5 l/min and unchanged ventilation (Komesaroff vaporizer, variation of the dial setting between positions 0.5 and 2).

as well as the injection method will remain the challenge of enthusiasts and, certainly, will not gain widespread use. The control of the volatile agent concentration and the continuous adaptation of fresh gas composition and volume to the nitrous oxide and oxygen uptakes is involved and imprecise, since the technical components for gas dosage are generally not designed for such low gas flows. Frequently, the systems are not sufficiently gas tight and are subject to leaks, while the function of older type anaesthetic ventilators may also be considerably impaired by the reduction of fresh gas flow.

According to current standards, the following technical requirements must be met to ensure reliable performance of closed system anaesthesia[31,32]:

- high grade gas tightness of the breathing system and the anaesthetic ventilator;
- precisely operating low flow control systems for nitrous oxide, air and oxygen;
- precisely operating dosage systems for administration of volatile anaesthetics, featuring an appropriate output and suitable for use with even the lowest fresh gas flows;

- an anaesthetic ventilator that features flow compensation, that is, one which operates independently of the fresh gas flow; and
- devices for continuous measurement and monitoring of the anaesthetic gas composition.

These requirements are only satisfied by the new generation of anaesthetic machines. The technical features of these machines are such that they enable the realization of closed system anaesthesia[33]. These technical pre-conditions provided, the delivery of fluid agent with the aid of a syringe pump directly into the breathing system, however, may become a practicable alternative, especially in nitrous oxide free closed system anaesthesia.

4.3.1   Non-quantitative closed system anaesthesia

Closed system anaesthesia, for instance, could be performed with the Cicero anaesthetic workstation (Dräger Medizintechnik, Lübeck, Germany), which features a flowmeter set especially designed for low flow anaesthesia[11]. By means of a computer, the nitrous oxide uptake ($\dot{V}_{N_2O}$) was calculated according to the Severinghaus formula, and the uptake of the anaesthetic selected ($\dot{V}_{AN}$) according to the Lowe formula at one minute intervals. The oxygen uptake ($\dot{V}_{O_2}$) was calculated by using the Brody formula and assumed to be constant during the course of anaesthesia (see Section 3.4). The respective adjustment of the vaporizer was obtained by calculation of following quotient:

$$100 \times \dot{V}_{AN}/(\dot{V}_{O_2} + \dot{V}_{N_2O}).$$

After an initial phase of between 5 and 15 min, during which a high fresh gas flow was used, the values calculated for the uptake were set at the flowmeter bank and the vaporizer, and were changed at 1-min intervals in accordance with the newly computed values. Possible imbalances in volume between calculated and actual gas uptake were compensated for automatically by the changing filling of the reservoir bag. If an average filling level of the reservoir was maintained, it could be assumed that the fresh gas flow more or less met the total gas uptake. Although in some cases the measured gas concentrations corresponded well to the chosen set points, and the anaesthetic gas composition did not change considerably during the course of anaesthesia (Figure 4.7a), in most of the cases undertaken with this procedure it was not possible to keep the gas composition as precisely constant as desired (Figure 4.7b). It is obvious that in the individual case there may be considerable differences between the actual and the calculated gas uptake.

Proceeding in the way described, it may be possible to achieve a fresh gas flow reduction down to just that gas volume which is taken up by the patient. This precludes any discharge of excess gas from the system. By definition, the procedure thus corresponds to closed system anaesthesia. However, this technique cannot be defined as being quantitative, since the changes observed in the anaesthetic gas composition can only be explained by an imbalance between the individual gas volumes fed into the system and the actual nitrous oxide, oxygen and anaesthetic uptake. The term

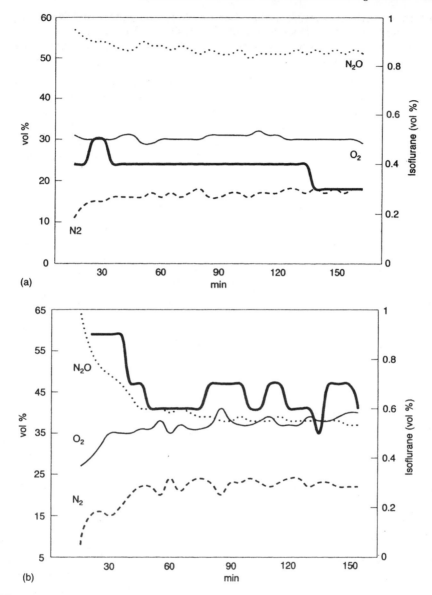

Figure 4.7 Oxygen, nitrous oxide, nitrogen and isoflurane concentrations during the course of two anaesthetics with closed system (Cicero, Dräger Medizintechnik, Lübeck, Germany). The accumulation of nitrogen results from slow nitrogen wash-out from the poor vessel group tissues. Also indispensable for performance of closed system anaesthesia, the sampling gas has to be led back into the system after its passage through the gas analyser. Thus, together with the anaesthetic gas, ambient air used as reference or calibration gas may flow into the breathing system and exacerbate nitrogen accumulation. Heavy line: expired isoflurane concentration. (a) 77-year-old patient, 1.62 m, 66.5 kg, nominal value for expired isoflurane concentration 0.5 vol%. (b) 49-year-old patient, 1.77 m, 96.5 kg, nominal value for expired isoflurane concentration 0.9 vol%

quantitative anaesthesia implies a constancy of composition as well as volume of circulating gas.

In addition, it is evident that in practice it will not be practicable for the anaesthetist to change the setting of the vaporizer and the flow control system continually.

4.3.2 Quantitative closed system anaesthesia

Quantitative closed system anaesthesia is practicable only if the dosage of the anaesthetic gases is electronically controlled by closed-loop feedback[11,34]. From the technical point of view this calls for precisely operating gas metering systems[35]. For the first time ever, such a technical concept has been realized in the form of the PhysioFlex machine (Dräger Medizintechnik, Lübeck, Germany)[36]. It was developed by a Dutch team headed by W. Erdmann from Rotterdam University. In this device oxygen is fed into the system at precisely that volume which will maintain a pre-set nominal inspiratory oxygen concentration. The constancy of the gas volume circulating in the system is guaranteed by an appropriate delivery of nitrous oxide, and the volatile anaesthetic is injected into the system in liquid form in just such an amount that a pre-selected expiratory set point is gained within a short time and kept constant at that level. Electronic control of gas metering with closed-loop feedback has proved to be very precise in clinical tests[33]. Provided that the system is absolutely gas tight and gas loss via leakage can be precluded, the gas volumes fed into the system correspond exactly to the respective uptake. The continuous measurement of oxygen uptake renders extensive monitoring of circulatory and metabolic functions possible.

Quantitative closed system anaesthesia is achieved only if the fresh gas composition and its volume correspond exactly to the patient's uptake of each individual component.

Only by this technique will it be possible to keep the anaesthetic gas composition and volume constant over the whole time course of an anaesthetic procedure, simultaneously dispensing completely with the discharge of any excess gas.

4.4   References

1. Baum JA and Aitkenhead AR. Low-flow anaesthesia. *Anaesthesia* 1995; **50** (Suppl.): 37–44.
2. Waters RM. Clinical scope and utility of carbon dioxide filtration in inhalation anaesthesia. *Anesth Analg* 1924; **3**, 20–22.
3. Foldes FF, Ceravolo AJ and Carpenter SL. The administration of nitrous oxide – oxygen anesthesia in closed systems. *Ann Surg* 1952; **136**, 978–981.
4. Virtue RW. Minimal flow nitrous oxide anesthesia. *Anesthesiology* 1974; **40**, 196–198.
5. White DC. Closed and low flow system anaesthesia. *Curr Anaesth Critical Care* 1992; **3**, 98–107.
6. Baker AB. Low flow and closed circuits. *Anaesth Intensive Care* 1994; **22**, 341–342.

7. Hargasser S, Mielke L, Entholzner E and Hipp R. Anästhesie mit niedrigem Frischgasfluß in der klinischen Routine. *Anästhesiol Intensivmed Notfallmed Schmerzther* 1995; **30**, 268–275.

8. Baxter A. Low and minimal flow inhalation anaesthesia. *Can J Anaesth* 1997; **44**, 643–653.

9. Foldes FF and Duncalf D. Low flow anesthesia: a plea for simplicity. In Lawin P, van Aken H and Schneider U, eds, *Alternative Methoden in der Anästhesie. INA-Schriftenreihe*, Bd. 50. Thieme, Stuttgart, 1985, pp. 1–7.

10. Virtue RW. Toward closed system anesthesia. *Anaesthesist* 1977; **26**, 545–546.

11. Baum J. Clinical applications of low flow and closed circuit anesthesia. *Acta Anaesth Belg* 1990; **41**, 239–247.

12. Grote B, Adolphs A and Merten G. Inhalationsnarkose im Low-Flow-System. In *Geschlossenes System für Inhalationsnarkosen*, Internationales Symposium, Düsseldorf, 7–8 May 1982, Abstract.

13. Spieß W. Narkose im geschlossenen System mit kontinuierlicher inspiratorischer Sauerstoffmessung. *Anaesthesist* 1977; **26**, 503–513.

14. Spieß W. Minimal-Flow Anästhesie – eine zeitgemäße Alternative für die Klinikroutine. *Anaesth Reanim* 1980; **5**, 145–149.

15. Spieß W. Sauerstoffverbrauch und Aufnahme von Lachgas und volatilen Anästhetika. In Lawin P, van Aken H and Schneider U, eds, *Alternative Methoden in der Anästhesie. INA-Schriftenreihe*, Bd. 50. Thieme, Stuttgart, 1985, pp. 8–18.

16. Baum J. Klinische Anwendung der Minimal-Flow Anästhesie. In Jantzen JPAH and Kleemann PP, eds, Narkosebeatmung: *Low Flow, Minimal Flow, Geschlossenes System*. Schattauer, Stuttgart, 1989, pp. 49–66.

17. Nunn JF. Techniques for induction of closed circuit anesthesia. In Aldrete JA, Lowe HJ and Virtue RW, eds. *Low Flow and Closed Circuit Anesthesia*. Grune & Stratton, New York, 1979, pp. 3–10.

18. Barton F and Nunn JF. Totally closed circuit nitrous oxide/oxygen anaesthesia. *Br J Anaesth* 1975; **47**, 350–357.

19. Ernst EA. Closed circuit anesthesia. In List FW and Schalk HV, eds, *Refresher-Kurs ZAK 85*. Akademische Druck- und Verlagsanstalt, Graz, 1985.

20. Weingarten M. Low flow and closed circuit anesthesia. In Aldrete JA, Lowe HJ and Virtue RW, eds, *Low Flow and Closed Circuit Anesthesia*. Grune & Stratton, New York, 1979, pp. 67–74.

21. Lowe HJ and Ernst EA. *The Quantitative Practice of Anesthesia*. Williams & Wilkins, Baltimore, 1981.

22. White DC. Injection of liquid anaesthetic agents into breathing circuits. In *Geschlossenes System für Inhalationsnarkosen*, Internationales Symposium, Düsseldorf, 7–8 May 1982, Abstract.

23. Droh R. Inhalationsnarkose im geschlossenen System. In *Geschlossenes System für Inhalationsnarkosen*, Internationales Symposium, Düsseldorf, 7–8 May 1982, Abstract.

24. Jordan MJ and Bushman JA. Closed-circuit halothane and enflurane using an in-circle Goldman vaporizer. *Br J Anaesth* 1981; **53**, 1285–1290.

25. Komesaroff D. Low flow anaesthesia – an Australian devotee's perspective. *Anaeth Intensive Care* 1994; **22**, 343–344.

26. Rucklidge M. Ultimate low flow anaesthesia. In Harper N, ed., *Proceedings of the Low Flow Anaesthesia Symposium*, Manchester, 1994.

27. Nunn G. Different types of vaporiser in circuit. Abstracts of the Annual Meeting of The Association for Low Flow Anaesthesia, Gent, 18–19 September 1998.

28. Morris LE. Closed carbon dioxide filtration revisited. *Anaesth Intensive Care* 1994; **22**, 345–358.

29. Stokes J. Low flow and closed system anaesthesia in Australasia: monitoring and other perspectives. *Appl Cardiopulmonary Physiol* 1995 (Suppl. 5); **2**, 75–81.
30. Baum J. Practical use of a vaporizer in-circuit. Abstracts of the Annual Meeting of The Association for Low Flow Anaesthesia, Gent, 18–19 September 1998.
31. Wallroth CF. Technical conception for an anesthesia system with electronic metering of gases and vapors. *Acta Anaesth Belg* 1984; **35**, 279–293.
32. Baum J. Quantitative anaesthesia in the low-flow system. In van Ackern K, Frankenberger H, Konecny E and Steinbereithner K, eds, *Quantitative Anaesthesia: Low Flow and Closed Circuit. Anästhesiologie und Intensivmedizin*, Bd. 204. Springer, Berlin, 1989, pp. 44–57.
33. Versichelen L and Rolly G. Mass-spectrometric evaluation of some recently introduced low flow, closed circuit systems. *Acta Anaesth Belg* 1990; **41**, 225–237.
34. Westenskow DR and Wallroth CF. Closed-loop control for anesthesia breathing systems. *J Clin Monit* 1990; **6**, 249–256.
35. Wallroth CF, Jaklitsch R and Wied HA. Technical realisation of quantitative metering and ventilation. In van Ackern K, Frankenberger H, Konecny E and Steinbereithner K, eds, *Quantitative Anaesthesia: Low Flow and Closed Circuit. Anästhesiologie und Intensivmedizin*, Bd. 204. Springer, Berlin, 1989, pp. 96–108.
36. Erdmann W, Veeger AI and Verkaaik APK. Narkosebeatmungsgeräte: Gegenwart und Zukunft. In Jantzen JPAH and Kleemann PP, eds. *Narkosebeatmung: Low Flow, Minimal Flow, Geschlossenes System.* Schattauer, Stuttgart, 1989, pp. 5–17.

Control of inhalational anaesthesia

The essential principles of anaesthesia management with reduced fresh gas flow can be demonstrated and rules for the control of inhalational anaesthesia established with the aid of computer simulations. Two computer programs for simulation of inhalational anaesthesia are discussed.

5.1 Computer simulation programs

5.1.1 NARKUP

This program, developed by White and Lockwood[1], runs on old-fashioned IBM-compatible AT computers with CGA, EGA, VGA or Hercules graphics card and also on modern Pentium computers.

Following selection of the breathing system, the figures for the settings at the anaesthetic machine and the patient's parameters can be widely varied in accordance with the desired simulation. The calculated concentrations of nitrous oxide and volatile anaesthetics are displayed numerically at any time, while concentration trends are simultaneously displayed as a line graph during the simulation. In addition to simulation of anaesthesia with all inhalational anaesthetics, this program enables simulation with anaesthetics such as cyclopropane or xenon. Depending on the menu selected, the individual uptake of anaesthetics is displayed numerically as well as in a line graph.

5.1.2 Gas Man

The Gas Man simulation program, developed by Philip[2], runs with the 4.1 or later operating system on all Macintosh computers including MacintoshPlus, SE and II series, which are equipped with 800 kbyte RAM. Alternatively, a Microsoft Windows version (Gas Man 2.0) is available.

It is an interactive teaching program which explains the pharmacokinetic rules of uptake and distribution of volatile anaesthetics. The display is clear-cut and straightforward. Following selection of the breathing system, the values for fresh gas flow, alveolar ventilation and cardiac output are entered. The data can be varied during simulation. The gas concentrations in the gas-containing compartments and in different tissues can be comprehensively displayed either in the form of a bar graph or as a line graph.

5.1.3   Clinical relevance of anaesthesia simulation by computer software

It must be admitted that anaesthesia simulation programs for personal computers are based upon simplified presuppositions:

- The oxygen consumption and the carbon dioxide production are assumed to be constant over the entire period of simulation, unless the pre-selected cardiac output has been changed.
- No consideration is given to the effects that changes in fluid balance (resulting from infusion or transfusion therapy or current loss of blood) have on the uptake and distribution of volatile anaesthetics.
- Loss of volatile anaesthetic by absorption in the breathing system's components, by diffusion via the skin and mucous membranes or by metabolism, are not given consideration in the calculations.
- The solubility of volatile anaesthetic in blood and in tissues is assumed to be constant.
- The saturation of breathing gas with water vapour is assumed to be 100%.
- No consideration is given to the effects of temperature, haemoglobin content and pH blood value on the solubility of oxygen and carbon dioxide.
- Cardiac output, pulmonary and systemic shunt and dead space are assumed to be constant at the values entered at the beginning of simulation, unless they have subsequently been changed.
- Pharmacodynamic processes occurring during an inhalational anaesthetic are not considered during pharmacokinetic calculations.

It must be pointed out that, notwithstanding the complexity of pharmacokinetic algorithms, computer simulations are based on simplified process and compartment models. However, these programs are perfectly suited to illustration of the pharmacokinetics of uptake and distribution of volatile anaesthetics in a graphic manner. The great number of procedure, machine and patient-specific factors which affect the composition of anaesthetic gases in a breathing system can be illustrated individually via comparative simulations, so that their particular significance on anaesthetic management can be evaluated. To this end, simulation programs are not only a perfect teaching aid for the on-the-job training of physicians, but they also provide extensive information for experienced anaesthetists on the complex processes which determine the composition of anaesthetic gas in a breathing system. Only a sound understanding of the functions of anaesthesia machines and the interactions between patient and machine makes it possible to use the currently available sophisticated anaesthetic technology to its full potential.

5.2   Control of inhalational anaesthesia

During the course of a surgical intervention, the concentration of the volatile anaesthetic selected for inhalational anaesthesia must be continuously adapted to the individual reactions and clinical requirements.

The anaesthetic concentration which is finally administered to the patient derives from a complex process which takes place in the breathing system, determined by a number of factors:

- by technical parameters such as the type of the breathing system, its technical design, the fresh gas utilization and the system's volume;
- by the individual gas uptake of the patient which is determined by pharmacokinetic and pharmacodynamic characteristics;
- by the selected fresh gas flow rate and the adjustment of the fresh gas composition; and
- by equipment-inherent conditions, such as the loss of anaesthetic gases or the entrance of air into the system as a result of leaks.

Therefore, the breathing system must not only be understood as being the technical conveyor of anaesthetic gases from the anaesthetic machine to the patient, but it is the essential interactive technical element by means of which the concentrations of anaesthetic gases are determined.

The following serves to explain to what extent the composition of anaesthetic gas is influenced by the fresh gas flow. This can clearly be demonstrated by means of computer simulation, since the fresh gas flow can be independently varied, while all the other simulation conditions remain unchanged.

Unless otherwise specified, the following simulations are all based on identical simulation conditions. The breathing system used is a rebreathing system, the circle absorption system. The vaporizer is mounted in the fresh gas supply and is thus used as a vaporizer outside the circuit (VOC). The volatile anaesthetic is isoflurane which is used on an adult patient of 75 kg body weight, with physiological circulatory conditions under normoventilation.

According to his own experience the author assumes that in the individual case the concentrations calculated by computer simulation may differ by about 10–15% from the values measured during clinical performance. Nevertheless, the simulated gas concentrations agree fairly well with the average values measured in larger clinical trials.

5.2.1   The induction phase

In the induction phase, a volatile anaesthetic is administered with the aim of obtaining an appropriate anaesthetic depth to permit commencement of a surgical intervention within an acceptable period of time. For this purpose, the desired anaesthetic concentration should not only be washed into the gas-carrying space, but also into the central nervous tissue.

In computer simulation of the induction phase (Figure 5.1a), the isoflurane concentration of the fresh gas is set to 1.5 vol% at different fresh

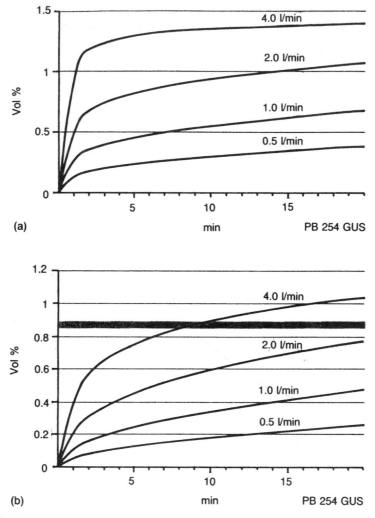

Figure 5.1   Induction phase: (a) inspired and (b) expired isoflurane concentration with different fresh gas flows, fresh gas isoflurane concentration 1.5 vol%

gas flows of 0.5, 1.0, 2.0 and 4.0 l/min. The lower the fresh gas flow, the more delayed is the rise in the inspired isoflurane concentration.

However, it is the end-tidal anaesthetic concentration which allows an estimate of the concentration in the blood and hence judgement of the depth of anaesthesia, since this corresponds approximately to the alveolar and thus arterial concentration[4]. With identical isoflurane concentration in the fresh gas, the rise in the expired anaesthetic concentration is similarly the more delayed, the lower is the fresh gas flow (Figure 5.1b). If the intended expired isoflurane concentration is 0.8–0.9 vol% – in addition to the MAC fraction of 60–70 vol% of nitrous oxide, this corresponds approximately to the AD_{95} for isoflurane – this value can only be

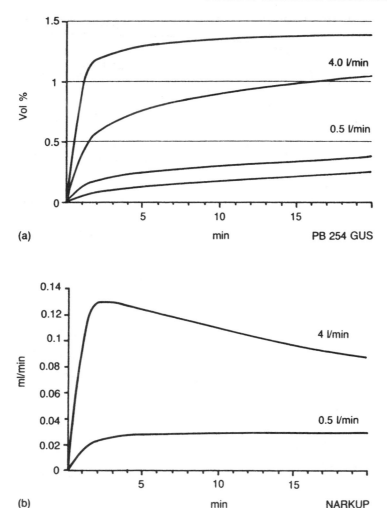

Figure 5.2   Induction phase: (a) inspired and expired isoflurane concentration with fresh gas flows of 4.0 versus 0.5 l/min, fresh gas isoflurane concentration 1.5 vol%; (b) corresponding isoflurane uptake (ml liquid isoflurane)

attained within an acceptably short initial period of 10–15 min with a fresh gas flow of 4 l/min.

This can be explained as follows (Figure 5.2a and b): with a given fresh gas flow of 4.0 l/min, the rebreathing fraction is comparatively low, so that a high portion of fresh gas is administered to the patient with each cycle. The isoflurane concentration of the inspired gas is therefore high. Correspondingly, a high alveolar–arterial partial pressure gradient is restored with each breath. This results in a high uptake which in turn leads to a fast increase in the expired isoflurane concentration.

On the other hand, with a low fresh gas flow of 0.5 l/min the rebreathing fraction increases considerably: the inspired isoflurane concentration is

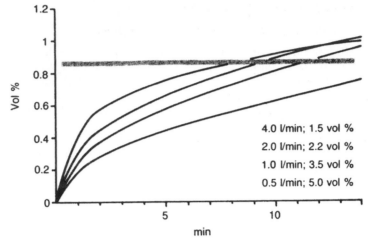

Figure 5.3   Induction phase: expired isoflurane concentration with different fresh gas flows and differing isoflurane admixture

now essentially determined by the composition of the isoflurane-depleted exhaled gas and, thus, increases only very slowly. The alveolar–arterial partial pressure gradient after each inspiration is therefore low, as is the uptake, which in turn slows down the increase in the expired isoflurane concentration.

The increase in the expired anaesthetic concentration can be accelerated if, with the reduction of the fresh gas flow, the isoflurane concentration in the fresh gas is raised (Figure 5.3). The target concentration between 0.8 and 0.9% can thus be achieved within an approximately short period of time even with a fresh gas flow of only 1.0 l/min. However, this approach may not be practicable at a fresh gas flow of only 0.5 l/min, since the desired concentration cannot be attained within an acceptable time, especially if the output of the vaporizer is limited to 5%.

The low solubility of the newer inhalational anaesthetics sevoflurane and desflurane and the corresponding low individual uptake of these agents result in a correspondingly short induction phase[5,6]. The initial desired anaesthetic concentration will be gained in a comparatively short time after induction. Thus, when using one of these low solubility agents, the initial high flow phase can be kept comparatively short, in low and minimal flow anaesthesia around 10 min[7,8] (see Chapter 10.3).

In summary, the following statement is justified: over a period of about 10–15 min a rather high fresh gas flow, approximately 4 l/min, has to be selected for induction of anaesthesia with conventional anaesthesia machines equipped with circle absorption systems and vaporizers outside the circuit, whereby the concentration of the anaesthetic in the fresh gas must be set approximately 0.5–1.0% higher than the target expired concentration. This is a reasonable way to increase the depth of inhalational anaesthesia within an appropriate period of time and to attain the desired anaesthetic gas composition.

5.2.2   Maintenance of anaesthesia

5.2.2.1   Adapting the fresh gas flow to the uptake

Since, after completion of the induction phase, the uptake decreases com-
plementary to the increase in expired anaesthetic concentration, the fresh
gas flow can now be adapted to the reduced uptake. According to his
concept of minimal flow anaesthesia[9], Virtue recommends reducing the
fresh gas flow to 0.5 l/min after an induction phase of about 15 min.
Only by an adequate reduction of the fresh gas flow will it be possible
to reduce the discharge of excess gas from the system and, thus, to increase
the rebreathing fraction. This is the only way to fully realize the advantages of rebreathing systems.

In another simulation (Figure 5.4), following a 15-min induction phase
with a fresh gas flow of 4.5 l/min and fresh gas isoflurane concentration of
1.5 vol%, the flow is reduced to 2.0, 1.0 or 0.5 l/min, respectively, while the
anaesthetic concentration is maintained. The greater the reduction of the
fresh gas flow, the greater the decrease in isoflurane concentration. This
can be attributed to the fact that the amount of anaesthetic vapour
delivered into the system, which, for its part, is reduced to 30, 15 or
even only 7.5 ml/min as a result of flow reduction, is not able to
replenish the volume of isoflurane vapour which is taken up by the
patient or discharged with the excess gas.

However, if the isoflurane concentration is increased to 2.5 vol% at the
same time as the fresh gas flow is reduced to 0.5 l/min, the target expired
isoflurane concentration of about 0.9 vol% can be maintained in spite of
an insignificant initial decrease.

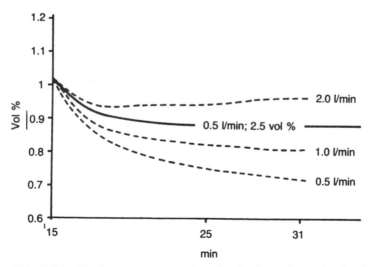

Figure 5.4   Expired isoflurane concentration after fresh gas flow reduction from 4.5
to 2.0, 1.0 or 0.5 l/min while fresh gas isoflurane concentration remained unchanged
at 1.5 vol%. For comparison: expired isoflurane concentration after fresh gas flow
reduction from 4.5 to 0.5 l/min, with simultaneous increase of the isoflurane concentration from 1.5 to 2.5 vol%

A standardized concept for control of inhalational anaesthesia according to the Virtue scheme can thus be derived from the simulation results. During the induction phase of 10–20 min, 1.5 vol% isoflurane is added to a fresh gas flow of about 4.0 l/min. Following flow reduction to 0.5 l/min, the isoflurane concentration is increased to 2.5 vol%. An average expired isoflurane concentration of 0.85 vol% can be attained with these standard settings. If such a dosage pattern is applied on a clinical trial, the measured anaesthetic concentrations correspond fairly well to the values predicted using computer simulation[9]. It should, however, be pointed out that these dosage schemes can only be regarded as guidelines for clinical practice. It goes without saying that this scheme has to be adjusted from case to case in line with individual reactions and clinical requirements.

5.2.2.2   Influence of the individual uptake

There is another characteristic of inhalational anaesthesia with low fresh gas flow that has considerable influence on the control of the volatile anaesthetic concentration (Figure 5.5a and b).

Due to the larger fraction rebreathing, the gas concentration in the breathing system is affected to a larger extent by the composition of the exhaled gas, i.e. by the individual uptake, than is the case with a high fresh gas flow.

The uptake of heavyweight and strong patients is greater than that of lightweight and slender ones. This means that in minimal flow anaesthesia, using an identical fresh gas concentration of 2.5 vol% isoflurane, the expired isoflurane concentration of a 75 kg patient is lower than that of a 55 kg patient. Such differences in concentration were also observed in clinical trials on patients of different body weight[10]. With a comparatively high fresh gas flow of 4.4 l/min, however, the expired isoflurane concentration is only insignificantly influenced by the body weight of the patient (Figure 5.5a).

Furthermore, the individual uptake is correlated to the cardiac output. Once again, a computer simulated anaesthesia on a normal weight adult patient can be used as an illustration (Figure 5.5b). After 30 min of simulation, the cardiac output is reduced by 50%, from 5.1 l/min to 2.5 l/min. While, under the conditions of high flow anaesthesia, the inspired concentration does not change at all and expired concentration only insignificantly, there is a distinct increase in both the inspired and expired isoflurane concentration in minimal flow anaesthesia.

5.2.3   The time constant

The inertia of the system increases considerably with reduction of the fresh gas flow, which can be demonstrated by means of comparison between high flow and minimal flow anaesthesia (Figure 5.6a and b).

For anaesthesia with high fresh gas flow, the flow remains constant at 4.4 l/min over the entire period of anaesthesia. During the first 25 min, an isoflurane concentration of 1.5 vol% is set at the vaporizer. The clinical situation at that time calls for an increase of the anaesthetic depth and so

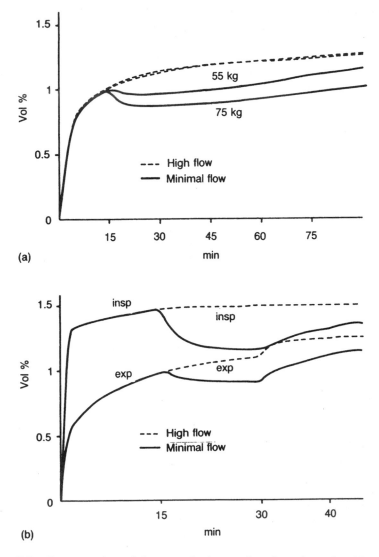

Figure 5.5 Concentration of the anaesthetic as a function of uptake: (a) expired isoflurane concentration as a function of body weight; (b) inspired and expired isoflurane concentration as a function of cardiac output

the isoflurane concentration in the fresh gas is increased to 2.5 vol%. After 40 min, the vaporizer is switched off.

In this example of high flow anaesthesia, the changes in the fresh gas concentration result in a rapid corresponding change in inspired and expired anaesthetic concentration in the breathing system.

During the initial phase of minimal flow anaesthesia, which is shown for comparison, an isoflurane concentration of 1.5 vol% is set with a fresh gas flow of 4.4 l/min. With fresh gas flow reduction to 0.5 l/min, the isoflurane

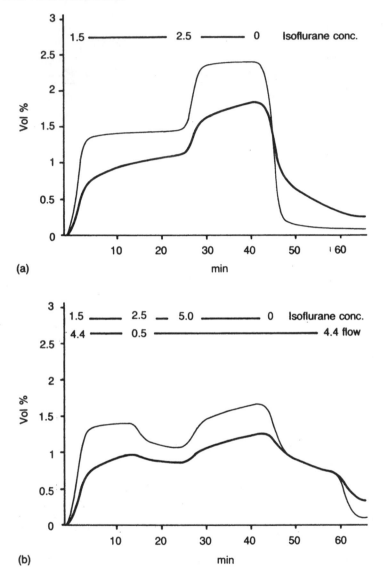

Figure 5.6   Time constants for comparison: high flow anaesthesia (4.4 l/min) versus minimal flow anaesthesia (0.5 l/min)

concentration in the fresh gas is increased to 2.5 vol%. In spite of the insignificant decrease in inspired and expired anaesthetic concentration, the latter stabilizes at the target value of between 0.8 vol% and 0.9 vol%. In this example, the clinical situation also calls for an increase of the anaesthetic depth after 25 min. While maintaining a flow of 0.5 l/min, the vaporizer is therefore set to its maximum output of 5 vol% isoflurane, and switched off again after 40 min.

In the case of minimal flow anaesthesia, even drastic changes of the

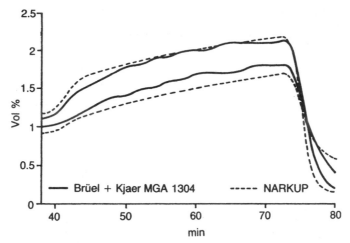

Figure 5.7   The long time constant of minimal flow anaesthesia in a clinical example (patient aged 41 years, weight 76 kg, height 1.79 m). At 40 min, the isoflurane fresh gas concentration is increased to 5 vol%. After 75 min, the system is flushed with pure oxygen (4 l/min)

fresh gas concentration will cause only delayed and slow changes of the inspired and expired anaesthetic concentrations in the breathing system.

Quantitatively, this phenomenon can be determined by calculation of the time constant T, which is a measure for that time in which concentration changes in the fresh gas result in corresponding concentration changes in the breathing system. According to Conway[11], the time constant can be calculated by the division of the total gas-containing volume ($V_L + V_S$) by the difference between the amount of agent (or anaesthetic gas) delivered into the system with the fresh gas flow ($\dot{V}_{Del}$) and the amount of agent (or anaesthetic gas) taken up by the patient ($\dot{V}_U$) at the same time:

$$T = (V_L + V_S)/(\dot{V}_{Del} - \dot{V}_U)$$

This means that with a given uptake and given system volume, the time constant of a breathing system is inversely proportional to the fresh gas flow.

As a numerical value, the time constant quantifies the speed of wash-in and wash-out processes. After time T has passed, the anaesthetic concentration in the breathing system attains 63% of the final concentration, after $2 \times T$ about 86.5% and after $3 \times T$ about 93%. The extended time constants have to be borne in mind during the use of low flow techniques.

The long time constant of a rebreathing system used with low fresh gas flow can be verified by another clinical example (Figure 5.7). A minimal flow anaesthesia is performed on a male patient (aged 41, weight 76 kg, height 179 cm) according to the standardized dosing scheme. After 40 min, the isoflurane concentration in the fresh gas is increased to 5 vol% while the flow of 0.5 l/min is maintained. During the following 30 min, both the inspired and expired isoflurane concentration (measured by means of a Brüel and Kjaer gas analyser MGA 1304) rise but very slowly, in accordance with the long time constant. The correspondence between the values calculated by computer simulation and the actually measured concentrations is once more convincingly demonstrated in this example.

With respect to the time constant, sevoflurane and desflurane, likewise, do have favourable properties if compared with the other conventional volatile agents: both agents, besides their low solubility, feature a comparatively low anaesthetic potency. For safety reasons, in general, the maximum output of most of the modern concentration calibrated vaporizers is limited to a value $5 - 3 \times$ MAC of the respective inhalational anaesthetic. Thus, the output of the sevoflurane vaporizer is limited at 8 vol%, that of the desflurane vaporizer even at 18 vol%. This means that even if an extremely low fresh gas flow as low as 0.5 l/min is used, the amount of agent, delivered into the system, can be increased considerably. While, when using enflurane or isoflurane, the maximum amount of agent delivered into the breathing system can be increased to only 26 ml/min vapour, it can be increased to 43.5 ml/min with sevoflurane, and even to 110 ml/min when desflurane is used. As, simultaneously, the individual uptake with just these agents is comparatively small, the difference $\dot{V}_{Del} - \dot{V}_{U}$ increases, resulting in a comparatively short time constant[7,8].

If judicious use is made of the comparatively wide range of the agent-specific sevoflurane or desflurane vaporizers, the agent concentration can be increased with short time constants even if the fresh gas flow is maintained at a very low rate. Due to the specific pharmacodynamic and pharmacokinetic properties of these anaesthetic agents, the time constants are comparatively short even in the low flow range.

5.2.4   Emergence from anaesthesia

The emergence phase of anaesthesia is aimed at a rapid reduction of anaesthetic depth until the patient wakes up. The anaesthetic concentration in the breathing system should therefore be rapidly reduced (Figure 5.8a and b).

Following an anaesthetic of 45 min duration with high fresh gas flow and an isoflurane concentration of 1.5 vol%, the vaporizer is switched off and the system flushed with oxygen flows of 0.5, 1.0, 2.0 and 4.0 l/min. As can be expected in accordance with the respective time constants, the expired isoflurane concentration decreases more slowly with the lower oxygen flows (Figure 5.8a).

Only if the system is flushed with a high oxygen flow of 4.0 l/min, the rebreathing fraction is comparatively low and the inspired oxygen concentration correspondingly high. The high alveolar–capillary partial pressure gradient causes a rapid discharge of the anaesthetic and a correspondingly rapid decrease in the expired isoflurane concentration (Figure 5.8b).

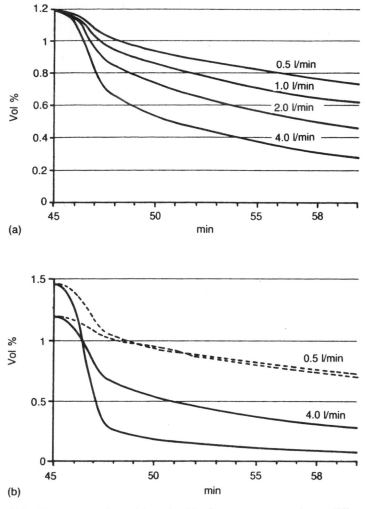

Figure 5.8 Emergence phase: (a) expired isoflurane concentration at different flows of pure oxygen; (b) inspired and expired isoflurane concentration during flushing of the system with pure oxygen at 4.0 versus 0.5 l/min

5.3 Characteristics of anaesthesia management as a function of fresh gas flow

According to the intended use, rebreathing systems can be operated with either high or low fresh gas flows[12,13]. The advantages of the rebreathing technique can only be realized provided that during the course of anaesthesia the fresh gas flow is adapted to the uptake. However, in varying the flow, the characteristic of the breathing system, i.e. the dynamics of volatile anaesthetic administration, may be subject to considerable changes.

With a high fresh gas flow, the composition of the anaesthetic gas corresponds approximately to that of the fresh gas. The greater portion of the exhaled gas is discharged via the exhaust port, the rebreathing fraction is insignificant. Since a high fresh gas portion is insufflated into the lungs with each ventilation stroke, a high alveolar–arterial partial pressure gradient, which is essentially determined by the fresh gas composition, is newly re-established with each breath. This results in an accelerated gas exchange between the gas and the blood compartment and a correspondingly rapid wash-in and wash-out of the anaesthetic. Only if the partial pressures between alveolar and blood compartment are balanced will the uptake or wash-out of the volatile anaesthetic decrease in accordance with the lower partial pressure gradient.

On the other hand, the discharge of excess gas volume from the system decreases significantly at low fresh gas flow rates. The greater part of the exhaled gas remains in the system, is mixed with a small amount of fresh gas and then routed back to the patient during the next inspiration. The composition of the anaesthetic gas is, thus, essentially determined by the composition of exhaled gas. But approximately 85% of the exhaled breath consists of alveolar gas. This means that in previous ventilation cycles the partial pressures of this gas have already been aligned to those of the blood compartment. The partial pressure gradient between the alveolar and blood compartments established with each inspiration is accordingly low, and the same has to be assumed for the uptake or discharge of the volatile anaesthetic.

5.4   Rules on anaesthetic management

Whenever the concentration of the anaesthetic in the gas-containing compartment is to be rapidly increased or reduced, the time constant of the breathing system has to be short. According to Conway's formula, at a given time, only the time constant can be influenced by an alteration of the amount of anaesthetic vapour delivered into the system with the fresh gas. Using the conventional volatile anaesthetics halothane, enflurane and isoflurane, this can only be accomplished to a significant degree by increasing the fresh gas flow rate. The inspired gas composition will more equal the composition of the fresh gas, the higher is the fresh gas flow rate. When the flow is nearly similar to the minute volume, the anaesthetic fresh gas concentration can equal the desired nominal value. When the new volatiles sevoflurane and desflurane are used, the amount of vaporized anaesthetic ($\dot{V}_{Del}$) can be significantly increased, even if the low fresh gas flow rate is maintained, if use is made of the wide dial range of the vaporizers. The shortening of the time constant will be the more pronounced, as at the same time the individual uptake ($\dot{V}_{U}$) just of these anaesthetics is comparatively low, and the resulting difference $\dot{V}_{Del} - \dot{V}_{U}$ correspondingly big. A rapid decrease of the anaesthetic concentration within the breathing system, however, can be accomplished exclusively by an increase of the flow rate, as adequate acceleration of the wash-out can only be effected exclusively by completely discharging the exhaled gas.

When anaesthesia, however, has reached the desired depth, and the uptake has reached low values in steady state, long time constants, i.e. low fresh gas flow, can be used. The difference between the fresh gas anaesthetic concentration and the inspired concentration has to be assumed to be the greater the lower is the fresh gas flow, and the higher is the agent's solubility.

If, while maintaining low fresh gas flow rates, the anaesthetic level is to be deepened or lightened – thus, the anaesthetist intends to work with long time constants – the agent concentration in the fresh gas must be adjusted to values distinctly above or below the target inspired concentration. The composition of the inspired gas will differ distinctly from that of the expired gas only if the amount of anaesthetic fed into the system by the low fresh gas volume is sufficiently increased or reduced. The resulting increase of the alveolar–capillary partial pressure gradient will enhance the gas exchange between the gas and the blood compartment. However, it must be considered that, as the output of the vaporizers is limited, this procedure is subject to distinct limitation as a function of the fresh gas flow selected.

5.5   References

1. White DC and Lockwood L. Narkup (Ver. 4.11). Northwick Park Hospital and Clinical Research Centre, Harrow, Middlesex HA1 3UJ, UK, 1989. Actual address: Dr G.G. Lockwood, Hammersmith Hospital, Du Cane Rd., London W12 0NN, UK.
2. Philip JH. Gas Man. Med Man Simulations, P.O. Box 67–160, Chestnut Hill, MA 02167, USA, 1991.
3. Philip JH. Closed circuit anesthesia. In Ehrenwerth J and Eisenkraft JB, eds, *Anesthesia Equipment: Principles and Applications.* Mosby, St Louis, 1993, pp. 617–635.
4. Zbinden AM. *Inhalationsanästhetika: Aufnahme und Verteilung.* Wissenschaftliche Verlagsabteilung, Deutsche Abbott, Wiesbaden, 1987.
5. Eger EI. New inhaled anaesthetics. *Anesthesiology* 1994; **80**, 906–922.
6. Conzen P and Nuscheler M. Neue Inhalationsanästhetika. *Anaesthesist* 1996; **45**, 674–693.
7. Baum J, Berghoff M, Stanke HG, Petermeyer M and Kalff G. Niedrigflußnarkosen mit Desfluran. *Anaesthesist* 1997; **46**, 287–293.
8. Baum J, Stanke HG. Low Flow und Minimal Flow Anästhesie mit Sevofluran. *Anaesthesist* 1998; **47** (Suppl. 1), S70–S76.
9. Virtue RW. Minimal flow nitrous oxide anesthesia. *Anesthesiology* 1974; **40**, 196–198.
10. Baum J. Klinische Anwendung der Minimal-Flow-Anästhesie. In Jantzen JPAH and Kleemann PP, eds, *Narkosebeatmung. Low Flow, Minimal Flow, Geschlossenes System.* Schattauer, Stuttgart, 1989, pp. 49–66.
11. Conway CM. Closed and low flow systems. Theoretical considerations. *Acta Anaesth Belg* 1984; **34**, 257–263.
12. Baum J. Narkosesysteme. *Anaesthesist* 1987; **36**, 393–399.
13. Bergmann H. Das Narkosegerät in Gegenwart und Zukunft aus der Sicht des Klinikers. *Anaesthesist* 1986; **35**, 587–594.

Advantages of the rebreathing technique in anaesthesia

6.1 Reduced consumption of anaesthetic gases

The extent to which the consumption of anaesthetic gases can be reduced by appropriate reduction of the fresh gas flow will be explained by the example of minimal flow anaesthesia. During performance of an isoflurane anaesthetic on a 75 kg patient, the fresh gas volume is reduced to 0.5 l/min after an initial 15-min phase with high flow of 4.4 l/min. The duration of anaesthesia is assumed to be 2 h and the target expired isoflurane concentration is about 1.0%, the target inspired concentration of oxygen about 35%, that of nitrous oxide about 65%. This minimal flow anaesthetic will be compared with an anaesthetic of identical duration and identical anaesthetic concentration, but with the high flow of 4.4 l/min maintained throughout. Total nitrous oxide consumption is reduced by 294 litres, oxygen consumption by 115.5 litres, and the consumption of isoflurane vapour by 5.62 litres (Figure 6.1). Even more pronounced is the reduction of anaesthetic agent consumption if desflurane is used: assuming an inspiratory desflurane concentration of 6.0%, with high flow anaesthesia (4.4 l/min) 161 litres desflurane vapour are consumed, with minimal flow anaesthesia this is reduced to just 33 litres[1].

Between 1984 and 1989, P. Feiss made a consistent switch in his clinic from non-rebreathing to rebreathing systems used with low fresh gas flow. In spite of a 25% increase in the number of anaesthetics undertaken, the annual nitrous oxide consumption was reduced by about 40% from 9200 to 5880 kg. With this drastic change in management, the isoflurane consumption could be reduced by as much as 90–93%[2].

Comparing high flow (Mapleson D) with low flow (circle absorber system) isoflurane–nitrous oxide anaesthesia, Pedersen et al.[3] found, in procedures lasting 2 h, mean isoflurane consumptions of 40.8 and 7.9 ml, respectively. A 54.7% reduction in the consumption of isoflurane and a 55.9% reduction in that of enflurane are reported by Cotter[4]. He made his investigation in entirely unselected clinical trials. The fresh gas flows compared were about 6.5 l/min in the 'high flow' group, but were only a little below 3 l/min and somewhat inconsistent in the 'low flow' group.

In Germany, about 5 million anaesthetic procedures are performed each year, and in the UK about 3.5 million[5]. If it is assumed that 20% are regional blocks, 20% total intravenous techniques or operations of short

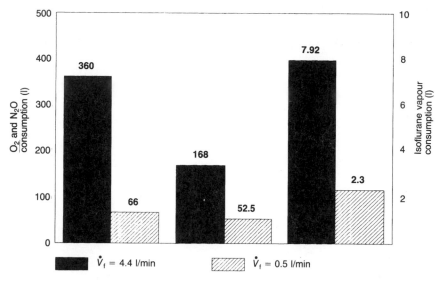

Figure 6.1   Anaesthetic gas consumption in litres over a period of 120 min. High flow anaesthesia ($\dot{V}_f = 4.4\,l/min$) versus minimal flow anaesthesia ($\dot{V}_f = 0.5\,l/min$).

duration, in which low flow anaesthesia would not be practical, then there are potential savings to be made in about 5 million cases in these two countries alone. Let us assume that enflurane is used in 50% of these cases, and isoflurane in the remaining 50%, and that the average end-expiratory concentration is $0.8 \times MAC$. Let us also assume that 50% of these anaesthetics last for 1 h, 33% for 2 h and 17% for 3 h, and that it would be common practice in each case to use a fresh gas flow rate of 4.5 l/min for a total of 30 min, so as to facilitate wash-in and wash-out of the anaesthetic gases at appropriate times. If, with these preconditions, low flow technique (1 l/min) is compared with high flow anaesthesia (4.5 l/min), the reduction of gas and anaesthetic consumption can be projected to be about 350 million litres of oxygen, 1000 million litres of nitrous oxide, 33 000 litres of liquid isoflurane and 46 000 litres of liquid enflurane per year (Table 6.1). By consistent educational efforts to establish low flow techniques in routine clinical practice it was possible to reduce the consumption of inhalational agents by 65%[6], and Namiki and co-workers even succeeded in reducing sevoflurane expenditure in paediatric anaesthesia by 86%[7].

6.2 Reduced costs

6.2.1   Anaesthetic gases

It is self-evident that reduction of anaesthetic gas consumption is accompanied by a reduction of costs. Based on the previous example of a 2-h

Table 6.1   Estimation of annual anaesthetic gas consumption and reduction of costs which could result from concomitant changes from high to low flow anaesthesia in Germany and the UK

	Consumption (l/year) *(Fresh gas flow rate 4.5 l/min)*	Consumption (l/year) *(Fresh gas flow rate 1.0 l/min)*	Cost savings *(US$/year)*
Oxygen	700×10^6	350×10^6	510 000
N$_2$O	1.5×10^9	0.5×10^9	12 200 000
Isoflurane	61 650	28 500	31 800 000
Enflurane	89 500	43 250	20 850 000

Values for isoflurane and enflurane represent volume of liquid (litres)[5].

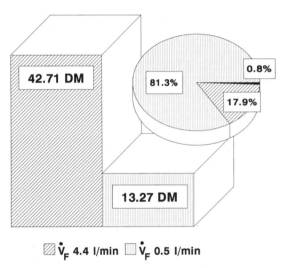

$\boxtimes \dot{V}_F$ 4.4 l/min $\square \dot{V}_F$ 0.5 l/min

Figure 6.2   Costs for anaesthetic gases used during 120 min anaesthesia. High flow anaesthesia (4.4 l/min) versus minimal flow anaesthesia (0.5 l/min). Pie chart indicates the breakdown of cost savings: isoflurane 81.3%, nitrous oxide 17.9%, oxygen 0.8%

isoflurane anaesthetic, performed according to the standardized scheme used routinely in the author's own hospital, the reduction of the fresh gas flow from 4.4 to 0.5 l/min results in cost savings of 72.4%, which means that about 33.90 DM (22.60 US$) can be saved. Based on the German prices for anaesthetic gases, approximately 83.7% of the savings can be attributed to the reduction of isoflurane consumption, 15.6% to that of nitrous oxide and only 0.7% to the reduction of oxygen consumption (Figure 6.2). The cost savings depend on the duration of the anaesthetic procedure and the price of the agent selected (Figure 6.3) and of course, on the extent of flow reduction (Figure 6.4).

The different calculations concerning the saving of costs by flow reduction[4,5,9,10] are hardly comparable as all are based on quite different

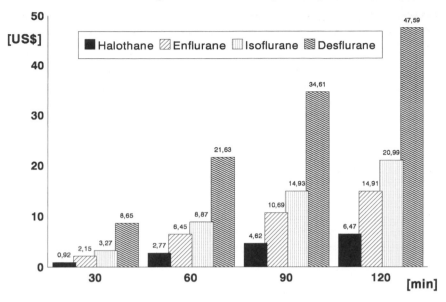

Figure 6.3   Cost savings by flow reduction as a function of duration of procedure and choice of anaesthetic agent

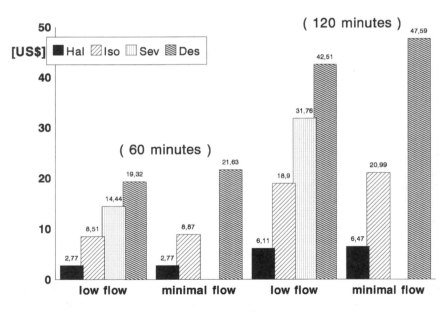

Figure 6.4   Cost savings as a function of degree of flow reduction

assumptions. Nevertheless, if an attempt is made to compile the different results, depending on the extent of flow reduction and the choice of the anaesthetic agent, a saving in costs due to reduced anaesthetic gas consumption of between 50 and 75% may be assumed for 1 h of anaesthesia

Table 6.2   Costs for anaesthetic gases as a function of the fresh gas flow (1 h anaesthesia)

	$\dot{V}_F \approx 6\,l/min$	$\dot{V}_F \approx 4\,l/min$	$\dot{V}_F \approx 3\,l/min$	$\dot{V}_F \approx 1\,l/min$
Baum[5]				
Isoflurane		28.50 DM		11.20 DM
		19.00 US$		7.47 US$
Enflurane		18.00 DM		8.30 DM
		12.00 US$		5.53 US$
Cotter *et al.*[4]				
Isoflurane	£11.40		£5.16	
	17 US$		7.70 US$	
Enflurane	£5.62		£2.48	
	8.40 US$		3.70 US$	
Loke *et al.*[9]				
Isoflurane	12 $Aus		6 $Aus	2 $Aus
	8 US$		4 US$	1.30 US$
Enflurane	8.64 $Aus		4.30 $Aus	1.44 $Aus
	5.80 US$		2.90 US$	0.96 US$
Pedersen *et al.*[3]				
Isoflurane	107 DKK		48.50 DKK	21 DKK
	14.50 US$		6.50 US$	2.90 US$

DM: German mark;   US$: US dollar;   £: Pound sterling; $Aus: Australian dollar;   DKK: Danish kroner (as at 1996).

(Table 6.2). Several authors emphasize that, in calculating the real costs of anaesthesia, the expenses for the soda lime, the supplementary intravenous drugs, the choice of the breathing system, expenses for acquisition and maintenance of the equipment, and last but not least the staff salaries, have also to be considered. Although the arguments are quite justified, these factors, except the soda lime consumption, are not directly linked to the setting of the fresh gas flow. One must not forget that every day many anaesthetic procedures are performed with technically advanced anaesthetic machines equipped with rebreathing systems and comprehensive monitoring, but using fresh gas flows which surely prevent the realization of any rebreathing. A more efficient use of available equipment by changing clinical practice alone would result in considerable savings.

Cost savings of between 55% and 75%[8,10] appear to be absolutely realistic if minimal flow anaesthesia is used consistently. Ernst has compared the cost involved in anaesthesia management with non-rebreathing systems with those in which closed rebreathing systems were used. If 10 000 anaesthetics are performed with rebreathing systems (60% of 1 h, 30% of 2 h and 10% of 3 h), this results in cost savings of 6930 US$ if halothane is used, 36 670 US$ for enflurane and 63 560 US$ if isoflurane is used[11]. Cotter[4] comes to the conclusion that routine use of low flow anaesthesia (4–3 l/min!!) could result in annual savings of £26 870 at his hospital, and Matjasko[12] reported annual savings of about 16 800 US$ by performance of isoflurane anaesthesia using low flow at his department. Herscher and Yeakel estimated that, in 1977, the financial loss in the USA resulting from the unnecessary discharge of unused excess gas out of breathing systems was about 80 million US$[13]. For an average procedure such as a cholecystectomy, the costs involved for a neurolept anaesthesia with non-rebreathing system, for an enflurane anaesthesia via a semi-closed rebreathing system with a fresh gas flow of about 4l/min, and for minimal flow anaesthesia with isoflurane are almost identical[14].

If the preconditions detailed in Section 6.1 are assumed, the annual financial savings resulting from reduced gas and anaesthetic consumption in Germany and the UK would total more than 65.4 million US$ if low flow anaesthetic techniques were performed consistently (Table 6.1).

According to Ernst[11], the efficiency of fresh gas utilization, i.e. the cost–benefit ratio of an anaesthetic method, can be described with the aid of the efficiency coefficient Q_{eff} by dividing the amount of agent taken up by the patient $\dot{V}_U$ by the amount delivered into the system at the same time $\dot{V}_{Del}$:

$$Q_{eff} = \dot{V}_U / \dot{V}_{Del}$$

This quotient, thus, has to be calculated separately for nitrous oxide, oxygen and the volatile anaesthetic. If the fresh gas flow and composition are kept constant, it is self-explanatory that during the course of anaesthesia the efficiency quotient varies with changes in uptake. The values established in a comparison between an anaesthetic with a high fresh gas flow of 4.4l/min and a minimal flow anaesthetic of a normal-weight adult patient over a period of 30 min after induction are illustrated in Table 6.3.

The efficiency of fresh gas utilization increases considerably with reduction of the fresh gas flow. This quotient for oxygen, nitrous oxide and the volatile anaesthetic can only reach its maximum value of 1 in the case of quantitative closed system anaesthesia.

An ether structure and halogenation exclusively by fluorine are the characteristics of the newer volatile anaesthetics desflurane and sevoflurane. The molecular structure of these agents result in low solubility and low anaesthetic potency. Thus, the pharmacokinetic and pharmacodynamic properties result in a low uptake, although a comparatively high

Table 6.3 Efficiency quotient

Fresh gas flow:	4.4 l/min	0.5 l/min
Fresh gas composition:	32% O_2, 68% N_2O	60% O_2, 40% N_2O
	1.1 vol% isoflurane	2.3 vol% isoflurane
	3.5 vol% desflurane	4.5 vol% desflurane
Isoflurane	0.23	0.96
Desflurane	0.09	0.52
Oxygen	0.18	0.85
Nitrous oxide	0.06	0.91

Uptake 30 min after induction (target expired isoflurane concentration 0.85%, target expired desflurane concentration 3.2%, weight of patient 75 kg): isoflurane 11.1 ml/min, desflurane 11.7 ml/min, O_2 254.9 ml/min, N_2O 182.6 ml/min.

partial pressure must be established and maintained in the breathing system and the alveolar space to gain a sufficiently deep anaesthetic level. If high flow anaesthesia is performed using these agents, a considerable amount of anaesthetic is vented to the atmosphere together with the exhaled air. Thus, only a small amount of the inhaled anaesthetic is actually taken up by the patient, but a considerably greater share is wasted after expiration, and the corresponding high amount of agent which has to be delivered into the system is needed to re-establish the required high alveolar concentration rather than meet the patient's uptake. The wastage of anaesthetic is the higher, the less potent the anaesthetic agent. By contrast, using a low flow system, the savings in consumption of these anaesthetic agents will be significant, as the amount wasted is considerably reduced, and only small amounts need be supplied into the breathing system to meet the small individual uptake together with a volume equivalent to that small amount vented to the atmosphere. The low uptake of desflurane and sevoflurane, furthermore, permits an early reduction of the anaesthetic fresh gas concentration (see Sections 10.3.1 and 10.3.2).

The lower the solubility and the lower the anaesthetic potency of an inhalational anaesthetic agent, the higher will be the increase in efficiency which can be gained by flow reduction[5]. The awareness of the problem, that the anaesthetic agent is wasted senselessly with the venting of great amounts of excess gas out of the system, leads directly to adequate flow reduction[15].

The greater economy of anaesthesia methods with reduced fresh gas flow cannot be denied. However, it must be emphasized that these techniques can only be considered as being advantageous provided that they are just as safe for the patient as methods performed with high fresh gas flows.

6.2.2   Soda lime consumption

In a number of publications it was assumed that the savings in anaesthetic gases resulting from flow reduction may be offset by increased soda lime consumption[16,17]. In calculating the costs involved for low flow anaesthesia, only a few publications gave consideration to the costs for increased soda lime consumption, whereby calculations were based on theoretically derived carbon dioxide production and the soda lime's absorption capacity. With a consistent reduction of the fresh gas flow to 0.5 l/min, the costs for soda lime will increase by a factor of 3–7[14,17,18].

However, under clinical conditions, the actual consumption of soda lime by carbon dioxide absorption is not only influenced by the fresh gas flow, but by many other factors too, which can hardly be comprehensively included in the calculation. These include individual metabolic variations (net carbon dioxide production), ventilation and equipment parameters (fresh gas utilization), and the type, frequency and duration of the anaesthetic procedures.

In the author's own department the absorption capacity of soda lime was measured under clinical conditions with different fresh gas flows of 4.4 and 0.5 l/min using various anaesthetic machines: AV 1, Cicero and Sulla

800 V (Dräger Medizintechnik, Lübeck)[19]. The AV 1 and Sulla 800 V were equipped with a single absorber canister of 1 litre volume and the Cicero with an absorber of 1.5 litres capacity and pelleted soda lime (ICI-Pharma, Plankstadt) was used. Consideration has to be given to the fact that, depending on the duration of anaesthesia and frequency of surgical interventions during an unselected daily list, it was by no means possible to work with a flow of 0.5 l/min continuously. The flow has to be high during induction and emergence phases, and a number of procedures, such as anaesthesia using a face mask, cannot be performed with reduced flow. This means that, prior to evaluation of the results, an accurate analysis had to be established to assess the percentage of time during which a fresh gas flow of 0.5 l/min was actually used. Soda lime was considered as being exhausted if the inspired carbon dioxide concentration had reached a value of 1%.

If a fresh gas flow of 4.4 l/min was used exclusively, the utilization time, until soda lime was completely exhausted, amounted to 99 h (Cicero), 62 h (AV 1) or 43 h (Sulla 800 V). Based on the current German price of 7.25 DM ($\approx$ 4.83 US$) per litre soda lime, the costs involved for soda lime under these conditions range between 0.11 DM ($\approx$ 0.07 US$) (Cicero) and 0.17 DM ($\approx$ 0.13 US$) (Sulla 800 V) per hour of anaesthesia.

If, whenever possible, the fresh gas flow was reduced to 0.5 l/min, the time of minimal flow anaesthesia with respect to total anaesthetic time ranged from 45% to 75%. The time during which anaesthesia can actually be performed with a low fresh gas flow essentially depends on the duration and the frequency of anaesthetic procedures. Even if a large proportion of anaesthetics are of long duration and reduction of the fresh gas flow is effected consistently, the share that minimal flow phases have in the entire time of absorber operation under clinical conditions can hardly be extended above 75–85%. The utilization time of soda lime up to complete exhaustion is then reduced to 20–30% of the utilization period measured for a fresh gas flow of 4.4 l/min (Figure 6.5).

Thus, with the greatest possible use of minimal flow anaesthesia, the costs for soda lime rise by a factor of four. With a view to the earlier example of a 2-h isoflurane anaesthetic, this means that the costs for soda lime rise from 0.30 DM ($\approx$ 0.20 US$) to about 1.20 DM ($\approx$ 0.80 US$). Compared with the savings in anaesthetic gases which amount to 33.90 DM ($\approx$ 22.60 US$), the additional costs for soda lime, about 0.90 DM ($\approx$ 0.60 US$), are insignificant. The same conclusion was drawn by Cotter et al.[4].

In recently performed trials we used soda lime, which does not contain potassium hydroxide (Spherasorb, Intersurgical Ltd, Berkshire, UK), as sodium and especially potassium hydroxide are implicated in the degradation of volatile agents[20–24]. Spherasorb is a mixture of sodium and calcium hydroxide and water compressed to globes with a mean diameter of 4 mm. It was found to generate significantly less compound A when exposed to sevoflurane, and due to the admixture of zeolites it is nearly dust free. This brand of soda lime was found to be especially effective, as, even with the flow at 0.5 l/min for an average of 76% of the time, the mean lifetime of 1.5 l of this absorbent was 33.4 h.

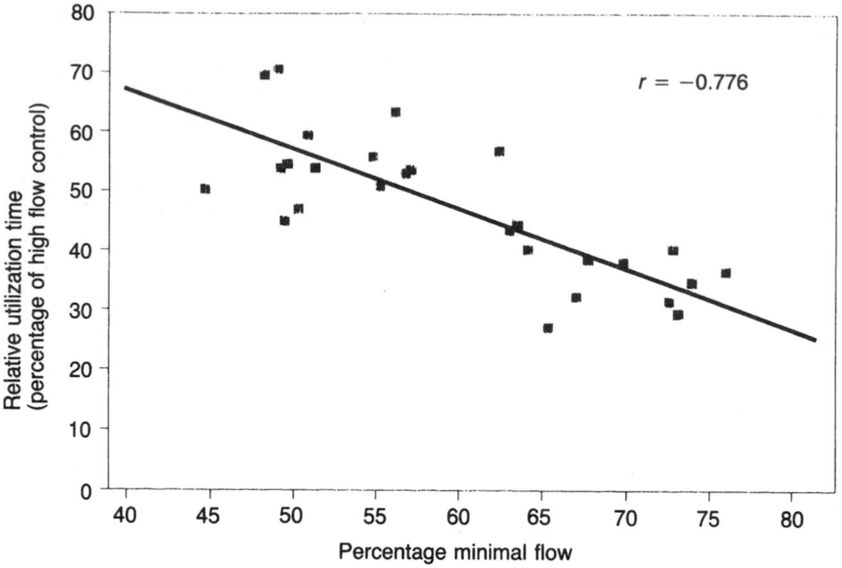

Figure 6.5   Utilization time of soda lime (depicted as percentage of utilization time, using a flow of 4.4 l/min), as a function of the percentage of time during which anaesthesia was actually performed with 0.5 l/min fresh gas flow

In summer 1999, an absorbent became available that contains neither potassium nor sodium hydroxide (Amsorb, Armstrong Medical Ltd., Coleraine, Northern Ireland) and does not react with desflurane or sevoflurane even if desiccated[25,26]. It contains predominantly calcium hydroxide with the addition of calcium chloride and calcium sulphate to retain water, mechanically stabilize the granules, and facilitate proper scavenging of carbon dioxide. To distinguish it from soda lime containing alkali metal hydroxides, this absorbent is referred to as calcium hydroxide lime. The scavenging capacity of calcium hydroxide lime is somewhat less than that of soda lime, nevertheless it is quite sufficient to be used in daily routine clinical practice.

With flows at 0.5–0.25 l/min for an average of 75–80% of the time, the mean lifetime of 1.5 l of this absorbent was 17–20 h. This absorbent is thus less effective than soda lime, and its consistent use will increase the costs over currently used absorbents. However, for safety reasons, especially when low flow techniques with sevoflurane are performed consistently, calcium hydroxide lime should preferably be routinely used in the future. The more so, as the costs for absorbents represent a minute portion of total peri-operative costs and might even be more cost-effective after considering medicolegal implications[25].

6.3   Reduced environmental pollution

6.3.1   Workplace exposure to anaesthetic gas

Although neither harmfulness nor harmlessness of sub-anaesthetic gas

Table 6.4   Workplace concentration limits (ppm) of inhalation anaesthetics*

	N_2O	Halothane	Enflurane	Isoflurane
Austria	–	5	–	–
Belgium	50	50	50	50
Denmark	50	5	2	–
Finland	–	–	10 (20)†	10 (20)†
France (?)	–	50	75	–
Germany	100 (400)†	5 (20)†	20 (80)†	10 (40)†
Italy (?)	50	–	–	–
Netherlands	80	5	20	20
Norway	100 (150)†	2 (4)†	2 (4)†	2 (4)†
Sweden	100 (500)†	5 (10)†	10 (20)†	10 (20)†
Switzerland	–	5 (10)†	–	–
UK	100	10	50	50
USA (NIOSH)	25	2 (0.5)†	2 (0.5)†	–
USA (TLV-list)	50	50	75	75

*The author owes a debt of gratitude to Prof. Dr J. Hobbhahn, University of Regensburg, an acknowledged expert in this field. He compiled the data given in this table by consulting the scientific societies of anaesthetists of the different countries. The data for France and Italy are given with reservation, as exact figures could not be obtained. (State: February 2000).
† Short time limits of workplace concentration, e.g. Finland and Norway: 15 min; Germany: 4×15 min/8 h.
‡ Limits of workplace concentration if the respective agent is applied together with nitrous oxide.

concentrations have yet been demonstrated[27–30], workplace exposure to anaesthetic gases is gaining more importance with growing environmental awareness. Thus, in nearly all industrial nations today comparatively low thresholds for maximum workplace concentrations of anaesthetic gases and vapours are defined[30,31] (Table 6.4). In the USA, the following threshold limit values have been adopted by the National Institute of Occupational Safety and Health (NIOSH): for nitrous oxide 25 ppm, for all volatile anaesthetics 2 ppm, and for all volatile anaesthetics used together with nitrous oxide 0.5 ppm[32]. The TLV list (Table of Threshold Limit Values) assesses a value of 50 ppm for nitrous oxide and for halothane, and 75 ppm ($= 575 \, mg/m^3$) for enflurane. Where the newest German MAK value list 1998 (MAK = Maximale Arbeitsplatz-Konzentration = maximum workplace concentration) is concerned, halothane is listed with a MAK of 5 ppm ($= 40 \, mg/m^3$), enflurane with 20 ppm, isoflurane with 10 ppm, and nitrous oxide with 100 ppm[33]. The authorities for occupational safety and health in three German states even defined a MAK value for nitrous oxide as low as 50 ppm ($= 91 \, mg/m^3$)[34].

Virtue[35] demonstrated that only by reduction of the nitrous oxide flow to 0.5 or 0.2 l/min could the nitrous oxide workplace concentration be reduced to 29 or 15 ppm, respectively (Figure 6.6). These values would even satisfy the stringent NIOSH requirements. As far as intubation anaesthesia is concerned, minimizing of emissions according to the 'state of the art', as is also sought by the German national regulations on harmful

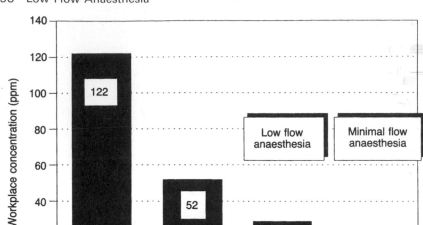

Figure 6.6   Reduction of workplace contamination with nitrous oxide by reduction of nitrous oxide flow. At a flow of 0.2 l/min (minimal flow anaesthesia), the value falls below the stringent NIOSH threshold. (From Virtue[35], by permission)

substances, could be realized on its own simply by means of adequate reduction of the fresh gas flow and judicious use of rebreathing systems.
    It is obvious that workplace contamination with anaesthetic gases can be considerably reduced by the use of gas scavenging systems, so that this problem is essentially overcome. Nevertheless, in the direct vicinity of anaesthetic machines the concentration of anaesthetic gases was found to be 40–150% higher in high flow anaesthesia (fresh gas flow > minute volume) than at a flow of 1.5 l/min[36]. Furthermore, it must be considered that at present the anaesthetic waste gases are discharged into the atmosphere.

6.3.2   Reduction of atmospheric pollution

6.3.2.1   Nitrous oxide

Every year the nitrous oxide concentration in the troposphere increases by 0.25%. This gas contributes to the continued warming of the atmosphere, the so-called 'greenhouse effect'[37–40]. Nitrous oxide molecules are extremely stable and during their lifetime of some 150 years they may ascend up to the stratosphere and contribute to the destruction of the ozone layer by generating nitric oxides (Figure 6.7)[32,41]. However, it must also be considered that vastly more nitrous oxide is generated in fertilized agricultural soil by bacterial nitrate decomposition. Only about

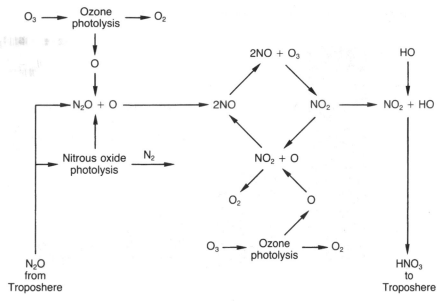

Figure 6.7 The reaction of nitrous oxide with stratospheric ozone. (From Waterson[32], by permission)

1% of the emitted volume of nitrous oxide is estimated to derive from medical sources[37,42].

6.3.2.2 Halogenated hydrocarbons

The volatile anaesthetics halothane, enflurane and isoflurane belong to the chlorofluorocarbon (CFC) group, which is held to be mainly responsible for the destruction of the ozone layer[37,41]. But the chlorofluorocarbons used as inhalational anaesthetics are only partially halogenated: that is, not all valencies of the carbon atoms are occupied by halogens. According to the ozone convention of Vienna and the protocol of Montreal, these partially substituted chlorofluorocarbons are held to be less noxious, as the ozone-destroying potential is less than 5% of that exerted by fully sub-stituted molecules[43]. Furthermore, these molecules have a comparatively short lifetime of only about 2–6 years and are, thus, already being destroyed in the troposphere[37,44,45]. This statement, however, is not undis-puted as just the CFCs with short lifetime, to which the volatile agents belong, shall have a significantly higher even though only short lasting ozone-destroying potency[46]. Last but not least, the quantity of volatile anaesthetics is estimated to be not more than 0.1% of the yearly produc-tion of industrially used CFCs[37,43]. However, it has to be considered critically that the figures describing the quantity of yearly global volatile agent production range widely from 100 tons[43] to 6400 tons[45]. The same criticism applies to the quoted figures for the amount of industrially produced and emitted CFCs, which differ considerably between publica-tions. Thus, for the time being it seems to be nearly impossible to quantify exactly the contribution that the emission of volatile anaesthetics exerts on the destruction of the ozone layer[47].

According to the results of the Montreal conference, the production of partially halogenated CFCs – to which belong halothane, enflurane and isoflurane – is to be reduced stepwise and finally brought to an end by the year 2030[48]. Inhalational anaesthetics that are partially substituted with fluorine only, i.e. desflurane and sevoflurane, are not CFCs and their ozone-depleting potential though not, however, their contribution to the greenhouse effect, is negligible. Neither agent is covered by the decisions of the Montreal conference.

Even though atmospheric pollution occurs with anaesthetic gases, their contribution to the greenhouse effect and the destruction of the ozone layer seems to be of minor importance. However, any environmental contamination with inhalation anaesthetics should be avoided conscientiously[37,45,49]. This goal seems to be all the more justified, as environmental pollution with anaesthetic gases can be considerably reduced so easily by the judicious use of the available modern, technically advanced rebreathing systems[32,37,42].

6.4   Improved anaesthetic gas climate

In terms of clinical relevance, the anaesthetic gas climate can be improved if the share of cold dry fresh gas is reduced, while at the same time the proportion of recirculating, already humidified and warmed exhaled gas is increased[50-54]. The significance that appropriate humidification and warming of anaesthetic gases have on the function of the ciliated epithelium and its mucociliary clearance has been convincingly proved. Given a relative humidity of 50% for inspired gas at room temperature, a cessation of ciliary movement can already be observed 10 min after commencement of ventilation. Considerable morphological damage to the epithelium of the respiratory tract is caused by 3 h of ventilation with dry gases. Together with the drying up of secretions, which results from inadequate humidification and warming of the inspired gas, this leads to mucus retention with partial obstruction of the bronchioles, which in turn supports the development of microatelectases. In addition, the improvement of the tracheobronchial climate helps in reducing fluid and heat loss via the respiratory tract.

During anaesthetic ventilation, the absolute humidity of the inspired gas should preferably range between 17 and 30 mgH$_2$O/l, and the breathing gas temperature between 28°C and 32°C[53-58]. Rathgeber, however, even demands a temperature of the inspired gases between 30°C and 37°C and a water content of 30–35 mgH$_2$O/l to optimize the climatization[59].

Climatization of breathing gases is determined by the technical design of the breathing system, the size of the absorber, length and heat conduction of patient hoses, the ambient temperature, ventilation patterns and the fresh gas flow, i.e. rebreathing fraction. This explains why a great number of investigations were carried out at quite different starting conditions. In addition, humidity was measured by various measuring methods so that a comparison of the published results remains very difficult.

6.4.1   Breathing gas temperature

Kleemann *et al.*[54,57] showed that after 2 h of anaesthesia with a fresh gas flow of 0.6 l/min, the inspired breathing gas temperature had increased to an average of 31.5°C. Although this high value is only achieved after about 90 min, the gas temperature rises to about 28°C within the first 30 min. The temperatures measured during low flow anaesthesia were at all times distinctly higher than those measured with a high fresh gas flow (Figure 6.8). Buijs points out that the high breathing gas temperature of 36–40°C which is measured directly downstream of the carbon dioxide absorber with low flow anaesthesia is rapidly reduced to 20–24°C by heat losses in the inspired limb of the patient hose system[60]. And yet, using a circle rebreathing system with a fresh gas flow of 0.5 l/min, Bengtson measured gas temperatures of 28.5°C, which were about 6.8°C above room temperature after a period of 30 min. These temperatures were higher than those measured with non-rebreathing systems, even though these were additionally equipped with heat and moisture exchangers (HME)[52]. In another comparative examination with absorber canisters of 4.7 and 0.9 litres volume, Bengtson comes to the conclusion that the breathing gas temperature with low flow anaesthesia is favourably influenced by absorber canisters of comparatively small volumes[52].

Recently we finished investigations on anaesthetic gas temperature during performance of inhalational anaesthesia with a Cicero EM anaesthetic machine (Dräger Medizintechnik, Lübeck, Germany) equipped with

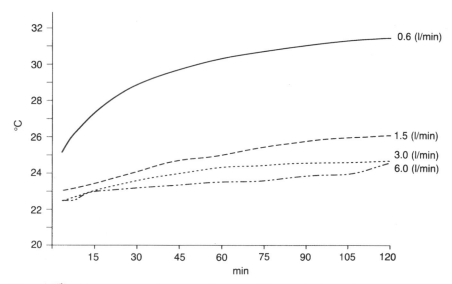

Figure 6.8   Temperature of anaesthetic gas at different fresh gas flows during 2 h of anaesthesia. (From Kleemann[53], by permission)

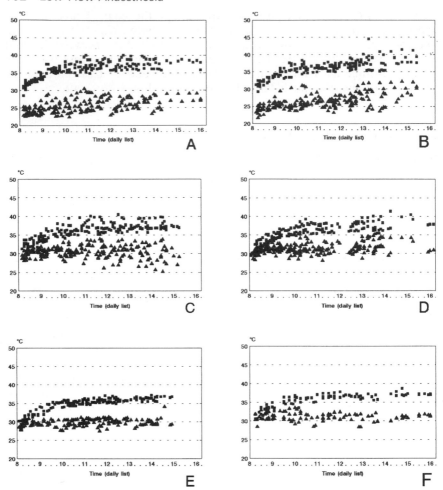

Figure 6.9 Inspired gas temperatures during the course of an all-day list, taken at the tube connector (▲) and the inspiratory outlet of the breathing system (■), using different fresh gas flows and hosings (Cicero EM anaesthetic machine). (A) Normal double limb hosing, $\dot{V}_F = 0.5\,l/min$; (B) coaxial system, $\dot{V}_F = 0.5\,l/min$; (C) heated double limb hosing, $\dot{V}_F = 0.5\,l/min$; (D) heated double limb hosing, $\dot{V}_F = 1.0\,l/min$; (E) heated double limb hosing, $\dot{V}_F = 2.0\,l/min$; (F) heated double limb hosing, $\dot{V}_F = 4.4\,l/min$

three different types of hoses: conventional corrugated silicon hoses, coaxial hoses and heated hoses, equally of 1.5 m length. The temperature of the anaesthetic gases at the inspiratory outlet of the heated breathing system of the Cicero machine was found to be independent of the fresh gas flow and the type of hose system: it started at 30°C in the early morning and rose after 60–90 min to 35–40°C (Figure 6.9). When conventional or coaxial hose systems were used, during minimal flow anaesthesia the temperature taken at the patient end of the inspiratory hose was about 10°C lower: mainly between 22 and 28°C, only in longer-lasting cases did it reach 28–30°C. A similar situation applies for the coaxial hose system: mainly the inspired gas temperature was between 22–28°C, only in longer-lasting cases did the temperature rise to values between 28 and 32°C. If heated hoses were used, however, the temperature loss was only 5°C: on average the temperature was between 28 and 35°C, from the very beginning of the list and independent of the fresh gas flow rate[58].

6.4.2   Breathing gas humidity

If anaesthesia is performed with a rebreathing system using low fresh gas flow, the humidity is considerably higher than with high fresh gas flows. Following 2 h anaesthesia with a fresh gas flow of 0.6 l/min, Kleemann found an average inspired humidity of 21 mgH$_2$O/l in the breathing gases. However, it takes a certain latency period (Figure 6.10), comparable to the rise in temperature of the breathing gases, for the humidity in the breathing gas to rise to sufficient values[53,57]. While Kleemann established 60–75 min for this latency period in his measurements, it amounted to just 30 min in Bengtson's investigations. He measured an absolute humidity of 28 mgH$_2$O/l in the breathing gases after 60 min with a fresh gas flow of 0.5 l/min[52]. The humidity values measured in the breathing gas after completion of the equilibrium period again correspond approximately to the values established if passive heat and moisture exchangers are used.

According to the author's own investigations with different types of patient hoses the humidity of the inspired gases is essentially influenced by the fresh gas flow[58] (Figure 6.11): using conventional hoses the humidity of the inspired gases rose after a short initial period of 15–30 min at the very beginning of the operation list to values higher

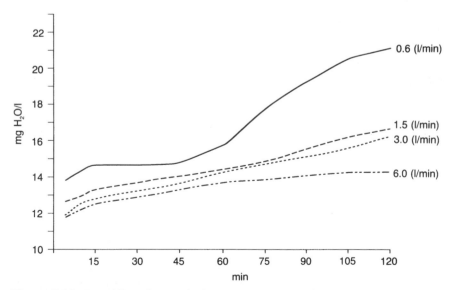

Figure 6.10   Humidity of anaesthetic gas at different fresh gas flows during 2 h of anaesthesia. (From Kleemann[53], by permission)

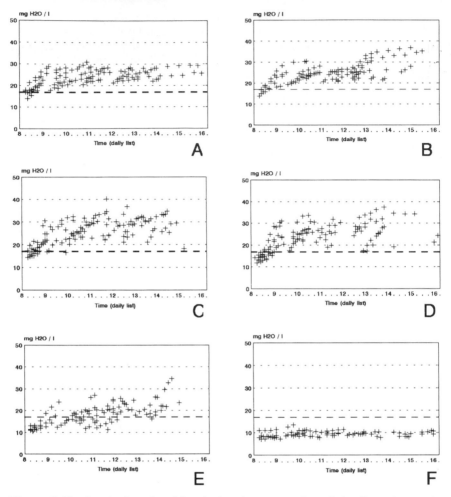

Figure 6.11 Inspired gas humidity during the course of an all-day list, taken at the tube connector, using different fresh gas flows and hosings (Cicero EM anaesthetic machine). (A) Normal double limb hosing, $\dot{V}_F = 0.5\,l/min$; (B) coaxial system, $\dot{V}_F = 0.5\,l/min$; (C) heated double limb hosing, $\dot{V}_F = 0.5\,l/min$; (D) heated double limb hosing, $\dot{V}_F = 1.0\,l/min$; (E) heated double limb hosing, $\dot{V}_F = 2.0\,l/min$; (F) heated double limb hosing, $\dot{V}_F = 4.4\,l/min$.

than $17\,mgH_2O/l$, and ranged on average between 25 and $30\,mgH_2O/l$ during the following whole time course of an all-day list. The same, in general, applies for the coaxial hose system. Only in very long-lasting cases at the end of the list did the humidity rise to values ranging from 30 to $35\,mgH_2O/l$. If the heated hose system was used, after a short initial period of 15–30 min the humidity of the inspired gases ranged from 25 to $35\,mgH_2O/l$. The same applies if this hose system was used at a fresh gas flow of $1.0\,l/min$. If the flow, however, was increased to $2.0\,l/min$ mean values were found to be considerably lower, between 14 and $25\,mgH_2O/l$, and when $4.0\,l/min$ were used, mean values were as low as

10 mgH$_2$O/l. These results are supported by the findings of Kleemann *et al.*[54]: using heated patient hoses they observed that the humidity of the inspired gases reached 27 mgH$_2$O/l and the temperature 33°C during longer-lasting low flow anaesthesia.

The results can be summed up as follows: the humidity of the inspired gases is essentially influenced by the flow, whereas the temperature is mainly influenced by the convective heat loss, and thus by the physical properties of the hose system[58]. Generally, by reducing the fresh gas flow, climatization of the anaesthetic gases can be improved and will reach acceptable values. The 25% better climatization which, according to Branson *et al.*[61,62], can be gained by the use of coaxial hoses, will only be realized in long-lasting anaesthetic procedures at the end of the all-day list. However, if the anaesthesia machine is equipped with a heated breathing system and heated hosing, climatization will reach optimal values which are similar to those gained by the use of heat and moisture exchangers[54].

6.4.3   Body temperature

Improved climatization of anaesthetic gases reduces the heat and fluid losses which occur in the respiratory tract when dry and cold gas is warmed up and humidified by the epithelium. The effect is to alleviate the decrease in body temperature that is usually observed[63–65]. There is just one clinical study available which confirms that the body temperature can be maintained merely by reduction of the fresh gas flow when closed system anaesthesia is performed[66]: after an initial average temperature drop of 0.8°C during the first 60 min, the body temperature rises within the next hour to the starting value established at the beginning of anaesthesia (Figure 6.12). However, in performing closed system anaesthesia, Buijs demonstrated a persistent drop of 1.6°C in oesophageal temperature within 120 min[60]. It must be remembered, though, that the heat losses with respiration amount to about 15 kcal/h for an uncovered narcotized patient, being only around 10% of the total net loss of energy amounting to about 150 kcal/h. Although the net heat loss can be reduced to 30 kcal/h if the narcotized patient is well protected by covers or is wrapped in reflective blankets, there remains 50% of heat losses which are absolutely unaffected by variation of the fresh gas flow.

6.4.4   Implications for anaesthetic practice

The following statements seem to be justified concerning improvement of anaesthetic gas climatization by reduction of the fresh gas flow:

- Temperature and humidity of anaesthetic gases increase if rebreathing systems are used with low fresh gas flow by leading back the already warm and moist exhaled gases to the patient.
- If minimal flow anaesthesia is performed with a fresh gas flow of 0.5 l/min, the values of anaesthetic gas temperature and humidity, attained after an equilibrium period, come very close to values between 28 and

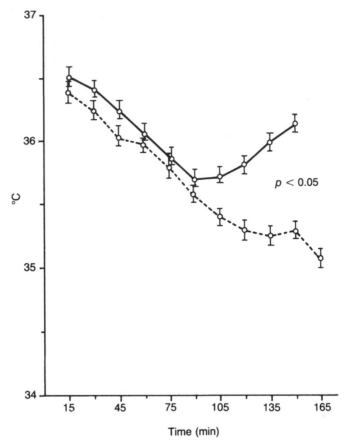

Figure 6.12 Average oesophageal temperature: (—) closed system anaesthesia;
(– –) anaesthesia with semi-closed rebreathing system using 5 l/min fresh gas flow.
(From Aldrete[66], by permission)

32°C and 17 and 30 mgH₂O/l, values which are considered as being
sufficient.

- The protection of morphological integrity and function of the tracheobronchial ciliated epithelium, as a result of improved breathing gas
  climatization by flow reduction, was impressively verified by animal
  experiments and clinical examination.
- Warming and humidification of breathing gases can be additionally
  improved if the breathing system and the patient hose system are
  heated. Under these technical preconditions the temperature of
  the inspired gases will increase to 30–35°C, the water content to
  30–35 mgH₂O/l, thus the climatization will become optimal and
  equals the use of heat and moisture exchangers.
- Even under optimal technical preconditions, sufficient humidification is
  necessarily bound to fresh gas flow reduction and can only be gained
  with flows ≤1.0 l/min.
- Adequate climatization of the breathing gas is a valuable contribution

with respect to maintaining the body temperature of a narcotized patient.

• The advantages of improving the anaesthetic gas climate by anaesthesia management with low fresh gas flow will be most marked in prolonged anaesthetics.

6.5   Extended potentials of patient monitoring and improved knowledge of machine functions

Before starting to practice low flow or even closed system anaesthesia the anaesthetist must be confident in his knowledge of the uptake and distribution of all anaesthetic gases, the function of the different breathing systems, and he has to carefully analyse the technical concept of the anaesthetic machine in use. Although the significance of these advantages can hardly be quantified it is self-evident that improved knowledge about the basics of inhalation anaesthesia and about the function of the technical equipment will enhance safety. In addition, the reduction of fresh gas flow calls for careful equipment maintenance which is itself beneficial for patients. A commitment to closed system anaesthesia and anaesthesia management with low fresh gas flows discloses new perspectives to the anaesthetist, leading to a better understanding of both patient and anaesthetic machine[17,67,68].

If the available technical equipment permits the performance of quantitative closed system anaesthesia, this will allow precise determination and continuous monitoring of oxygen consumption, uptake of volatile anaesthetics and carbon dioxide production, which in turn facilitates comprehensive evaluation of metabolic, respiratory and circulatory conditions[69–71].

6.6   References

1. Stanke HG and Baum J. CIA – Costs of inhalation anaesthesia. Computer program for calculation of costs of inhalation anaesthesia, Ver. 3.0E. Hosp. St. Elisabeth-Stift, Lindenstrasse 3–7, D-49401 Damme, May 1999.
2. Feiss P, Demontoux MH and Colin D. Anesthetic gas and vapour saving with minimal flow anesthesia. *Acta Anesth Belg* 1990; **41**, 249–251.
3. Pedersen FM, Nielsen J, Ibsen M and Guldager H. Low-flow isoflurane–nitrous oxide anaesthesia offers substantial economic advantages over high-flow and medium flow isoflurane–nitrous oxide anaesthesia. *Act Anaesth Scand* 1993; **37**, 509–512.
4. Cotter SM, Petros AJ, Doré CJ, Berber ND and White DC. Low-flow anaesthesia. *Anaesthesia* 1991; **46**, 1009–1012.
5. Baum JA and Aitkenhead AR. Low flow anaesthesia. *Anaesthesia* 1995 (Suppl); **50**, 37–44.
6. McKenzie AJ. Reinforcing a 'low flow' anaesthesia policy with feedback can produce a sustained reduction in isoflurane consumption. *Anaesth Intens Care* 1998; **26**, 371–376.

7. Igarashi M, Watanabe H, Iwasaki H and Namiki A. Clinical evaluation of low-flow sevoflurane anaesthesia for paediatric patients. *Acta Anaest Scand*, 1999, **43**, 19–23.

8. Baum J. Die Narkose mit niedrigem Frischgasfluß: Darstellung des Verfahrens in Frage und Antwort. Bibliomed, Med. Verl. Ges., Melsungen, 1993.

9. Loke J and Shearer WAJ. Cost of anaesthesia. *Can J Anaesth* 1993; **40**, 472–474.

10. Droh R and Rothmann G. Das geschlossene Kreisystem. *Anaesthesist* 1977; **26**, 461–466.

11. Ernst EA and Spain JA. Closed-circuit and high-flow systems: examining alternatives. In Brown BR, ed., *Future Anesthesia Delivery Systems. Contemporary Anesthesia Practice*, vol. 8. F. A. Davies, Philadelphia, 1984, pp. 11–38.

12. Matjasko J. Economic impact of low-flow anaesthesia. *Anesthesiology* 1987; **67**, 863–864.

13. Herscher E and Yeakel AE. Nitrous oxide – oxygen based anesthesia: the waste and its cost. *Anaesth Rev* 1977; **4**, 29.

14. Bengtson JP, Sonander H and Stenqvist O. Comparison of costs of different anaesthetic techniques. *Acta Anaesthesiol Scand* 1988; **32**, 33–35.

15. Euliano TY, van Oostrom JH and van der Aa J. Waste gas monitor reduces wasted volatile anesthetic. *J Clin Mon Comp* 1999; **15**, 287–293.

16. Christensen KN, Thomsen A, Jorgensen S and Fabricius J. Analysis of costs of anaesthetic breathing systems. *Br J Anaesth* 1987; **59**, 389–390.

17. Edsall DW. Economy is not a major benefit of closed-system anesthesia. *Anesthesiology* 1981; **54**, 258–259.

18. Buijs BHMJ. Herwardering van het Gesloten Ademsysteem in de Anesthesiologie. Dissertationsschrift der Erasmus-Universität, Rotterdam, 1988.

19. Baum J, Enzenauer J, Krausse Th and Sachs G. Atemkalk – Nutzungsdauer, Verbrauch und Kosten in Abhängigkeit vom Frischgasfluß. *Anaesthesiol Reanimat* 1993; **18**, 108–113.

20. Funk W, Gruber M, Wild K and Hobbhahn J. Dry soda lime markedly degrades sevoflurane during simulated inhalation induction. *Br J Anaesth* 1999; **82**, 193–198.

21. Förster H and Dudziak R. Über die Ursachen der Reaktion von trockenem Atemkalk und halogenierten Inhalationsanästhetika. *Anaesthesist* 1997; **46**, 1054–1063.

22. Förster H, Warnken UH and Asskali F. Unterschiedliche Reaktion von Sevofluran mit einzelnen Komponenten von Atemkalk. *Anaesthesist* 1997; **46**, 1071–1075.

23. Förster H. Das Soda lime-Problem. *Anaesthesist* 1999; **48**, 409–416.

24. Neumann MA, Laster MJ, Weiskopf RB, Gong DH, Dudziak R, Forster H and Eger EI. The elimination of sodium and potassium hydroxides from desiccated soda lime diminishes degradation of desflurane to carbon monoxide and sevoflurane to compound A but does not compromise carbon dioxide absorption. *Anesth Analg* 1999; **89**, 768–773.

25. Kharasch ED. Putting the brakes on anesthetic breakdown. *Anesthesiology* 1999; **91**, 1192–1194.

26. Murray JM, Renfrew CW, Bedi A, McCrystal CB, Jones DS and Fee JPH. Amsorb, a new carbon dioxide absorbent for use in anesthetic breathing systems. *Anesthesiology* 1999; **91**, 1342–1348.

27. Pothmann W, Shimada K, Goerig M, Fuhlrott M and Schulte am Esch J. Belastungen des Arbeitsplatzes durch Naroksegase. *Anaesthesist* 1991; **40**, 339–346.

28. Spence AA. Environmental pollution by inhalation anaesthetics. *Br J Anaesth* 1987; **59**, 96–103.

29. Conzen P. Gesundheitliche Risiken von Inhalationsanästhetika. *Anästhesiol Intensivmed Notfallmed Schmerzther* 1994; **29**, 10–17.
30. Schulte am Esch J. Gefahren der Narkosegasbelastung am Arbeitsplatz. *Anästh Intensivmed* 1994; **35**, 154–161.
31. Huber E. Rechtliche Aspekte und MAK-Werte. *Anästh Intensivmed* 1994; **35**, 162–165.
32. Waterson CK. Recovery of waste anesthetic gases. In Brown BR, ed., *Future Anesthesia Delivery Systems. Contemporary Anesthesia Practice*, vol. VIII. Davies, Philadelphia, 1984, pp. 109–124.
33. Deutsche Forschungsgemeinschaft: Maximale Arbeitsplatzkonzentrationen und biologische Arbeitsstofftoleranzwerte, 1994.
34. Amt für Arbeitsschutz: Merkblatt für den Umgang mit Narkosegasen, Stand, August 1990. Freie und Hansestadt Hamburg, Behörde für Arbeit, Gesundheit und Soziales, Hamburg, 1990.
35. Virtue RW. Low flow anesthesia: advantages in its clinical application, cost and ecology. In Aldrete JA, Lowe HJ and Virtue RW, eds, *Low Flow and Closed System Anesthesia*. Grune & Stratton, New York, 1979, pp. 103–108.
36. Imberti R, Preseglio I, Imbriani M, Ghittori S, Cimino F and Mapelli A. Low flow anaesthesia reduces occupational exposure to inhalation anaesthetics. *Acta Anaesthesiol Scand* 1995; **39**, 586–591.
37. Logan M and Farmer JG. Anaesthesia and the ozone layer. *Br J Anaesth* 1989; **53**, 645–646.
38. Dale O and Husum B. Nitrous oxide: from frolics to a global concern in 150 years. *Acta Anaesth Scand* 1994; **38**, 749–750.
39. Schirmer U. Lachgas – Entwicklung und heutiger Stellenwert. *Anaesthesist* 1998; **47**, 245–255.
40. James MFM. Nitrous oxide: still useful in the year 2000? *Curr Opin Anaesthesiol* 1999; **12**, 461–466.
41. Graul EH, Forth W. Das 'gute' Ozon. *Dt Ärztebl* 1990; **87**, 2284–2291.
42. Sherman SJ and Cullen BF. Nitrous oxide and the greenhouse effect. *Anesthesiology* 1988; **68**, 816–817.
43. Hoechst: Umweltwirkung der Fluor-Chlor- Kohlenwasserstoffe (FCKW) und ihre Bedeutung für die Anästhesie. Stellungnahme der Fa. Hoechst, Frankfurt a. M., vom 4 September 1989.
44. Hutton P and Kerr JA. Anaesthetic agents and the ozone layer. *Lancet* 1989; **8645**, 1011–1012.
45. Pierce JMT and Linter SPK. Anaesthetic agents and the ozone layer. *Lancet* 1989; **8648**, 1011–1012.
46. Solomon S and Albritton D. Time-dependent ozone depletion potentials for short and long-term forecasts. *Nature* 1992; **357**, 33–37.
47. Radke J and Fabian P. Die Ozonschicht und ihre Beeinflussung durch N_2O und Inhalationsanästhetika. *Anaesthesist* 1991; **40**, 429–433.
48. Deutscher Bundestag: Umfang der Reduktion von Produktion und Verbrauch der FCKW und Halone nach den Beschlüssen der 4. Vertragsstaatenkonferenz in Kopenhagen. Drucksache 12/8555, 1994.
49. Noerreslet J, Frieberg S, Nielsen TM and Römer U. Halothane anaesthetic and the ozone layer. *Lancet* 1989; **8640**, 719.
50. Aldrete JA, Cubillos P and Sherrill D. Humidity and temperature changes during low flow and closed system anaesthesia. *Acta Anaesthesiol Scand* 1981; **25**, 312–314.
51. Wick C, Altemeyer KH, Ahnefeld FW and Kilian J. Vergleichende Feuchtigkeitsmessungen in halbgeschlossenen und halboffenen Systemen unter zusätzlicher Verwendung von künstlichen Nasen. *Anaesthesist* 1987; **36**, 172–176.
52. Bengtson JP, Bengtson A and Stenqvist O. The circle system as a humidifier. *Br J Anaesth* 1989; **63**, 453–457.

53. Kleemann PP. Tierexperimentelle und klinische Untersuchungen zum Stellenwert der Klimatisierung anästhetischer Gase im Narkosekreissystem bei Langzeiteingriffen. Wissenschaftliche Verlagsabteilung Abbott GmbH, Wiesbaden, 1989.
54. Kleemann PP, Schickel BK and Jantzen JPAH. Heated breathing tubes affect humidity output of circle absorber systems. *J Clin Anaesth* 1993; **5**, 463–467.
55. Bengtson JP, Sonander H and Stenqvist O. Preservation of humidity and heat of respiratory gases during anaesthesia – a laboratory investigation. *Acta Anaesthesiol Scand* 1987; **31**, 127–131.
56. Chalon J, Ali M, Turndorf H and Fischgrund GK. *Humidification of Anesthetic Gases*. Charles C. Thomas, Springfield, 1981.
57. Kleemann PP. Humidity of anesthetic gases with respect to low flow anaesthesia. *Anaesth Intens Care* 1994; **22**, 396–408.
58. Baum J, Züchner K, Hölscher U, Sievert B, Stanke HG, Gruchmann T and Rathgeber J. Klimatisierung von Narkosegasen bei Einsatz unterschiedlicher Patientenschlauchsysteme. *Anaesthesist* 2000; **49**, 402–411.
59. Rathgeber J. Konditionierung der Atemgase bei intubierten Patienten in Anästhesie und Intensivmedizin [Habilitationsschrift]. Georg-August-Universität, Göttingen, 1997, p. 105.
60. Buijs BHMJ. Herwardering van het Gesloten Ademsysteem in de Anesthesiologie. Dissertationsschrift der Erasmus-Universitt, Rotterdam, 1988.
61. Branson RD, Davis K and Porembka DT. Reassessment of humidification supplied by the circle system using ISO 9360: conventional versus co-axial circuit. *Anesthesiology* 1995; **83**, A401.
62. Branson RD, Campbell RS, Davis K and Porembka DT. Anaesthesia circuits, humidity output, and mucociliary structure and function. *Anesth Intensive Care* 1998; **26**, 178–183.
63. Imrie MM and Hall GM. Body temperature and anaesthesia. *Br J Anaesth* 1990; **64**, 346–354.
64. Newton DEF. The effect of anaesthetic gas humidification on body temperature. *Br J Anaesth* 1975; **47**, 1026.
65. Stone DR, Downs JB, Paul WL and Perkins HM. Adult body temperature and heated humidification of anesthetic gases during general anesthesia. *Anesth Analg* 1981; **60**, 736–741.
66. Aldrete JA. Closed circuit anesthesia prevents moderate hypothermia occurring in patients having extremity surgery. *The Circular* 1987; **4**, 3–4.
67. Baum J. Quantitative anaesthesia in the low-flow system. In Van Ackern K, Frankenberger H, Konecny E and Steinbereithner K, eds, *Quantitative Anaesthesia: Low Flow and Closed Circuit. Anaesthesiology and Intensive Care Medicine*, vol. 204. Springer, Berlin, 1989, pp. 44–57.
68. Cullen SC. Who is watching the patient? *Anesthesiology* 1972; **37**, 361–362.
69. Spieß W. Narkose im geschlossenen System mit kontinuierlicher inspiratorischer Sauerstoffmessung. *Anaesthesist* 1977; **26**, 503–513.
70. Van der Zee H and Verkaaik APK. Cardiovascular implementations of respiratory measurements. *Acta Anaesth Belg* 1990; **41**, 167–175.
71. Verkaaik APK and Erdmann W. Respiratory diagnostic possibilities during closed circuit anesthesia. *Acta Anaesth Belg* 1990; **41**, 177–188.

Technical requirements for anaesthesia management with reduced fresh gas flow

7.1 Technical regulations and standards

In several countries there are binding national regulations concerning technical features and mandatory safety devices for inhalational anaesthetic machines, the neglect of which may be subject to medicolegal consequences in the event of any complication.

In the German-speaking countries, different national standards on technical features of anaesthetic machines were in force until 1998: DIN 13252 in Germany, ÖNORM K2003 in Austria and SN 057 600 in Switzerland[1,2]. Due to the intention to harmonize these national standards, since 13 June 1998 a common European standard EN 740: 'Anaesthetic Workstations and their Modules – Essential Requirements' is binding for all manufacturers and anaesthetists in the countries of the European Union[3]. Anaesthetic machines, like all medical products which comply with the harmonized European standards, are certified and marked with the CE label indicating approval for unrestricted distribution in all the EU countries.

Before starting with low flow anaesthetic techniques, the anaesthetist should be aware whether this anaesthetic technique is covered by the specification of the particular anaesthetic machine given by the manufacturer. Furthermore, it should be checked whether the technical features of the anaesthetic apparatus meet the technical preconditions for safe performance of low flow anaesthesia. Generally, all modern anaesthetic machines will comply with these demands. Excellent aids in checking the technical features and details of anaesthetic machines are the newer technical monographs from J. T. B. Moyle, A. Davey and C. Ward[4], J. Ehrenwerth and J. B. Eisenkraft[5] and J. A. Dorsch and S. E. Dorsch[6].

7.2 Technical requirements for the anaesthetic equipment with respect to the extent of fresh gas flow reduction

7.2.1 Medical gas supply systems

All techniques of anaesthesia management with reduced fresh gas flow place no special technical requirements on the gas supply system. Both medical gas pipeline systems and gas cylinders complete with a pressure regulator can be used likewise. The gas delivery system of the anaesthetic machine has to feature a nitrous oxide cut-off and an audible oxygen failure signal, both devices being mandatory technical safety facilities for inhalation anaesthetic machines under EN 740.

7.2.2 Gas flow control systems

Nitrous oxide, air and oxygen are either controlled individually at the respective flow control system or as pre-mixed gas, having passed a calibrated blender. In the majority of machines, the gas flow is adjusted at fine needle valves and measured with conventional flowmeter tubes. Alternatively, the gas flow can be measured electronically and may be displayed either numerically or by an analogue scale. The requirements placed on the valve function and the calibration and graduation of gas flow control systems increase in line with the degree of flow reduction[7,8].

Low flow anaesthesia, in general, can be performed with flow control systems of all common types of anaesthetic machines. Even where older machines are concerned, the nitrous oxide and oxygen flow can be accurately set down to 500 ml/min at the controls. However, not all the older anaesthetic machines are additionally equipped with a flow control system to deliver air, or the flowmeter tubes are not graduated in the low flow range, but start with a minimum flow of 0.8 l/min or even higher.

Performance of minimal flow anaesthesia calls for more precisely calibrated flowmeter tubes which, starting with a gas flow of 50–100 ml/min, should be graduated in increments of 50 ml/min, but at worst 100 ml/min. This requirement is satisfied by the new generation of anaesthetic machines, the majority of which are equipped with two flowmeter tubes in tandem for exact control of oxygen and nitrous oxide even over the lowest flow range. The flowmeter tube for air should start at least with a minimum flow of 200 ml/min and should be graduated in increments of 50 ml/min. The accuracy of gas measurement readings in the low flow range is quoted as being 10% by the different standards[3,9]. For performance of minimal flow anaesthesia, which is by no means a quantitative method, this error is acceptable for use in clinical routine.

In this context, the reader's attention is drawn to an incident observed by the author himself. Using a brand new anaesthetic machine it was noticed that, after about 15 min of anaesthesia, the float in the flowmeter tube was no longer spinning freely. The rotating movement of the float ceased, then it dropped down in the unchanged gas flow, and it was clear that it was partially tilted and jammed in the metering tube. On checking these flowmeter tubes, we noticed that in this case of malfunction the oxygen volume supplied was 100–150 ml/min higher than that indicated by the bobbin. Inaccuracies in calibration of the flowmeter tubes up to a maximum of 50% have also been described by Saunders et al.[10]. On the other hand, the precision of flowmeter tubes was judged satisfactorily by Rügheimer[11]. It was later demonstrated that the malfunction, which could likewise be observed in all anaesthetic machines of that series, was attributable to a manufacturing fault.

In dealing with this case of malfunction, a fundamental problem deserves emphasis. Since most anaesthetists and anaesthetic nurses are accustomed to using high excess gas volumes, routine technical maintenance and checks to verify that the flow control systems conform to the tolerances in the low flow range specified by the manufacturer are often neglected. It is important that, prior to performance of low flow anaesthesia, the flow control systems should be carefully tested for accurate function, especially in the low flow range.

Flowmeter tubes only display precisely the actual flow if the float is spinning freely in the gas stream.

Quantitative closed system anaesthesia can only be realized provided that the anaesthetic machine is fitted with gas flow control systems which, starting at 50–100 ml/min, are graduated in increments of 10 ml over the low flow range to a flow of 300 ml/min. This would be the only way to ensure that gas volumes, which correspond to the actual oxygen and nitrous oxide uptake of the patient, could be appropriately adjusted at the machine. Low flow tubes with such accurate graduation are available for instance as an option for the Cicero anaesthetic machine (Dräger Medizintechnik, Lübeck, Germany) (Figure 7.1).

With such low gas flows, however, the imprecise performance of needle valves presents a problem[9]. The repeated correction of oxygen and nitrous oxide settings would take a lot of time and attention on the part of the anaesthetist.

It is not the limited precision of the flowmeter tubes but rather the imprecise function of the mechanical fine needle valves which mostly impedes an exact setting of gas flows in increments in the range 10 or even 50 ml/min.

There is an additional problem to be considered: the different technical standards demand anti-hypoxic devices as safety features of the gas delivery systems. In most of the modern anaesthetic machines the oxygen and the nitrous oxide flow are linked to prevent the delivery of a fresh gas mixture containing less than 25% of oxygen. Technically that can be realized by mechanical, pneumatic or electronic coupling of the oxygen to the nitrous oxide flow. Other flow control systems maintain an oxygen flow of at least 200–300 ml/min to guarantee the metabolic needs and, thus, don't allow the flow to be reduced to lower values. It must be strongly emphasized, however, that these anti-hypoxic devices can prevent the development of hypoxic gas mixtures only if high fresh gas flows are used. In low flow anaesthesia, these devices are completely unsuited to safely prevent hypoxia. Additionally, all these anti-hypoxic devices hinder significantly the independent and precise setting of very low gas flows, or even render it impossible. While the mechanical coupling of the oxygen to the nitrous oxide flow with the aid of a chain link (Link 25, Ohmeda, Madison, USA) allows the precise setting of very low gas flows (Figure 7.2), the pneumatic link of the gas flows (Figure 7.3), which is often referred to as oxygen ratio controller (ORC), especially in older types of machines, makes it difficult or even impedes the precise setting of flows lower than 300–250 ml/min[13]. In some machines slow shifts of the membrane of the oxygen ratio controller can lead to spontaneous alteration of the gas flows by up to 100–150 ml/min although the settings of the fine needle valves are kept unchanged.

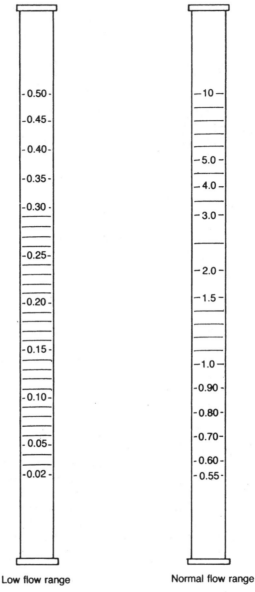

Figure 7.1   Set of special low flow tubes for metering nitrous oxide and oxygen; the graduation in the low flow range permits precise reduction down to closed system anaesthesia (From Frankenberger and Wallroth[12], by permission)

Special problems also result from the fresh gas control by a gas mixer, as was realized for example in one of the older German machines, the AV 1 anaesthetic machine (Dräger Medizintechnik, Lübeck, Germany)[14]. Once oxygen and nitrous oxide have been mixed in the desired ratio, the flow of mixed gas has to be adjusted by the aid of a flowmeter calibrated

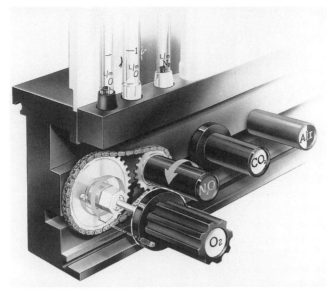

Figure 7.2 Link 25 anti-hypoxic device: the needle valves are connected via a chain to ensure a fresh gas oxygen concentration of at least 25%. (By courtesy of Ohmeda, Madison, USA)

for a defined gas mixture (consisting of 40% O_2 and 60% N_2O). However, the density of the mixed gas is reduced with increasing oxygen portion, so that the resultant gas flow is actually higher than that indicated by the flowmeter. Although this fault can be tolerated in low flow and minimal flow anaesthesia, the accuracy of the mixed-gas flowmeter tube would not satisfy the requirements for quantitative closed system anaesthesia. However, as the calibration of the AV 1 mixed-gas flowmeter tube started only at a minimum flow of 400 ml/min, this machine could not be used with flows less than 500 ml/min. The same applies for instance to the Siemens Anesthesia System (Siemens–Elema, Solna, Sweden): once the fresh gas has passed the blender, it is not possible to select a flow less than 500 ml/min with the required accuracy[15].

The precision of gas blending, which is quoted for the Dräger gas mixer as being ±4% with arbitrary nitrous oxide–oxygen mixtures, and for the Siemens Elema blender ±5%, is suitable for performance of low flow and minimal flow anaesthesia in routine clinical practice.

Not only conventional gas blenders but also very modern electronic flow control and blending devices, like the one in the Julian anaesthetic machine (Dräger Medizintechnik, Lübeck, Germany), may render impossible the use of fresh gas flows lower than 500 ml/min[14]. Thus, even an apparatus as modern as this one may not meet the technical requirements for closed system anaesthesia.

One should be aware of the fact, that the 90 years old technical concept of the flow control systems consisting of fine needle valves and flowmeter tubes – as it was used for the first time in 1910 by M. Neu in his oxygen nitrous oxide apparatus[16] (see Section 2.1.2.2) – is limited in its precise

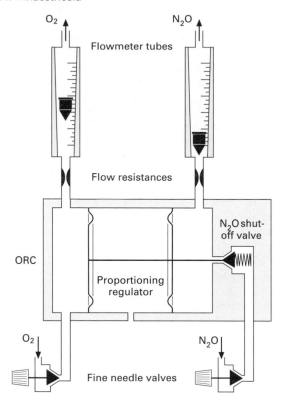

Figure 7.3   Oxygen ratio controller (ORC), the anti-hypoxic device of the Dräger anaesthetic machines: the nitrous oxide flow pneumatically is linked to the oxygen flow to ensure a fresh gas oxygen concentration of at least 25%. (By courtesy of Dräger Medizintechnik, Lübeck, Germany)

function at gas flows of 200–300 ml/min, particularly when fitted with an anti-hypoxic device.

7.2.3   Vaporizers

The technical modules by which inhalational anaesthetics are converted from the liquid to the vapour state and mixed with the fresh gas are universally referred to as vaporizers. From a technical point of view, however, one should differentiate between evaporation, generation of the vapour without supply of energy, and vaporization, that is, generation of the vapour with supply of energy. Only in the TEC 6 vaporizer (Ohmeda, Madison, USA) is desflurane really vaporized with the aid of electric energy, whereas the vapour of halothane, enflurane, isoflurane and sevoflurane is generated by evaporation.

7.2.3.1   Precision

It is general practice today that volatile anaesthetics are admixed to the fresh gas, i.e. the vaporizers are connected into the fresh gas supply (VOC, vaporizer outside the circle). For performance of low flow anaesthesia, use should be made of precision plenum vaporizers. In addition to pressure and temperature compensation, they should deliver the pre-set concentration reliably even at very low fresh gas flows. In conventional plenum vaporizers this is guaranteed by their laminar flow characteristics[17]. The high flow constancy of the Vapor 19.n vaporizers (Dräger Medizintechnik, Lübeck, Germany) (Figure 7.4) was confirmed by Züchner[18] and Gilly[19], even for extremely low gas flows down to 20 ml/min. These devices, of course, can be used safely in all low flow techniques. The same applies, likewise, for the TEC 4 and TEC 5 vaporizers (Ohmeda, Hatfield, UK) and – with reservations – for the Penlon PPV Sigma vaporizers (Penlon, Abingdon, UK) which are also adequate for performance of low flow anaesthesia. The TEC 6 desflurane vaporizer (Ohmeda, Madison, USA) equally features a precisely working flow compensation[6,20,21]. Sometimes, however, the concentration delivered by the TEC 6 vaporizer was observed to be somewhat higher than the dialled one[22]. As desflurane has a comparatively low anaesthetic potency, clinically this will not be significant, especially in low flow anaesthesia. Although the Ohio vaporizers (Ohio Medical Products, Wisconsin, USA) maintain the dialled concentration less precisely in case of flow variation, they can be used safely in low flow and minimal flow anaesthesia. If older type vaporizers like the TEC 2 are still used, however, depending on the fresh gas flow rate the delivered

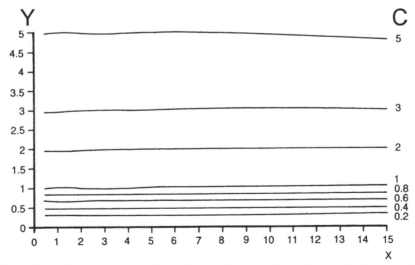

Figure 7.4   Flow constancy of the Vapor 19.n vaporizer (Dräger Medizintechnik, Lübeck, Germany): precise performance over a flow range of 0.4–15 l/min (C: concentration set on isoflurane vaporizer, vol%; X: fresh gas flow rate; Y: isoflurane fresh gas concentration, vol%). (By courtesy of Dräger Medizintechnik, Lübeck, Germany)

concentration may differ considerably from the dialled one. During controlled ventilation this pronounced flow dependency may even be augmented by the pumping effect.

The so-called 'pumping effect' (effect of pressure change during controlled ventilation) on the concentration supplied by the vaporizer can be reduced by taking care that the vaporizer chamber is always adequately filled if low concentrations are dialled during low flow anaesthesia[17].

The precision of the concentration supplied is also a function of the fresh gas composition; this dependency decreases with low fresh gas flow rates and dialling higher concentrations.

In summarizing the results of his investigations, Gilly[19] points out that the concentration supplied even from modern plenum vaporizers may vary greatly as a function of flow, dialled concentration and composition of the carrier gas. The nominal and delivered value of anaesthetic agent concentration may differ by up to 20% if several parameters are varied simultaneously. These vaporizers are, nevertheless, suitable for use in low flow anaesthesia: differences between the dialled anaesthetic concentration and that actually supplied are buffered by the gas volume of the breathing system which is large in relation to the fresh gas volume. Furthermore, changes in anaesthetic gas composition occur only gradually in low flow anaesthesia, due to the particularly long time constant. If the requirements imposed on the precision of vaporizer performance are solely evaluated in terms of patient safety, however, with decreasing fresh gas flow the specification need not be so demanding. Quantitative closed system anaesthesia, however, cannot be performed with conventional plenum vaporizers. Their inadequate precision allows neither exact metering and supply of defined quanta of the anaesthetic, nor a sufficiently accurate determination of the amount of anaesthetic being taken up by the patient.

The vaporizer's dependency on gas composition and flow can be reduced with the aid of an alternative technical concept in which the anaesthetic is fed into the fresh gas flow in defined quanta. The Gambro–Engström anaesthetic delivery systems employ this principle[23,24]. In the Elsa and the EAS 9010 anaesthetic machines (Gambro–Engström, Bromma, Sweden), the liquid anaesthetic is injected under pressure into a heated vaporizer chamber. The anaesthetic vapour is then admixed to the fresh gas in defined boluses via an electronically controlled pulsating valve whose frequency is related directly to the fresh gas flow (Figure 7.5).

The performance of the Servo Anaesthesia System's vaporizer (Siemens-Elema, Solna, Sweden) is also flow independent[15]: the liquid agent is sprayed by gas pressure via a nozzle directly into a fresh gas stream of intermittent flow (Figure 7.6). Corresponding to its calibration to 400 or 350 kPa (4 and 3.5 bar), the exact performance of this type of vaporizer essentially depends on the precise control of the gas pressure at 450 ± 30 kPa or 360 ± 30 kPa, respectively. If the piped medical gas is supplied with a higher pressure of about 520–550 kPa (nominal pressure in central gas piping systems: Germany and Austria 500 kPa, ANSI (USA, Australia, Canada, France, Japan) 345 kPa, ISO (Italy, Scandinavia, South Africa, Spain, Switzerland) 414 kPa) unexpected high concentrations,

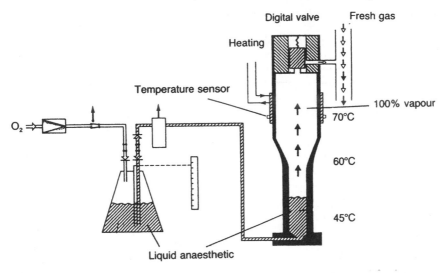

Figure 7.5 Electronically controlled device for supply of anaesthetic vapour in defined boluses. (By courtesy of Gambro–Engström, Bromma, Sweden[23])

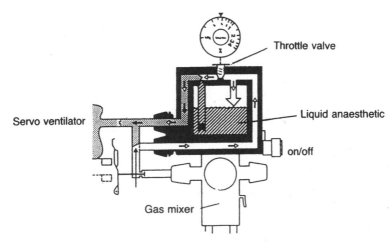

Figure 7.6 Siemens vaporizer 950: the liquid anaesthetic agent is sprayed by gas pressure via a nozzle directly into the fresh gas stream. (By courtesy of Siemens–Elema, Solna, Sweden[15])

60–100% higher than the dial setting, may be delivered by this vaporizer. In this case, the use of an additional pressure regulator switched into the pipeline connections to the gas mixer is required[25].

However, Gilly remarks critically on this subject that, although the amount of anaesthetic supplied to the fresh gas may be more accurately metered with such improved dosing systems, the inaccuracies of the flow control systems counteract the precision potentially offered by such devices[19].

7.2.3.2   Limitation of vaporizer output

Anaesthesia management with low fresh gas flows is rendered difficult in so far as the maximum concentration delivered by most of the vaporizers is limited to a value of about $5 - 3 \times$ MAC (minimal alveolar concentration), commonly in halothane vaporizers to 4 or 5 vol%, in those for enflurane and isoflurane to 5 vol%, in sevoflurane vaporizers to 8 vol%, and in desflurane vaporizers to 18 vol%. Due to this limitation the maximum output of the vaporizers outside the circuit decreases in direct proportion to the extent of fresh gas flow reduction. A fresh gas flow of 0.5 l/min assumed, not more than 21 ml/min halothane vapour or 26 ml/min enflurane or isoflurane can be delivered into the breathing system even if the maximum output of the vaporizers is dialled. The amount of anaesthetic vapour, however, can be increased to 43.5 ml/min if sevoflurane is used, or even to 110 ml/min if desflurane is used. The difficulty mentioned applies to all situations in which a comparatively large amount of anaesthetic vapour is to be supplied into the breathing system. This can only be accomplished with comparatively high fresh gas flow rates: for instance during the induction phase with its wash-in processes and initial high uptake or during the course of anaesthesia, if the anaesthetic depth is to be increased within a short period of time. If the demand for anaesthetic vapour is high, the limited amount being supplied by an output-limited vaporizer may be too low at low fresh gas flow, this holds especially for halothane, enflurane and isoflurane. The limitation of the maximum output of the vaporizers outside the circle is the main cause for the significant prolongation of the time constants after fresh gas flow reduction.

The anaesthetic concentration can only be rapidly increased in spite of a low fresh gas flow rate, if the following procedures and technical alternatives are adopted:

- demand-specific supply of the anaesthetic agents by direct injection of the liquid anaesthetic into the breathing system;
- use of precision injection systems, working independently of the fresh gas flow;
- use of vaporizers which are switched into the breathing system (VIC – vaporizer inside the circuit) so that the anaesthetic can be supplied without being influenced in any way by the adjustment of the fresh gas flow; and
- increase of the output limits of vaporizers which are connected into the fresh gas flow (VOC).

Intermittent manual injection of the volatile anaesthetic into the system can not be recommended for clinical practice, as has already been pointed out. It is extremely involved, especially during the initial phase of anaesthesia, and rapid changes of the agent's concentration in the circle may occur.

Switching the vaporizer into the breathing system must be seen critically with respect to patients' safety, unless stringent monitoring standards are met (see Section 4.3). Particularly in the case of controlled ventilation, the use of VICS may create problems as high anaesthetic concentrations may be rapidly achieved, especially in low flow anaesthesia. Nevertheless, with the overall availability of reliable gas monitors, the low flow enthusiasts seriously discuss anew the reconsideration of the use of even the most simple in-circuit vaporizers like the Komesaroff or the classic Goldman vaporizer[66-70].

At present, the only anaesthetic machines which are equipped with precisely operating injection systems for metering the volatile agents are Elsa and EAS 9010 (Gambro–Engström, Bromma, Sweden), the Julian and the PhysioFlex (Dräger Medizintechnik, Lübeck, Germany). According to investigations by Versichelen and Rolly and the author's own experiences, the vapour delivery devices of these machines work accurately and reliably in clinical use[26].

The use of vaporizers with increased output would be the most simple and practicable alternative, the more so as in low flow techniques even drastic changes in anaesthetic fresh gas concentration result in only slow alterations of the agent concentration within the breathing system. Thus, such vaporizers would not present an increased risk for the patient, especially as a mechanical device, which needs to be unlocked before the dialled vaporizer concentration exceeds a $3 \times MAC$ limit, could be an additional safeguard against accidental overdose. Plenum vaporizers with an increased maximum output will be available in the near future. The new generation of Dräger vaporizers, Vapor 2000, will deliver following maximum concentrations: halothane 6%, enflurane 8%, isoflurane 6%, whereas the maximum output of the sevoflurane and desflurane vaporizers will not be changed. Currently, the Elsa and EAS 9010 machines are the only devices in which the output of the agent metering system has been increased to 8% for halothane, enflurane and isoflurane.

At present, since conventional plenum vaporizers outside the circle are in general use, anaesthetists have to change from low to high fresh gas flow rates whenever a large amount of anaesthetic vapour is to be supplied into the system rapidly.

7.2.3.3 Specified range of operation

The operation range specified by the manufacturer for reasons of liability may be another impediment to the user and, sometimes, seems to be substantially unjustified. For instance, in accordance with its Instructions for Use, the Vapor 19.1 (Dräger Medizintechnik, Lübeck, Germany)[14] is approved for its use in anaesthesia with rebreathing and non-rebreathing systems. The flow range is quoted as being between 0.3 and 15 l/min. However, according to the Instructions for Use of April 1986, the usage range of the Vapor 19.n is restricted as follows: 'The Vapor is approved for use with semi-closed and semi-open systems, but should not be used with closed, or nearly closed breathing systems', leaving absolutely unexplained, what is meant by the term 'nearly closed'. The arbitrary establishment of the vaporizer's lower flow range limit to 0.5 l/min seems especially unfounded if they are attached to machines which are equipped with the optionally available low flow tubes. This fact has been considered in the latest version of the Instructions for Use, dated March 1991, where the lower limit of the vaporizer's operation range is again quoted as being 250 ml/min, and its use with even lower flows is not definitively precluded.

7.2.3.4   The Tec 6 desflurane vaporizer

Due to the low solubility of desflurane in the blood, this agent is especially suitable for its use in low flow anaesthesia (see Section 10.2.1)[27,28]. Due to the high vapour pressure of desflurane at room temperature, 669 mmHg at 20°C, the desflurane vaporizer features a completely new technology (Figure 7.7). The TEC 6 vaporizer (Ohmeda, Madison, USA), unlike the other conventional plenum vaporizers, is an electronically controlled device. The fluid desflurane is heated to 39°C, thus providing a constant vapour pressure of 1460 mmHg. An electronic controlled regulator delivers just that amount of vaporized desflurane which, mixed with the actual carrier gas flow, results in the pre-set fresh gas concentration. Several safety features are incorporated into this device. A shut-off valve only opens the connection between the vaporizing chamber and the regulator if the device is operational, electrically powered and placed correctly on the back bar of the anaesthetic machine. In case of angular displacement exceeding 15° from the vertical position, a 'tilt switch' activates the shut-off valve, thus preventing liquid desflurane from leaving the sump. A flow from 0.2 to 10 l/min is the specified working range of the desflurane vaporizer. Using pure oxygen as carrier gas the desflurane concentration delivered may differ in a range within 15% relative or 0.5 vol% absolute from the dialled concentration. At flow rates less than 2 l/min, the desflurane concentration is generally about 8% lower than at higher carrier gas flow rates, but is still within the above limits. If the dialled concentration exceeds 12 vol%, in the fresh gas flow range less than 1 l/min, the output concentration can be up to 1 vol% higher than the dial setting. Due to the lower viscosity, with 70 vol% nitrous oxide in oxygen the output concentration can be 20% less than the dial setting[20,21]. The output

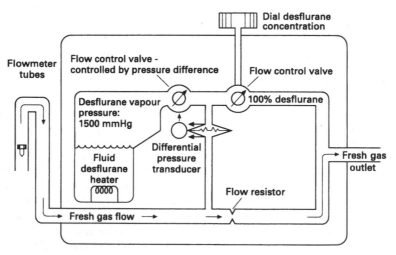

Figure 7.7   Technical sketch of a TEC 6 desflurane vaporizer

performance of the TEC 6 desflurane vaporizer, as specified, satisfies the requirements for safe performance of low and minimal flow anaesthesia.

7.2.4 Breathing systems

For rebreathing techniques, use can generally be made of both the to-and-fro and the circle absorption system. To-and-fro absorption systems are rarely used today since working with a carbon dioxide absorber mounted near the patient is awkward and carbon dioxide absorption may become inadequate with increasing duration of anaesthesia[29]. Circle systems can be used in all different techniques of anaesthesia with low fresh gas flow. However, the technical demands placed on the rebreathing systems increase with decreasing fresh gas flow.

7.2.4.1 Gas tightness

Virtually all anaesthetic machines should be suitable for anaesthesia with a fresh gas flow as low as 1 l/min, assuming they are well maintained. It is necessary, however, to check the breathing systems for leaks in accordance with the manufacturer's instructions to ensure that quoted leakage tolerances are not exceeded. Under these provisions, low flow anaesthesia can be undertaken without any further technical effort.

The requirements concerning the gas tightness of the systems are higher in minimal flow anaesthesia. With a pressure of 2 kPa ($\approx 20\,cmH_2O$) within the system, gas loss resulting from leaks should not exceed 100 ml/min. The required gas tightness can be achieved by careful cleaning of rubber seals and replacement if they are brittle, as well as careful tightening of screw connections in the circle system. Plastic components must be checked for brittleness and cracks, and have to be replaced if required. In addition, attention must be paid to the proper mounting of carefully cleaned taper connections (Figure 7.8).

Manufacturers quote the following leakage tolerances for their respective breathing systems. The leakage rate of the 8 ISO breathing system (Dräger Medizintechnik, Lübeck, Germany) must not exceed 200 ml/min at an internal system pressure of 4 kPa ($\approx 40\,cmH_2O$)[14]; a leak rate of less than 50 ml/min is quoted for the Megamed 048 and 219 circle systems (Megamed, Cham, Switzerland) at a pressure of 3 kPa ($\approx 30\,cmH_2O$)[30]. The automatic leak test performed on the Cicero or Cato anaesthetic workstations (Dräger Medizintechnik, Lübeck, Germany) at 3 kPa ($\approx 30\,cmH_2O$)[14] results, according to the author's experience, in average values between 10 and 40 ml/min. An automatic leak test at 3 kPa ($\approx 30\,cmH_2O$) is also carried out by the Elsa and the EAS 9010 anaesthetic machines (Gambro–Engström, Bromma, Sweden)[23]. The compact circle absorber systems of the Aestiva 3000 and Ohmeda CD (Ohmeda, Madison, USA) or the AS/3 ADU (Datex–Ohmeda, Helsinki, Finland) anaesthesia machines also proved to be highly gas tight. With the Servo Anaesthesia Circle System 985 (Siemens–Elema, Solna, Sweden) the leak test of the breathing system and identification of leaks is quite difficult as the test cannot be performed under static conditions but only during operation of the ventilator. The author's own experiences confirm the

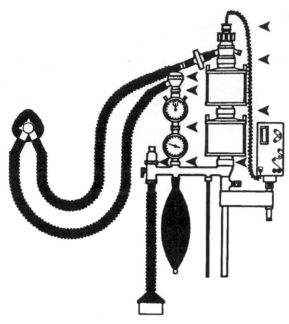

Figure 7.8 Points predisposed to leaks demonstrated on a conventional circle absorber system 8 ISO (Dräger Medizintechnik, Lübeck, Germany): all screw and plug connections and the valve and absorber seals. (Note: This circle absorption system would no longer meet the demands of the new technical norm, EN 740)

results of investigations concerning gas leakage of breathing systems published by Leuenberger *et al.*[31]. All circle absorption systems tested performed below the leakage limit of 150 ml/min at a pressure of 3 kPa ($\approx 30\,cmH_2O$) as demanded by the Common European Standard EN 740. The Authorities for Occupational Safety and Health, Hamburg, provides in its Instruction Sheet on the Handling of Anaesthetic Gases that the breathing system should be checked for leaks at a pressure of 3 kPa ($\approx 30\,cmH_2O$) several times per day, and that leaks in excess of 100 ml/min must not be accepted[32]. All breathing systems which indicate such low leakage loss satisfy the technical requirements placed on gas tightness for performance of anaesthesia even with the lowest fresh gas flows.

Performance of closed system anaesthesia requires a rebreathing system to be leakproof to the greatest possible extent. The connections between the individual components of older circle absorber assemblies, and the tapers in particular, must fit each other perfectly and may be coated with a sealing paste (e.g. Oxygenox 54, Dräger Medizintechnik, Lübeck, Germany). The number of connections should be restricted to a minimum. It is proven practice to mark all individual components of a gas tight circle absorber assembly and to fit the appropriate components of the same circle system together for reassembly[33]. On the other hand, the compact breathing systems of the new generation machines are in general so gas tight that, without further modification, they cope with the requirements for closed system anaesthesia, assuming appropriate maintenance[34].

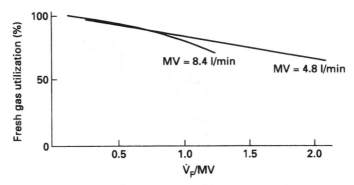

Figure 7.9 Fresh gas utilization of a conventional circle absorber system 8 ISO (Dräger Medizintechnik, Lübeck, Germany), illustrated as a function of the quotient of fresh gas flow ($\dot{V}_F$) and minute volume (MV). (From von dem Hagen and Kleinschmidt[59], by permission)

7.2.4.2 Fresh gas utilization

Utilization of fresh gas will be explained by the example of the 8 ISO circle absorption system (Drägerwerk, Lübeck, Germany). The degree of fresh gas utilization increases with reduction of the fresh gas flow and reaches about 100% in the minimal flow range. With a higher fresh gas flow this value amounts to only about 70% (Figure 7.9). Fresh gas utilization is also determined by the design of the system, for instance by the position of the fresh gas inlet in relation to the exhaust port, as well as by its flow characteristics (Figure 7.10). In the Cato and Cicero (Dräger Medizintechnik, Lübeck, Germany), for instance, fresh gas utilization is optimized by the position of the fresh gas inlet and active control of the opening of the exhaust valve[14]. In all circle absorber systems tested, a sufficiently high degree of fresh gas utilization could be gained if the fresh gas flow was decreased to 1.5 l/min or lower[36].

Equilibration will take longer, the lower is the fresh gas utilization, which, in turn, may have an adverse effect on the course of low flow and minimal flow anaesthesia when time constants are already long. However, the design of the system has no influence on anaesthesia management with closed breathing systems, since there is no discharge of excess gas and fresh gas utilization must amount to 100%.

Furthermore, it must be considered that in the case of the breathing system whose design imposes a low fresh gas utilization, the oxygen content of the fresh gas has further to be increased in order to ensure an adequate oxygen concentration[35].

7.2.4.3 Specified range of operation

According to its instructions for use[14], the older type conventional circle absorption system 8 ISO (Dräger Medizintechnik, Lübeck, Germany) can be used both semi-closed and closed. The same applies to all the different compact breathing systems of the new generation of anaesthetic machines.

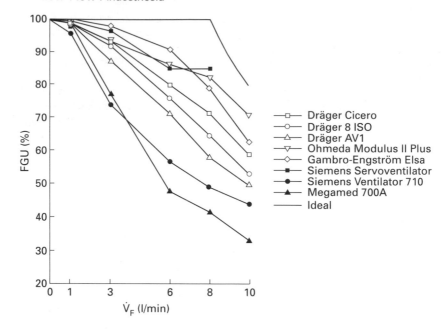

Figure 7.10 Fresh gas utilization (FGU) of different breathing systems as a function of fresh gas flow ($\dot{V}_F$). (From Zbinden and Feigenwinter[36], by permission)

Anaesthesia management with a closed, or virtually closed, system is especially included in the range of operation quoted for the following anaesthetic machines: AS/3 ADU (Datex–Ohmeda, Helsinki, Finland), Cato and Cicero (Dräger Medizintechnik, Lübeck, Germany), Elsa and EAS 9010 (Gambro–Engström, Bromma, Sweden), Megamed 700 and Mivolan (Megamed, Cham, Switzerland).

7.2.5   Carbon dioxide absorbers

Today's common use of double carbon dioxide absorbers, containing about 1 kg absorbent each[37], or of one Jumbo canister, containing 1.5–2 kg absorbent, satisfies the requirements of all low flow techniques. Adequate absorption capacity is ensured, especially if pelleted soda lime is used which is evaluated as being very effective[38,39]. According to Dräger and ICI, the absorption capacity of 1 litre of soda lime amounts to at least 120 litres of carbon dioxide[40]. If the entire exhaled gas in closed system anaesthesia passes the absorber, a utilization period of about 5 h can be calculated for 1 litre of soda lime assuming a minute volume of 10 l/min and an expired carbon dioxide concentration of 4% by volume, which was confirmed in laboratory tests.

7.2.5.1   Utilization period

Accordingly, a utilization period of about 5 h for the soda lime filling of a

1 litre absorber canister is unanimously quoted, at least in German textbooks. This is the reason why double absorbers are frequently used. In the past the contents of the absorber proximal to the expiratory valve was disposed of after each working day and a newly filled absorber fitted into the system.

The utilization periods achieved in clinical use, however, are considerably longer[41]. In accordance with the results of the author's own investigations, the utilization period of 1 litre absorber canisters ranges between 40 and 60 h if anaesthesia is performed exclusively with a fresh gas flow as high as 4.4 l/min. If, however, whenever possible, the flow is reduced to 0.5 l/min, the maximum proportion using this flow will be some 70–80% of the total using time of the absorber (see Sections 6.2.2, 9.1.1.3 and 9.1.2.2.4). Under these conditions the utilization period of a 1 litre absorber canister decreases to around 10–15 h. The difference between the figures given in the textbooks and the measured values can be explained as follows: using a semi-closed rebreathing system, depending on the fresh gas flow rate and the fresh gas utilization, only a certain part of the exhaled air really passes the absorber (see Figure 4.1). Furthermore, under clinical conditions the soda lime is not exposed continuously to the expired gas, but only intermittently. During the load-free interim periods, the absorbed carbon dioxide penetrates from the surface into the core of the soda lime granules, at which the external layers are regenerated to hydroxide. In this way the surface of the granules become available again for carbon dioxide absorption[40], although this regeneration adds only insignificantly to the absorption capacity. Another factor, which has a specific favourable effect on the absorption capacity in performance of low flow anaesthesia, is the maintenance or even increase of the water content of the absorbent.

7.2.5.2 Implications for anaesthetic practice

In clinical practice, the utilization period measured for absorbers filled with soda lime is, depending on the fresh gas flow, considerably longer than that quoted in the literature. Routine disposal of the absorber filling, for instance after each working day, should be rejected, particularly for reasons of ecology and economy. If the inspired and expired carbon dioxide concentration is monitored, the absorption capacity can be utilized completely without impairing patient safety using only one single 1 litre absorber canister. However, if carbon dioxide monitoring is not available, the use of double or Jumbo absorbers should be mandatory. The contents of the absorber proximal to the expiratory valve should only be discarded if the dye of the second absorber signals the beginning of exhaustion of the soda lime[40]. The colour change of the indicator, however, cannot be taken as a very reliable sign of soda lime exhaustion, since it may be deactivated by intense ultraviolet light[42]. It is proven clinical practice to note down the filling date of the absorber on an adhesive label fixed to the canister as an additional safeguard. Even in very long-lasting anaesthetics with the flow reduced to its utmost extent, one can assume that the absorptive capacity of a newly filled double or

Jumbo absorber system will be sufficient for at least the whole working day.

The following has to be considered if single use absorbers are used which are offered, for example, by Anmedic, Datex–Ohmeda and Gambro–Engström: each absorber should be wrapped separately with a material impermeable to water and should be labelled with the charge number and the expiry date. These measures should prevent the undetected use of accidentally desiccated soda lime[43]. Dry soda lime, containing alkali metal hydroxides, especially potassium hydroxide, reacts with all the inhalational anaesthetics, possibly generating toxic compounds like carbon monoxide or haloalkenes (see Sections 9.1.2.2.4 and 9.1.2.2.8).

7.2.6   Anaesthesia ventilators

In most of the modern anaesthetic machines the ventilator is an integral part of the complete device. Anaesthesia ventilators feature a lot of technical details (Table 7.1) which significantly influence the performance of low flow anaesthesia. This will be discussed comprehensively in the following chapter.

7.2.6.1   The gas reservoir

7.2.6.1.1   Anaesthetic machines without gas reservoir
The majority of the older conventional anaesthesia ventilators in Germany are bellows-in-box ventilators[6] with suspended bellows arrangement (Figure 7.11a and b). The expiratory expansion of the bellows is limited

Table 7.1   Differentiation of anaesthesia ventilators

A. *Ventilators differentiated according mechanical features*
- Bellows-in-box ventilators
    with hanging (suspended) bellows
    with standing (upright) bellows
    volume of the bellows limited to the tidal volume
    floating bellows
- Bag-in-bottle ventilator
- Piston pump ventilator
- Membrane chamber ventilator

B. *Ventilators with anaesthetic gas reservoir*
- Bellows-in-box ventilators with floating bellows
- Bag-in-bottle ventilators
- Ventilators equipped with a fresh gas decoupling valve, the manual bag serving as gas reservoir

C. *Ventilators featuring fresh gas flow compensation*
- Ventilators equipped with a fresh gas decoupling valve
- Electronic control of the ventilator performance according to the fresh gas flow
- Electronic control of discontinuous expiratory fresh gas supply
- Electronic control of discontinuous inspiratory fresh gas supply and ventilator performance

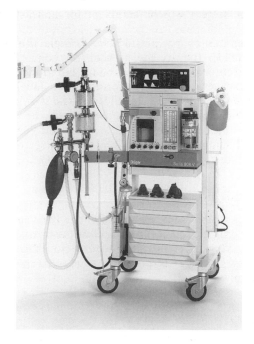

(a)

(b)

Figure 7.11   (a) Sulla 808 V anaesthetic machine. (b) Flow diagram of this conventional type anaesthetic machine. (By courtesy of Dräger Medizintechnik, Lübeck, Germany)

by a mechanical stop, the position of which is adjusted according to the desired tidal volume. Thus, at the end of expiration, the bellows are filled with just that gas volume which will be delivered to the patient. Surplus gas volumes, delivered into the breathing system, are immediately discharged via the exhaust valve. The box, containing the bellows, belongs to the driving system, which is referred to as the primary system. The bellows, which are connected to the breathing system by a hose, are filled with anaesthetic gas and thus belong to the secondary system. If the pressure within the primary system is increased, the bellows are squeezed and the gas contained in them delivered into the breathing system and hence to the patient. During expiration the exhaled gas again flows back to the system and fills the bellows, together with the continuously flowing fresh gas. If it reaches the limit stop, again all surplus gas will be vented out of the system as excess gas until the next inspiratory stroke begins. In some machines the expiratory expansion of the bellows is supported by an additional force, usually a weight fixed to its bottom (i.e. Ventilog, Dräger Medizintechnik, Lübeck, Germany) or, alternatively, by a negative pressure generated in the primary system during the expiratory phase (i.e. Pulmomat, Dräger Medizintechnik, Lübeck, Germany)[44].

The American AV-E ventilator of the Narkomed machines (North American Dräger, Telford, USA) is also a bellows-in-box ventilator; however, it is equipped with a rising bellows arrangement (Figure 7.12). During expiration, the bellows of this machine are expanding without any supporting force only by the small pressure generated by the fresh gas flow and the exhaled gas flowing back from the patient's lung into the breathing system. The expansion of the bellows is also limited by an adjustable stop, and if the bellows are filled with the pre-set tidal volume, all surplus gas is discharged out of the system via the excess gas valve, which closes no earlier than the beginning of the following inspiratory stroke[45].

7.2.6.1.1.1 Airway pressure and ventilation characteristics with fresh gas flow reduction. Using such bellows-in-box ventilators without gas reservoir, in low flow anaesthesia only a very small amount of fresh gas, together with the exhaled air, is available for filling the bellows during expiration. In machines in which the expansion of the bellows is supported by an additional force, a negative pressure resulting from this force will be maintained in the breathing system until the bellows has reached the adjustable stop. Generally, this phenomenon also can be observed in high flow anaesthesia, and provided this initial-expiratory negative pressure does not last longer than the first third of the total expiratory phase, this remains clinically irrelevant[47]. However, if patients suffering from chronic obstructive lung disease are anaesthetized, the exhaled gas flows back into the system markedly more slowly, resulting in a considerable prolongation of this early-expiratory negative pressure, in some cases requiring an adjustment to increase the fresh gas flow[48].

In the event that the gas loss via individual uptake and leakages is higher than the fresh gas volume, there will be a gas volume deficiency, the bellows will not be sufficiently filled any more and will not reach the

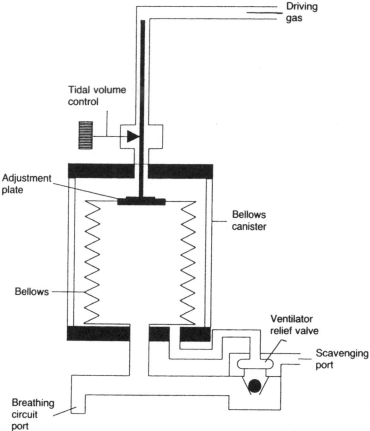

Figure 7.12   Technical sketch of the AV-E ventilator (North American Dräger, Telford, USA): the expiratory expansion of the bellows is limited by the position of an adjustable stop. (From Cicman *et al.*[45], by permission)

adjustable stop. In the next inspiratory stroke a somewhat smaller gas volume will be delivered to the patient, resulting in a decrease of the peak and plateau pressure and the tidal volume. If the expiratory expansion of the bellows is supported by an additional force, as long as the bellows can not reach the stop, the negative pressure becomes effective in the breathing system too, resulting in a change from intermittent positive pressure ventilation (IPPV) to alternating pressure ventilation (APV) (Figure 7.13).

In older-type anaesthesia ventilators without any gas reservoir, a positive end-expiratory pressure (PEEP) can only be built up if anaesthetic gas is available in excess. The PEEP valve is fitted directly to the exhaust port of the ventilator to prevent the discharge of any excess gas unless the pre-set PEEP is achieved. This is why in these ventilators a desired PEEP can only be built up if a surplus of fresh gas is supplied into the system (Figure 7.14).

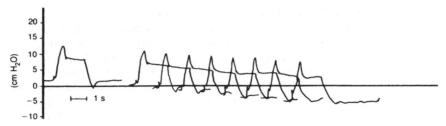

Figure 7.13 Course of the pressure within the breathing system at a fresh gas flow of 0.5 l/min and an actual leakage of 150 ml/min. Due to the resulting gas volume deficiency a decrease of inspired peak and plateau pressure and transition to alternating pressure ventilation can be observed. Fresh gas deficiency results in considerable alteration of the ventilation pattern if the expiratory expansion of the bellows is supported by an additional force. (From Baum and Schneider[46])

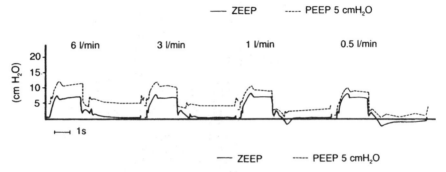

Figure 7.14 PEEP and fresh gas flow ($\dot{V}_F$) reduction using an older type anaesthetic ventilator, Dräger Pulmomat. Although the PEEP valve is set to its maximum, with decreasing $\dot{V}_F$ the expiratory pressure is lower the lower the fresh gas flow and may even drop to zero, indicating gas volume deficiency. The graph shows the course of the airway pressure of one ventilatory stroke each at different $\dot{V}_F$. (From Baum and Schneider[46])

According to Spieß[49], the increased demands with respect to leakproofness of such conventional-type anaesthesia ventilators without gas reservoir in low flow anaesthesia can be met by switching on the PEEP valve maximally at the moment the fresh gas flow is reduced. Thus, the unwanted expiratory discharge of excess gas via the exhaust valve, opening at 2 mbar, can be reduced. If, after flow reduction, an adequate gas volume is available, a PEEP will be slowly built up in the breathing system. In this case the PEEP-valve control should be re-adjusted to lower values, as the PEEP valve is only used for enhancing the leakproofness of the ventilator. This way of operating the ventilator should be restricted to the experienced anaesthetist.

In conclusion, when anaesthesia ventilators without gas reservoir are used, gas volume deficiency will occur whenever the fresh gas volume is lower than the gas volume lost via uptake and leakages. This will immediately result in an alteration of the tidal volume and airway pressure and may even change the ventilation patterns.

7.2.6.1.2 Anaesthetic machines with gas reservoir

7.2.6.1.2.1 Bellows-in-box ventilators with floating bellows. The alternative technical concept to the bellows-in-box ventilators with adjustable stop are the bellows-in-box ventilators with floating bellows. The prototype of this technique is the American Air-Shields ventilator with rising bellows (Figure 7.15). The bellows of this machine are installed standing upright in the pressure chamber. It features an extremely high compliance and its expiratory filling is effected exclusively by the inflow of the fresh gas and the gas volume, exhaled back into the breathing system. During inspiration, the driving gas flows into the pressure chamber (= box), in accordance with the ventilation parameters selected, and

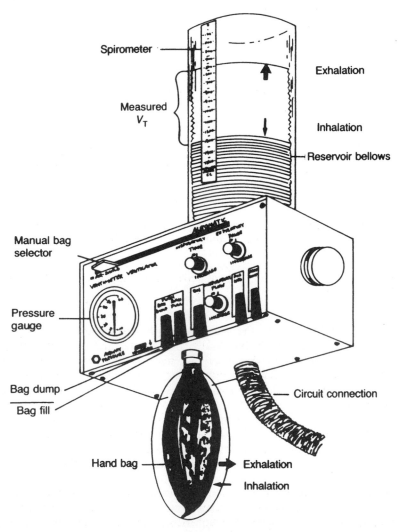

Figure 7.15 Air-Shields Ventilator with rising bellows, which serve as anaesthetic gas reservoir. (From Lowe and Ernst[50], by permission)

squeezes the bellows. Generally, the bellows are not completely compressed, but oscillate at an average filling level during the ventilation cycles. Imbalances between the fresh gas volume and the volume loss via uptake and leakages are compensated by a greater or lesser inspiratory emptying of the bellows. Thus, in case of gas volume deficiency, the floating bellows serve as an anaesthetic gas reservoir to cover the delivery of the desired tidal volume over a certain period of time during which adequate corrections at the flow control system can be made[50]. The tidal volume can be read from the amplitude of the bellows movement. The Ohmeda ventilators, the ventilator of the Siemens Servo Anaesthesia System and the ventilator of the Datex AS/3 ADU anaesthetic machine are of this type. The Dräger Julian anaesthetic machine is equipped with a bellows-in-box ventilator with floating bellows, but features a suspended bellows arrangement.

7.2.6.1.2.2 Bag-in-bottle ventilators. In bag-in-bottle ventilators a reservoir bag, containing a volume of about 2–4 litres anaesthetic gas and thus belonging to the secondary system, is enclosed by a cylinder functioning as the pressure chamber which belongs to the primary driving system. During inspiration the pressure within the cylinder is increased, compressing the reservoir bag. According to the pre-set tidal volume the content of the bag is partially delivered to the breathing system. The gas volume which remains stored in the bag at the end of the inspiratory phase serves as a gas reservoir. Imbalances between the fresh gas volume and the volume loss via uptake and leakages again can be compensated by a greater or lesser inspiratory emptying of the reservoir bag. The Engström anaesthetic machines Elsa and EAS 9010, and the Siemens Anesthesia System 711 are likewise equipped with such bag-in-bottle ventilators.

7.2.6.1.2.3 Ventilators with fresh gas decoupling valve   Generally, in older type machines a continuous flow of fresh gas is supplied into the breathing system. Nowadays, a considerable number of modern anaesthetic ventilators feature an alternative technique of fresh gas supply wherein a decoupling valve is switched into the fresh gas line (Figure 7.16). During the inspiratory stroke this valve cuts off the connection to the breathing system and directs the fresh gas to the manual bag, which serves as a gas reservoir. In the expiratory phase, the fresh gas decoupling valve opens again and the fresh gas and the gas contained in the manual bag can enter freely into the breathing system. Thus, not only the air exhaled back into the system and the fresh gas, but also the additional gas volume contained in the bag is available to the secondary system of the ventilator. By the function of this valve the fresh gas is delivered into the breathing system only during the expiratory phase. Different types of ventilators can be equipped with such a decoupling valve. Firstly there are the conventional bellows-in-box ventilators with suspended bellows arrangement, like the Dräger Sulla 909, the Heyer anaesthetic machines Access, Dogma and Narkomat, and the Megamed machines Megamed 700 and Mivolan. Secondly, there are the piston pump ventilators such as are used in the Dräger Cato and Cicero machines, equipped with a piston–cylinder unit with rolling seal (Figure 7.17). In these machines a piston is moving to and fro in a cylinder driven by an electronic control. During inspiration the piston is pushed forward and the gas contained in the cylinder is delivered to the patient, the fresh gas decoupling valve is closed to the breathing system and the fresh gas is directed into the manual bag. During expiration the piston is retracted according to the pre-set tidal volume, the fresh gas decoupling valve opens and the cylinder fills with a mixture of fresh gas and exhaled gas. Once the cylinder is filled, the exhaust valve is actively opened by its electronic control only if a pressure of 0.5 mbar is built up in the breathing system, thus ensuring a sufficient filling of the reservoir bag. If, in case of gas volume deficiency, the manual bag is completely emptied and the fresh gas flow very low, a negative pressure may develop in the cylinder during retraction of the piston. If that attains −0.5 mbar, the piston stops in its movement and the alarm message 'Gas Volume Deficiency' will be displayed.

The new Dräger machine Fabius is also equipped with a more simple electrically driven piston pump ventilator with rolling seal (Figure 7.16). Its compact breathing system 'Cosy' features a fresh gas decoupling valve, the manual bag again serving as an anaesthetic gas reservoir. In case of gas volume deficiency and an empty manual bag, however, an emergency air intake valve opens, allowing ambient air to enter the breathing system.

In conclusion, if a gas reservoir is available, small imbalances between the fresh gas volume and the volume loss via uptake and leakages can be compensated for by the surplus gas volume. Thus, in case of gas volume deficiency, the missing volume can be added from the reservoir to cover the delivery of the desired tidal volume over a certain period of time, during which adequate corrections at the flow control system can be made. The availability of a gas reservoir facilitates the performance of low flow anaesthetic techniques. Nevertheless, if in case of persisting gas volume deficiency the gas reservoir is emptied, the ventilator will not be filled sufficiently in the expiratory phase, resulting again in a decrease of the inspiratory, peak and plateau pressures and the minute volume.

7.2.6.2   Fresh gas flow compensation

7.2.6.2.1   Performance of ventilators without fresh gas flow compensation
In older conventional types of anaesthetic machines the fresh gas is delivered into the breathing system with a continuous gas flow during both the inspiratory and expiratory phases. Thus, the tidal volume is dependent on the fresh gas flow rate. In each inspiratory stroke of the ventilator not only the pre-set tidal volume, i.e. the volume contained in the bellows, but additionally the fresh gas volume supplied during the inspiratory phase will be delivered to the patient. This may be explained by taking the Ventilog anaesthetic ventilator (Dräger Medizintechnik, Lübeck, Germany) as an example. The ventilator is calibrated at a fresh gas flow of 4 l/min. Given a minute volume of 7000 ml/min, a respiratory frequency of 10 per minute, and an inspiratory–expiratory time ratio $I : E = 1 : 2$, the machine supplies a stroke volume of 567 ml which adds

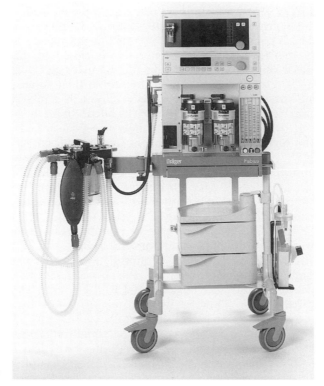

(a)

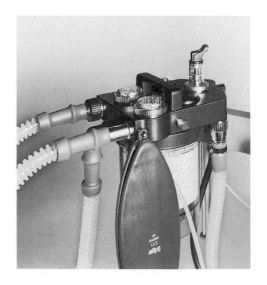

(b)

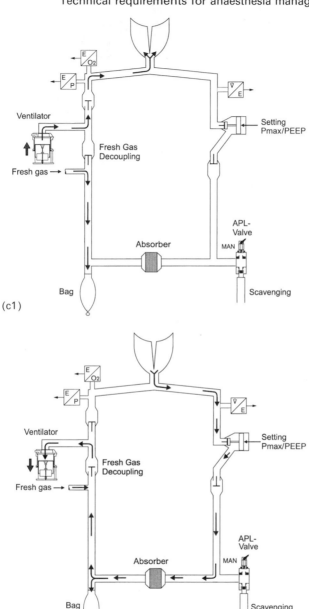

Figure 7.16 (a) Fabius anaesthetic machine equipped with the compact breathing system Cosy (b) (Dräger Medizintechnik, Lübeck, Germany). (c1 and c2) Flow diagrams for the Fabius. Technical feature: fresh gas flow compensation realized by the function of a fresh gas decoupling valve and discontinuous supply of fresh gas into the system. During inspiration (c1), the fresh gas is stored in the manual bag, which serves as an anaesthetic gas reservoir. (c2) The fresh gas together with the gas from the reservoir is fed into the system only during the expiratory phase. (By courtesy of Dräger Medizintechnik, Lübeck, Germany)

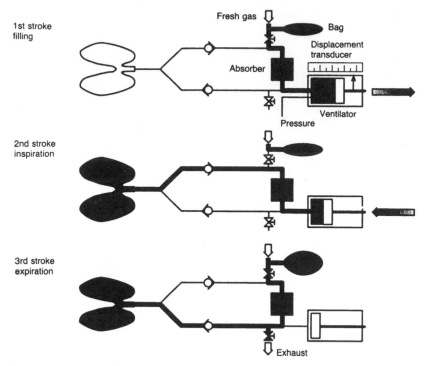

Figure 7.17   Flow diagram of the Cicero anaesthetic workstation depicting the function of the piston pump ventilator in different phases of a ventilatory stroke. (By courtesy of Dräger Medizintechnik, Lübeck, Germany)

to the inspiratorily delivered fresh gas volume of 133 ml to the desired tidal volume of 700 ml. If the fresh gas flow is reduced to 0.5 l/min, the volume fed into the system during inspiration is reduced to 17 ml, so that, together with the machine-supplied stroke volume, the tidal volume amounts to only 584 ml. The minute volume thus decreases by 1160 ml if the flow is reduced from 4.0 to 0.5 l/min. This phenomenon is referred to in the supplement to the instructions for use of the Sulla 808 under the heading 'Possibility of Metering Low Fresh Gas Volumes', as well as in other publications[4,51–53]. It was in 1988, in the third edition of the manual for the Dräger Ventilog 2 ventilator that, for the first time, a restriction was defined by the manufacturer not to use this device with fresh gas flows lower than 2 l/min. This seems hardly justified, as the anaesthetic machine Sulla, equipped with just this ventilator, is advertised to be especially suitable for low flow techniques.

The interdependence between minute volume and fresh gas flow can be simply corrected by increasing the tidal volume set at the machine according to and at the same time as flow reduction.

In the manual for the Ohmeda Modulus CD, equipped with the Ventilator 7800 (Figure 7.18), a formula is given to calculate the fresh gas volume V_{Fi} which is fed into the breathing system during inspiration:

$$V_{Fi} = \dot{V}_F / (f \times (1 + E : I).$$

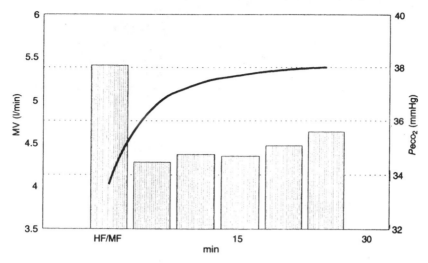

Figure 7.18   Increase of the expiratory carbon dioxide partial pressure (curve) due to decrease of minute volume (bars) resulting from fresh gas flow reduction using an Ohmeda 7800 anaesthesia ventilator without fresh gas flow compensation. HF/MF: MV and $PeCO_2$ taken just before flow reduction from 4.4 to 0.5 l/min

Generally, the minute volume (MV) delivered to the patient in such older type machines with constant fresh gas flow can be calculated by dividing the product of tidal volume (TV) and ventilation rate (f) plus the fresh gas flow rate ($\dot{V}_F$) by the sum of 1 plus $I : E$:

$$MV = TV \times f + \dot{V}_F / (1 + I : E)$$

In conclusion, in anaesthetic ventilators without fresh gas flow compensation the gas volume delivered to the patient is dependent on the fresh gas flow. Any alteration of the fresh gas flow rate will significantly influence the minute volume (Figure 7.19).

7.2.6.2.2   Technical possibilities to realize fresh gas flow compensation
Technically, the dependence of the tidal volume on the fresh gas flow rate can be overcome with fresh gas flow compensation[54]. If the ventilator features this property, the tidal volume remains unaffected by any variation of the fresh gas flow rate (Figure 7.19). Due to the increasing interest in low flow techniques, the manufacturers of anaesthetic machines became aware of this problem and so most of the modern ventilators are nowadays fresh gas flow compensated. Fresh gas flow compensation can be realized technically in the following ways:

7.2.6.2.2.1   Fresh gas decoupling valve.   The function of the fresh gas decoupling valve was described comprehensively beforehand (see Section 7.2.6.1.2.3). Fresh gas flow compensation is realized by the fact that, during the inspiratory phase, the fresh gas is not supplied into the breathing system itself but in-between is stored in the manual bag

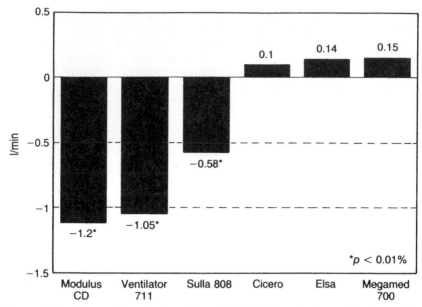

Figure 7.19 Change in minute volume (MV) with reduction of fresh gas flow: average values of differences in minute volumes, measured immediately prior to, and 15 min after, fresh gas flow reduction from 4.4 to 0.5 l/min. In all machines without fresh gas flow compensation the MV decreases significantly, whereas in all machines featuring flow compensation the MV remains unchanged or even increases slightly

serving as a gas reservoir. Thus, fresh gas flow compensation is realized by the function of the fresh gas decoupling valve effecting a discontinuous delivery of the fresh gas into the breathing system only in the expiratory phase. This principle of fresh gas flow compensation can be found in the Dräger machines Cato, Cicero, Fabius and Sulla 909, in the Heyer machines Access, Dogma and Narkomat, and the Megamed 700 and Mivolan.

7.2.6.2.2.2 Electronic control of the ventilator performance.   In the Datex machine AS/3 ADU, the Engström machines Elsa and EAS 9010 and the Ohmeda Ventilator 7900 fresh gas flow compensation is gained by a quite different technical solution. In all these machines the fresh gas is supplied continuously into the breathing system. The tidal volume, however, delivered to the patient is measured electronically and, once the pre-set gas volume is supplied, the ventilator stops the delivery of any further volume. Thus, by electronic control of the ventilator's performance the duration of the inspiratory phase is adapted to the fresh gas flow rate to deliver the pre-set tidal volume.

7.2.6.2.2.3 Electronic control of discontinuous fresh gas supply.   In the Dräger Julian anaesthetic machine the fresh gas is mixed and supplied to the breathing system with the aid of an electronically controlled delivery system. The pre-set fresh gas volume is delivered into the system in distinct quanta, adapted to the pre-set ventilation patterns. Thus, fresh gas flow compensation in this machine is realized by electronically controlled discontinuous fresh gas supply only during the expiratory phase. As the capacity of the electronic delivery system is limited, the fresh gas flow rate must not exceed 12 l/min, otherwise the gas will be delivered into the system during both the inspiratory and expiratory phases.

7.2.6.2.2.4   Electronic control of discontinuous fresh gas supply and ventilator performance.   Finally a fourth technique of fresh gas flow compensation will be described which is realized in the Siemens Servo Anesthesia System 985. In this machine the fresh gas is supplied into the breathing system in quanta adapted to the pre-set fresh gas flow and the pre-set ventilation patterns by an electronic delivery system only during the inspiratory phase. Thus, the performance of the ventilator has to be adapted simultaneously to the added fresh gas volume to ensure the delivery of just the pre-set tidal volume.

   In conclusion, using an anaesthesia ventilator featuring fresh gas flow compensation the tidal volume can be set and is delivered independently of the setting or alteration of the fresh gas flow.

7.3   Specific features of different anaesthetic machines

The following descriptions of the specific features and the performance of different anaesthetic machines are mainly based on the author's own experiences gained during clinical use of these apparatuses with low flow techniques.

7.3.1   Aestiva 3000 (Datex-Ohmeda, Madison, USA)

The Aestiva 3000 anaesthetic machine (Figure 7.20) is a conventional type machine[55]. It can be operated with gas supply from central gas piping system or gas cylinders. The flow control system consists of fine needle valves and flowmeter tubes. If a two flowmeter tubes in tandem arrangement is used, the low flow tubes for O_2, N_2O and air range from 0.05 to 0.95 l/min. The precise performance of the Link 25 anti-hypoxic device enables the setting of even the lowest fresh gas flows. The TEC 5 and TEC 6 vaporizers have proven to be sufficiently flow-compensated to deliver correctly the dialled concentration even at very low flows. The Aestiva 3000 ventilator is fresh gas flow-compensated by adapting the ventilator's performance to the fresh gas flow according to the gas volume supplied to the patient. Volume- and pressure-controlled ventilation modes are both available. As the gas volume is measured for both inspiration and expiration, a patient circuit leak alarm comes on if less than half of the inspired volume returns through the expiratory flow sensor during mechanical ventilation. The breathing system with a volume of 5.5 litres is made of plastic. After some practice it can be

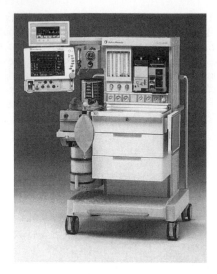

Figure 7.20   Aestiva 3000 anaesthetic machine (Datex-Ohmeda, Madison, USA). (By courtesy of Datex-Ohmeda, Madison, USA)

easily disassembled and remounted and is highly gas tight (total system leakage ≤ 300 ml/min at 3 kPa). A special drain valve allows condensed water which may accumulate in the breathing system to drain into the drain dish at the bottom of the absorber. A two-chambered Jumbo canister, containing 1.35 kg of soda lime in each chamber, is attached to the system. It has a drain plug which can be unscrewed to remove water condensate, which may be a help if very low flows are used in very long cases. When using the Aestiva machine in the author's own department, increased water condensation, however, was not a problem at all. The Aestiva 3000 anaesthetic machine is simple to operate and meets all technical preconditions to safely and easily perform all the different techniques of low flow anaesthesia.

7.3.2   AS/3 ADU Plus Anesthesia Delivery Unit (Datex Engström, Helsinki, Finland)

This machine is a highly integrated anaesthesia workstation (Figure 7.21). The flow control system consists of fine needle valves with electronic metering and digital display of the gas flows, which allows precise setting of even the lowest flows. The same holds for the control of air flows if an oxygen–air carrier gas mixture is used. The inhalation anaesthetics are delivered by cassettes (Figure 7.21b), the function of which is similar to conventional plenum vaporizers, although they are controlled electronically and the desired concentration is dialled digitally. The cassettes are absolutely safe if tilted and are comparatively lightweight. The compact breathing system has proven to be highly gas tight in clinical practice, and the same applies for the alternatively available Dameca circuit (Dameca, Denmark). The sampling gas, used for side-stream analysis of the anaesthetic gas composition, is fed back into the breathing system. The ventilator features an upright floating bellows arrangement. The gas volume still contained in the bellows at the end of inspiration is the reservoir by which small gas volume deficiencies can be balanced. The ventilator is flow-compensated by electronic adaptation of the ventilator's performance to the actual fresh gas flow. The in-built Datex monitoring is comprehensive and works reliably in clinical practice. All the dialled values for fresh gas delivery and ventilator performance as well as all monitoring parameters needed for comprehensive information about the machine's performance and the patient's condition are displayed on two almost freely configurable colour screens. As all these parameters are measured electronically in real time simultaneously, this machine offers optimal preconditions for data management and automatic record keeping. The AS/3 ADU is perfectly suitable for all different types of low flow techniques and even closed system anaesthesia. The succeeding model, AS/3 ADU plus, additionally features ventilation modes like SIMV and PCV (synchronized intermittent mandatory ventilation and pressure-controlled ventilation) and can be used with all inhalational anaesthetics, as a cassette for desflurane recently became available.

7.3.3 Cato and Cicero EM (Dräger Medizintechnik, Lübeck, Germany)

The anaesthetic machine Cato (Figure 7.22) and the Cicero EM anaesthesia workstation (Figure 7.23) are equipped with the same compact breathing system and a piston pump ventilator featuring fresh gas flow compensation by fresh gas decoupling. The breathing system is characterized by very high gas tightness which is checked automatically when switching on the machine. The ventilator can be used even in the smallest infants as the lowest tidal volume precisely delivered is only $20\,\mathrm{ml}$[56,70]. The fresh gas utilization is optimalized by the performance of the valves during expiration phase: at the moment that the piston starts to move backwards, the fresh gas decoupling valve is opened prior to the expiratory valve. Thus, the ventilator is filled preferentially with fresh gas, whereas it is mostly exhaled gas which is discharged as waste when the exhaust valve opens during the later expiratory phase. The gas tightness of the system is enhanced in so far as the exhaust port is not opened by a passively functioning non-return valve, as is the case with conventional systems, but the exhaust valve is actively opened at an end-expiratory pressure of more than $0.1\,\mathrm{kPa}$ ($\approx 1\,\mathrm{cmH_2O}$). The exhaust valve is already closed again as soon as the pressure drops to $0.05\,\mathrm{kPa}$ ($\approx 0.5\,\mathrm{cmH_2O}$). In this way, excess gas is only discharged if the gas reservoir, the manual bag, is sufficiently filled; thus the performance of the machine is automatically adapted to the fresh gas flow rate. Gas volume deficiency will not lead to the generation of any negative pressure in the ventilator as the retraction of the piston is immediately interrupted and a clear text message at the front panel of the machine indicates the problem.

Both machines are equipped with conventional flow control systems consisting of fine needle valves, flowmeter tubes and conventional

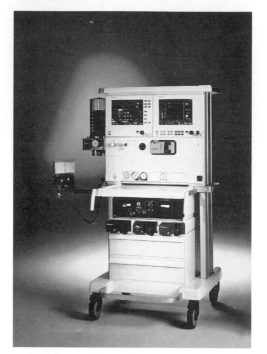

(a)

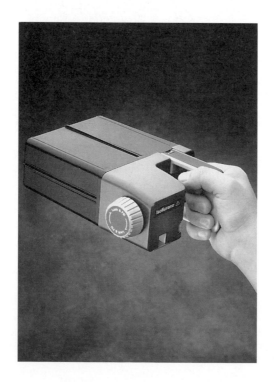

(b)

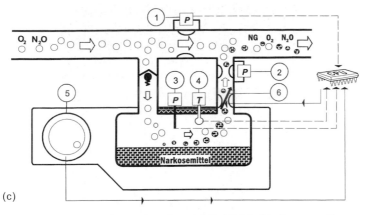

(c)

Figure 7.21 (a) Anaesthetic workstation AS/3 ADU. (b) Cassette (Datex unique anaesthetic vapour delivery module). (c) Flow diagram of a Datex cassette: 1 and 2: pressure difference transducers; 3 and 4: pressure and temperature sensors; 5: dial for agent concentration; 6: electronically controlled flow resistor. NG: vaporized anaesthetic agent; Narkosemittel: liquid anaesthetic agent. (By courtesy of Datex-Ohmeda, Madison, USA)

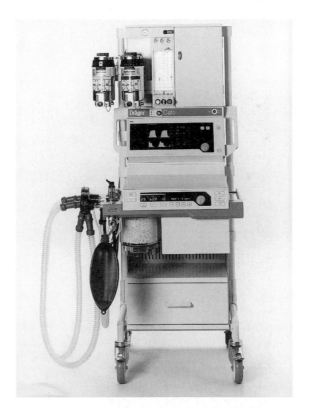

Figure 7.22 Cato anaesthetic machine. (By courtesy of Dräger Medizintechnik, Lübeck, Germany)

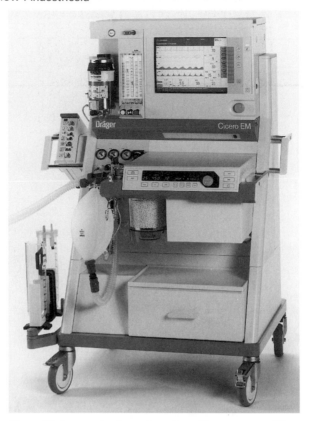

Figure 7.23   Cicero EM anaesthetic workstation. (By courtesy of Dräger Medizin-technik, Lübeck, Germany)

plenum vaporizers. While the vaporizers perform precisely in the very low flow range, the pneumatically controlled anti-hypoxic 'Oxygen Ratio Controller' (ORC) device renders it difficult and time-consuming to accurately dial very low flow rates. Frequently the flow changes spontaneously in a range between 50 and 100 ml/min as a result of slow oscillations of the membrane of the ORC. Both machines are especially suitable for use in low and minimal flow anaesthesia. If a mixture of oxygen and nitrous oxide is used as carrier gas flows lower than 500 ml/min can not be dialled due to the imprecise function of the ORC.

Cato and Cicero EM only differ in respect to the monitoring equipment: whereas the Cato meets only the needs of EN 740, in the Cicero EM a high grade of integration of monitoring and controls is gained, including all the essential patient monitoring. All parameters are displayed on one common data screen. Whenever a monitored parameter exceeds any alarm threshold or in case of any technical problem, an alarm message will be displayed instantly, rated according to its clinical significance by the alarm hierarchy.

The Cicero EM additionally is equipped with the monitoring tool

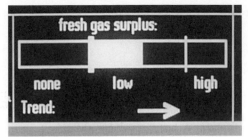

Figure 7.24   The monitoring module 'Econometer', continuously displaying the balance of fresh gas input and gas losses via uptake and leakages. (By courtesy of Dräger Medizintechnik, Lübeck, Germany)

'Econometer' which continuously provides information about the gas volume circulating within the breathing system. Thus, the anaesthetist gets continuous information on whether fresh gas flow is supplied in excess, just meets the gas loss via uptake and leakages, or whether gas volume deficiency may develop. The actual filling condition is displayed by a bar graph (Figure 7.24) and enables a precise adaptation of the fresh gas flow rate to the current needs, thus enhancing the safety in performance of flow flow anaesthesia. Without any doubt, such a monitoring device is an excellent educational tool increasing the readiness to reduce adequately the fresh gas flow[57].

7.3.4   Dogma, Access and Narkomat (Heyer, Bad Ems, Germany)

All the three apparatuses are similar in respect of their technical features. The ventilator is a bellows-in-box type with suspended and floating bellows arrangement. Their expiratory expansion, however, is supported by a 250 g weight fixed to its bottom. Fresh gas flow compensation is realized by the function of a fresh gas decoupling valve, the manual bag again serving as a gas reservoir (Figure 7.25a and b). The machines are all equipped with the same heated compact breathing system, carrying a Jumbo canister containing 1.5 kg of absorbent. A separate electric motor engages the breathing system; its active heating warms up the anaesthetic gases and reduces water condensation. The fine needle valves work somewhat imprecisely in the very low flow range, the flowmeter tubes are graduated to deliver even lowest flows. The design of the machines is exemplary as all connections between the anaesthetic machine itself and the breathing system are hidden in the interior of the machine. The same applies for all cable and tube connections needed for internal communication of the different modules and the technical equipment for power and medical gas supply: all these technical structures are hidden behind a smooth back. The machines impress as very tidy with smooth surfaces and so can easily be cleaned and disinfected.

Due to the support of the expiratory expansion of the bellows, in the event of gas volume deficiency a negative pressure will develop in the

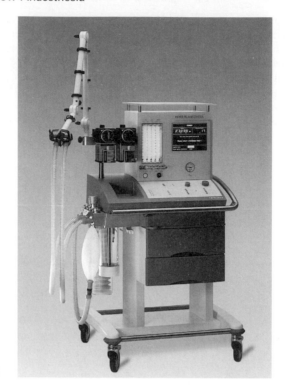

(a)

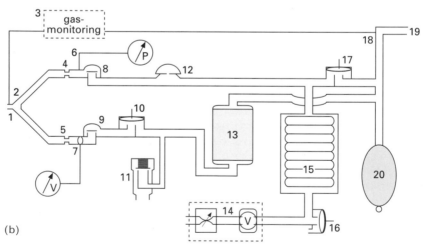

(b)

Figure 7.25   (a) Narkomat anaesthetic machine. (b) Flow diagram of the Access, Dogma and Narkomat anaesthetic machines. 1: Y-piece; 2: gas sampling tube; 3: gas analyser; 4: inspiratory port; 5: expiratory port; 6: airway pressure monitor; 7: spirometer; 8: inspiratory valve; 9: expiratory valve; 10: PEEP valve; 11: APL valve; 12: emergency air intake port; 13: carbon dioxide absorber; 14: ventilator control pneumatic; 15: bellows dome; 16: pressure control valve; 17: fresh gas decoupling valve; 18: gas sampling return tube; 19: fresh gas inlet; 20: reservoir/manual bag. (By courtesy of Heyer, Bad Ems, Germany)

breathing system, opening automatically an emergency air intake valve to allow air to enter the system until the bellows are completely filled with gas. Dogma and Access perform without any problem at a fresh gas flow of 1.0 l/min, whereas in minimal flow anaesthesia – at least in cases with high individual uptake and tidal volumes – the emergency air intake port frequently opens, resulting in an increase of the nitrogen and a decrease of the oxygen and nitrous oxide concentration. This air intake valve also opens frequently although the reservoir bag is still sufficiently filled with gas, which can only be explained by imprecise tuning of the performance of the valves and the gas flows within the breathing system. Dogma and Access, which only differ in respect of the monitoring equipment, are equally suitable for low flow, but have some limitations for minimal flow anaesthesia. The same may hold for the new machine, Narkomat, as the technical concept remains unchanged; however, the author has not yet had the chance to check and test the machine personally. Narkomat features compliance compensation and new ventilation modes such as PCV and SIMV.

7.3.5   Elsa and EAS 9010 (Gambro–Engström, Bromma, Sweden)

The Elsa anaesthetic machine (Figure 7.26b) operates with a classic bag-in-bottle ventilator. The 4-litre patient bag, which is placed in a cylindrical pressure chamber, is filled with fresh gas and exhaled air during expiration. During inspiration, driving gas flows into the pressure chamber in accordance with the set ventilation parameters, the bag is squeezed and part of its gas volume is delivered into the breathing system. In spite of the fact that the fresh gas is fed into the system continuously, the ventilator features fresh gas flow compensation. The inspired flow is measured electronically and the inspiration phase is completed once the set tidal volume has been supplied to the patient. The time cycle of the ventilator's control thus changes as a function of the fresh gas flow selected. Possible imbalances between fresh gas volume and gas loss via uptake and leaks are compensated for by greater or lesser evacuation of the reservoir bag. The tidal volume only decreases if this gas reservoir is no longer filled sufficiently. In the event of fresh gas deficiency, the unit signals this problem by displaying the message 'reservoir bag empty'.

The compact breathing system is highly gas tight, and a leak test is performed automatically. The electronic vaporizer can be set to a maximum output of 8 vol%; the machines, available for clinical tests, could only deliver the older inhalation anaesthetics halothane, enflurane and isoflurane. To facilitate precise adjustment of the gas flows in the low flow range, the electronic flowmeter bar graph display can be switched to high resolution. Thus, the Elsa anaesthetic machine meets all requirements for performance of anaesthesia with even the lowest fresh gas flows. The newer Gambro–Engström anaesthetic machine EAS 9010 (Figure 7.26a) is equipped with comprehensive monitoring in accordance with the requirements of the common European standard EN 740.

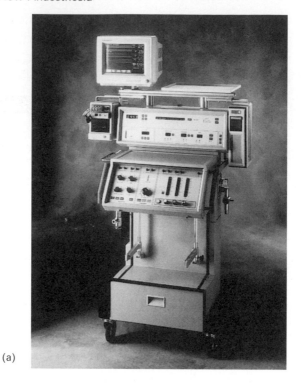

(a)

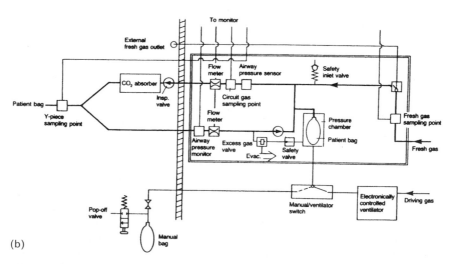

(b)

Figure 7.26   (a) EAS 9010 anaesthetic machine. (b) Flow diagram of the Elsa and EAS 9010. Specific technical features: electronic metering system for volatile anaesthetics, bag-in-bottle ventilator. (By courtesy of Gambro–Engstrom, Bromma, Sweden)

7.3.6 Fabius (Dräger Medizintechnik, Lübeck, Germany)

The Fabius is a comparatively simple, nevertheless remarkable, conventional anaesthetic machine (Figure 7.16a and b). The gas flow control system for oxygen, air and nitrous oxide consists of fine needle valves, including an ORC as an anti-hypoxic device, followed by flowmeter tubes in tandem which are calibrated and graduated even in the lowest flow range. The machine is equipped with conventional plenum vaporizers switched into the fresh gas line. The ventilator is a piston pump arrangement driven by an electric motor. Fresh gas flow compensation is realized by the function of a fresh gas decoupling valve. As long as the manual bag, serving as a gas reservoir, is filled sufficiently, ventilation patterns remain unchanged. In case of fresh gas deficiency the manual bag collapses completely and an emergency air intake valve opens during the expiratory retraction of the piston. Ambient air may then enter, thus diluting the other gases circulating within the system. The breathing system 'Cosy' is a compact system with high gas tightness. The Fabius anaesthetic machine is equipped only with that monitoring essentially needed to monitor the correct function of the machine: airway pressure, inspired oxygen concentration and minute and tidal volume. The machine performed perfectly in low and minimal flow anaesthesia. If fresh gas flow rates lower than 0.5 l/min were used, however, ambient air frequently entered the breathing system.

If anaesthetists renounce the use of nitrous oxide and use pure oxygen as carrier gas, performance of inhalational anaesthesia becomes extremely simple and safe, and can be realized even under extremely unfavourable conditions, such as in field or disaster medicine[58]. To operate the system with smallest amounts of gas and anaesthetics only compressed oxygen or oxygen supplied by an oxygen concentrator, fluid anaesthetic agent and electric current would be needed, thus eliminating otherwise existing logistical needs for compressed air and nitrous oxide (see Chapter 11 and Section 12.3.2).

7.3.7 Julian (Dräger Medizintechnik, Lübeck, Germany)

The anaesthetic machine Julian (Figure 7.27a and b) is the first commercially available Dräger device featuring electronically controlled fresh gas delivery. Superficially, an optimization of the technical design attracts the attention. Gas, control and power connections from the machine to the breathing system are hidden internally, similarly all the cable and tube connections between the different modules are hidden by a smooth back. When the power supply is switched on short initial test sequences run automatically and can be interrupted if necessary after 1 min. The electronically controlled fresh gas supply performs precisely down to a gas flow of 0.5 l/min, as it is needed in minimal flow anaesthesia. The carrier gas composition (air–oxygen or nitrous oxide–oxygen), the total fresh gas flow and its oxygen concentration are set at the controls. It is impossible to dial fresh gas flows lower than 0.5 l/min. During performance of low flow techniques, a fixed minimum oxygen flow of 250 ml/min and a fresh gas oxygen concentration of at least 25% are obstacles to the free

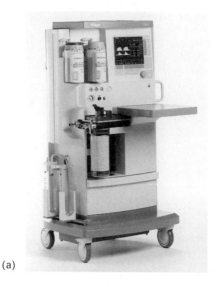

(a)

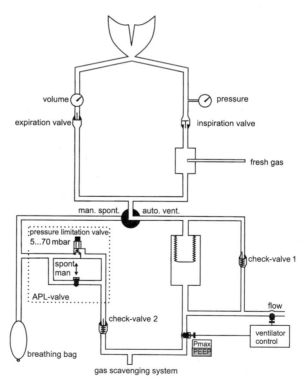

(b)

Figure 7.27 (a) Julian anaesthetic machine. (b) Flow diagram of the Julian anaesthetic machine. Specific technical features: electronic control of fresh gas flow and its composition, fresh gas flow compensation by discontinuous expiratory supply of the fresh gas into the breathing system. (By courtesy of Dräger Medizintechnik, Lübek, Germany)

adjustment of the gas composition within the breathing system in favour of nitrous oxide, in the event that the nitrous oxide concentration would be too low. If very low fresh gas flow rates are used, alteration of the fresh gas composition will only lead to delayed corresponding alterations of the gas composition within the breathing system. The electronically controlled metering system stores the fresh gas in a reservoir tank containing 0.5 l at a pressure oscillating between 0.6 and 1.2 bar. Not until the contents of the tank are delivered into the system will alterations of the fresh gas composition become effective. Furthermore, the long time constants resulting from the fresh gas flow reduction itself have to be considered. The compact breathing system, containing a gas volume of about 4.5 litres, is highly gas tight and equipped with a 1.5 litres absorber canister. The bellows-in-box ventilator with a floating suspended bellows arrangement features fresh gas flow compensation: corresponding to the ventilation patterns the fresh gas is delivered into the breathing system, only during the expiratory phase, in just such quanta to precisely meet the pre-set fresh gas flow. The gas volume contained in the bellows at the end of the inspiratory phase serves as a gas reservoir. If in case of gas volume shortage the bellows is not filled sufficiently and cannot reach the bottom of the box, the resulting negative pressure of −1 mbar is insignificant. The Julian anaesthetic machine is likewise suitable for easy and safe performance of low flow and minimal flow anaesthesia.

7.3.8   Megamed 700 and Mivolan (Megamed, Cham, Switzerland)

The Megamed 700 anaesthetic machine (Figure 7.28a–c) is equipped with a bellows-in-box ventilator with suspended bellows arrangement without support of its expiratory expansion. Fresh gas flow compensation is realized by the aid of a fresh gas decoupling valve directing the fresh gas into the breathing system discontinuously only during the expiratory phase. During inspiration the fresh gas is stored in the manual bag serving as a gas reservoir. In the Megamed 700 excess gas is not discharged via an automatically opening exhaust valve. Corresponding to the fresh gas flow rate, the exhaust valve must be adapted manually to ensure a sufficient gas filling of the manual bag. Once the valve is opened too much, the manual bag collapses, the bellows is not filled sufficiently and the tidal volume decreases. If, on the other hand, the valve is closed too much, the manual bag is overfilled and the pressure within the breathing system increases. Particular attention must be paid to correct manual adjustment of this valve if the fresh gas flow rate is changed. The correct setting of the adjustable pressure-limiting valve to a maximum pressure exceeding the peak pressure by only 10 mbar safely prevents accidental barotrauma of the lung[30]. In the succeeding anaesthetic machine Mivolan, which was not available for the author's own clinical trials, this disadvantage is overcome by automatic discharge of the excess gas. The breathing system 048NR makes it possible to switch from the rebreathing to a non-rebreathing function mode. If the non-rebreathing mode is used, the exhaled air is discharged completely out of the system. In this case, the fresh gas flow must at least equal the minute volume, the time constant of the system

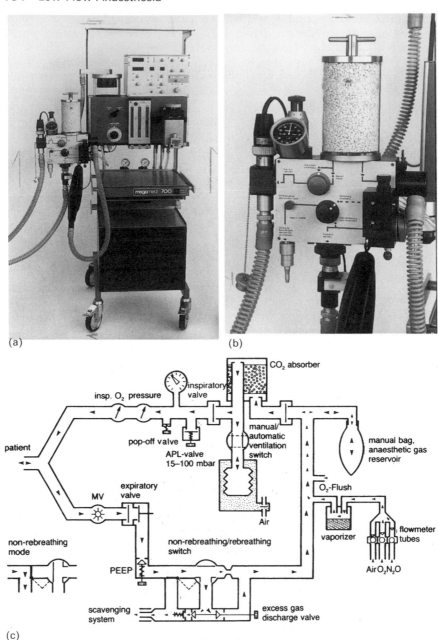

Figure 7.28 (a) Megamed 700 anaesthetic machine. (b) Compact circle absorption system of the Megamed 700. Specific technical features: the adjustable pressure-limiting valve has to be set manually; a switch enables a change from rebreathing to non-rebreathing mode. (c) Flow diagram of the Megamed 700: the manual bag serves as an anaesthetic gas reservoir; fresh gas decoupling valve, discontinuous fresh gas supply into the system only during expiratory phase. (By courtesy of Megamed, Cham, Switzerland)

becomes as short as possible and wash-in or wash-out of anaesthetic gases proceeds rapidly.

7.3.9   Modulus SE and Excel SE (Datex–Ohmeda, Madison, USA)

The Modulus SE (Figure 7.29) and Excel SE anaesthetic machines are suitable for the performance of anaesthesia even with lowest fresh gas flows. The flow control unit allows precise and easy adjustment even in the low flow range. Oxygen and nitrous oxide controls are connected by a chain, thus making it impossible to set a fresh gas oxygen concentration lower than 25 vol% (Figure 7.2). The Link 25 anti-hypoxic device does not hinder the precise setting of very low gas flows. Both Ohmeda machines are equipped with a GMS absorber utilizing a dual absorbent canister configuration. The machines may be equipped either with the Ohmeda 7800 or Ohmeda 7900 ventilator. Both are bellows-in-box type ventilators with floating ascending bellows arrangement. The bellows serves as an anaesthetic gas reservoir, by which small imbalances between the fresh gas volume and the gas loss via leakages and uptake can be compensated. The 7800 ventilator features no fresh gas flow compensation: the fresh gas is fed into the breathing system continuously and the tidal volume, being supplied to the patient, depends upon the fresh gas flow. The Ohmeda 7900 ventilator, however, features fresh gas flow compensation: the gas volume delivered to the patient is measured electronically. Once the pre-set tidal volume is supplied, the ventilator interrupts its inspiratory stroke,

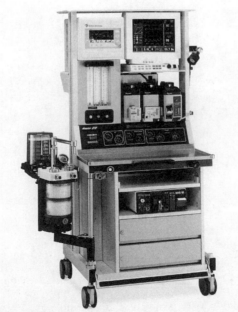

Figure 7.29   Modulus SE anaesthetic machine. (By courtesy of Datex-Ohmeda, Madison, USA)

thus the performance of the ventilator is adapted to the fresh gas flow rate and the tidal volume is not influenced by the flow.

7.3.10   Narkomed 4 (North American Dräger, Telford, USA)

The Narkomed 4 workstation offers comprehensive monitoring for safe performance of anaesthesia and computerized automatic record-keeping. However, the technical features of the flow control system, the breathing system and the anaesthesia ventilator are more conventional. The fresh gas flow is fed into the breathing system continuously, resulting in a dependency of fresh gas flow and inspired volume in the case of controlled ventilation. There is no anaesthetic gas reservoir available, as the expiratory expansion of the rising bellows is stopped by the pre-set position of the adjustment plate (Figure 7.12). Only if this stop is adjusted to its highest position at the top of the bellows canister can the ventilator be used with floating bellows which then may serve as the anaesthetic gas reservoir. Even though the breathing system features a high number of connections, it proves to be adequately gas tight. However, the anti-hypoxic safety device of the flow control system of older type Narkomed machines, the oxygen ratio controller (ORC), is so sensitive that precise control of the oxygen and nitrous oxide flow even in the range of low flow anaesthesia is nearly impossible and needs frequent corrections. Now optionally available is a low flow gas flow control system 'Low Flow Update Kit', which performs precisely down to a flow of 0.5 l/min with the following specifications: minimum oxygen flow 150–200 ml/min, maximum nitrous oxide flow with minimum oxygen flow 425–500 ml/min.

The successor model, Narkomed GS equipped with the AV 2 ventilator, was not available for clinical trial. It can be configured with optional low flow flowmeter tubes that provide a measuring scale for flows below 600 ml/min.

The new Narcomed 6000 is equipped with a piston pump ventilator and a compact breathing system completely identical to those of the Cicero and Cato anaesthetic machines. The technical properties and features were comprehensively described in Section 7.3.3.

7.3.11   SA 2 (Dräger Medizintechnik, Lübeck, Germany)

The SA 2 (Figure 7.30a and b) is an anaesthetic machine featuring fresh gas flow compensation by the aid of a fresh gas decoupling valve. The fresh gas is fed into the system only during the expiratory phase. During inspiration, the gas is stored in the manual bag, which functions as an anaesthetic gas reservoir. If equipped with the optional tandem flowmeter tubes for oxygen and nitrous oxide, the flow control system allows precise adjustment of gas flows down to 0.1 l/min. The pneumatically controlled ORC, however, impedes adjustment of the oxygen flow to values lower than 0.35 l/min. The compact breathing system, CU 1, is highly gas tight with a mean leakage loss lower than 50 ml/min at 4 kPa ($\approx 40\,cmH_2O$). The APL valve has to be adapted carefully to the airway pressure, otherwise an inspiratory loss of gas may occur. In the event of gas

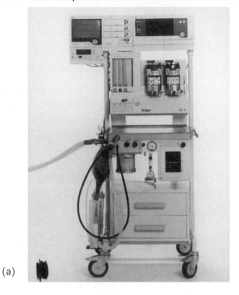

(a)

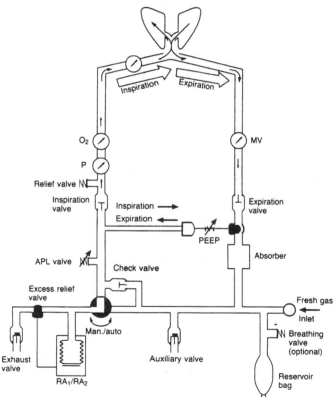

(b)

Figure 7.30   (a) SA 2 anaesthetic machine with RA1/RA2 electric ventilator and CU 1 compact breathing system. (b) Flow diagram of the SA 2 anaesthetic machine. (By courtesy of Dräger Medizintechnik, Lübeck, Germany)

deficiency and resultant negative pressure within the system during expiratory expansion of the bellows, room air can enter the system via the emergency air intake valve which opens at 200 to 400 Pa ($\approx$ −2 to 4 cmH$_2$O). In the CU 1 breathing system, the carbon dioxide absorber is attached to the expiratory limb of the breathing system. Optionally the machine is available with the absorber in the inspiratory limb in order to avoid water condensation within the CU 1 breathing system, which may be advantageous, especially in low flow anaesthesia. The RA 2 ventilator is electrically driven and equipped with a hanging bellows. The poor performance of the ORC in the low flow range is the deciding factor for the limited suitability of the SA 2 machine in using very low fresh gas flows. The anaesthetic machine SA 2, however, meets all the requirements for safe and simple performance of low flow anaesthesia.

7.3.12   Servo Anesthesia System (Siemens–Elema, Solna, Sweden)

The Servo Ventilator C and D equipped with an Anaesthesia Circle System 985 (Figure 7.31a and b) belongs to the group of machines featuring gas reservoir and discontinuous fresh gas supply into the system. The fresh gas is mixed by a blender and, having passed the Siemens vaporizer[15], it is fed into the system in defined quanta, adapted to the dialled fresh gas flow and the pre-set ventilation patterns, only during the inspiratory phase. Following carbon dioxide absorption, the re-circulating exhaled air is mixed with the fresh gas during the inspiratory stroke of the ventilator. The volume delivered by the ventilator is adapted to the additionally delivered fresh gas volume to just meet the pre-set tidal volume. The ventilator with ascending and floating bellows arrangement serves as a reservoir. According to the author's own experience, the flow transducer, measuring the expired gas volume, was extremely susceptible to malfunction, which was attributable to the frequently observed contamination of the sensor. Such contamination occurred in particular when leakage losses had to be compensated for by frequent actuation of the 'gas exchange button'. The leak test of this machine was cumbersome, as it could not be performed under resting conditions but only if the ventilator was working. For adequate performance, the machine required a fresh gas flow of at least 0.7–0.8 l/min.

7.3.13   Siemens Anesthesia System 711 (Siemens–Elema, Solna, Sweden)

Compared to the Servo Anaesthesia System, the Anesthesia System 711 (Figure 7.32) is a more conventional type of machine. It is equipped with a commonly used flow control system and plenum vaporizers, and the fresh gas is fed into the system continuously. The anaesthetic ventilator is a classic bag-in-bottle design, with a 3-litre reservoir bag. Thus, a sufficient amount of reservoir gas is available for initial compensation of gas volume imbalances. There is no fresh gas flow compensation. With this device, flow reduction down to 0.5 l/min could be realized in daily clinical practice.

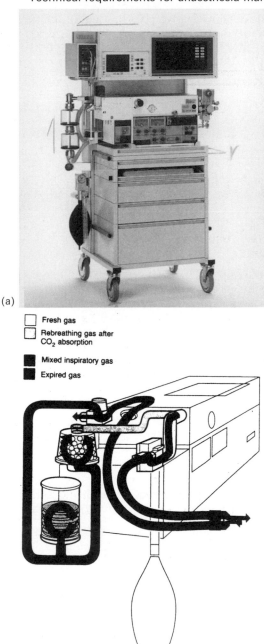

(a)

☐ Fresh gas

▨ Rebreathing gas after
   CO_2 absorption

■ Mixed inspiratory gas

■ Expired gas

(b)

Figure 7.31   (a) Siemens Servo Ventilator with Anaesthesia Circle System 985. (b) Flow diagram of the Siemens Servo Ventilator with Anaesthesia Circle System 985. Special technical features: discontinuous inspiratory supply of fresh gas into the breathing system, anaesthetic ventilator with rising bellows arrangement and electronic fresh gas flow compensation. (By courtesy of Siemens–Elema, Solna, Sweden)

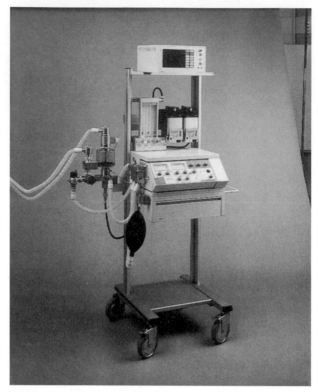

Figure 7.32 Siemens Anesthesia System 711. Technical feature: a conventional anaesthetic machine without fresh gas flow compensation and fitted with a bag-in-bottle ventilator. (By courtesy of Siemens–Elema, Solna, Sweden)

7.3.14 Sulla 909 (Dräger Medizintechnik, Lübeck, Germany)

The Sulla 909 (Figures 7.11a and 7.33) with respect to its technical design, in general equals the conventional Sulla 808 anaesthetic machine; however, the machine is equipped with a fresh gas decoupling valve and so features fresh gas flow compensation. The FGE (Frischgasentkoppelung = fresh gas decoupling) valve is connected to the bellows-in-box ventilator by two silicon tubes needed for pneumatic control of the fresh gas flow supply and the PEEP valve. During inspiration, the fresh gas is temporarily stored in the manual bag which serves as a gas reservoir, and is fed into the breathing system only during the expiratory phase. The anaesthetist, however, has to observe carefully the performance of the valve. Following thermo-disinfection with a washing machine, water may accumulate within the FGE valve or the control tubes, resulting in dangerous malfunction of this device. Alternating PEEP levels or even severe obstruction of the expiratory flow were observed. It cannot be overemphasized that this device should preferably be autoclaved and dried carefully after daily use. Provided that this procedure and a carefully performed leak test

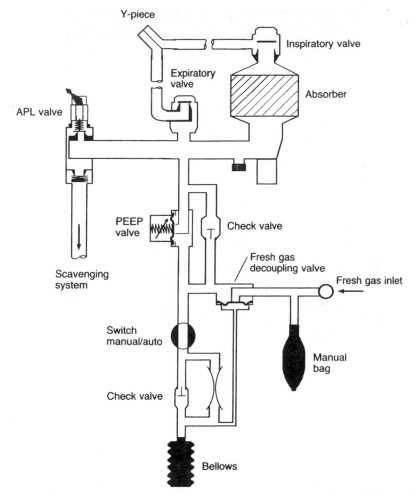

Figure 7.33 Flow diagram of the Sulla 909 V. Specific technical features: fresh gas flow compensation by fresh gas decoupling valve, manual bag serves as gas reservoir. (By courtesy of Dräger Medizintechnik, Lübeck, Germany)

are carried out, the Sulla 909 anaesthetic machine with FGE valve meets the technical requirements for low and even minimal flow anaesthesia.

7.3.15 System volumes of different anaesthetic machines

With constant uptake and fresh gas flow, the time constant is directly proportional to the volume of the entire gas-filled space (see Section 5.2.3). It is calculated from the sum of machine-related gas volumes and functional residual capacity. With high system volumes the time constant is long, and correspondingly short with small system volumes.

Table 7.2 lists the volumes of some newer anaesthetic machines. This compilation is based on the following conditions: the patient system

Table 7.2 Volumes (l) contained in the breathing systems of some newer anaesthetic machines

	Cicero	Elsa	Megamed	Sulla
Patient hose system	0.9	0.9	0.9	0.9
Breathing system	0.6	0.4	0.5	0.4
Absorber	2.0	1.0	1.0	1.0
Anaesthetic gas reservoir	1.5	3.0	1.5	–
Hose connections	0.5	0.4	0.4	0.5
Ventilator volume	0.7	–	0.7	0.7
Total volume	6.2	5.7	5.0	3.5

consists of two corrugated hoses of 1 m length, only one 1-litre carbon dioxide absorber or one Jumbo canister is fitted in the breathing system and the anaesthetic gas reservoirs – the 4-litre reservoir bag of the Elsa machine, and the 2.3-litre manual bag of the Cicero or Megamed machines – are only filled up to 75% of their maximum capacity. Under these conditions, the machine-related gas volume can be assumed to be 5.3 litres on average. Together with a functional residual capacity of 2.5 litres, the volume of the entire gas-filled space adds up to about 7.8 litres. The comparatively high gas volumes contained even in the newer anaesthetic machines result in considerable prolongation of the time constants in case of fresh gas flow reduction.

7.4   Anaesthetic machines with electronically controlled gas delivery systems

A fundamental problem of low flow anaesthetic techniques is the very slow but continuous alteration of the gas composition within the breathing system if the fresh gas flow and composition is maintained over a longer period of time. This is due to the slow but continuous alteration of the uptake of anaesthetic agents and gases during the course of anaesthesia. Even with frequent and careful alterations of the settings at the gas flow controls and the vaporizer, it is hardly possible to adapt the fresh gas volume and its composition precisely to the uptake and leakage loss, especially as all alterations in uptake will only become effective with a significant time delay. By manual control it is' impossible to keep constant the composition of the gas circulating within the breathing system when low flow techniques are performed. Furthermore, the lower the flow the greater is the difference between the gas composition within the breathing system and the fresh gas composition. It is only by clinical experience that the anaesthetist succeeds in setting a suitable fresh gas composition resulting in the desired, though quite different, anaesthetic gas composition which is to be delivered to the patient.

An alternative to the conventional manual operation of the gas flow and vaporizer controls could be the electronic control of gas and vapour supply by closed loop feedback[59-65]. Although this technical concept is already quite well developed, and prototypes have already worked reliably in clinical trials[60-62], there is at present only one anaesthetic machine commercially available realizing electronic control of the gas supply. Two different technical concepts for electronic control of the fresh gas and anaesthetic vapour supply can be distinguished.

Electronic control of the inspired gas composition: The anaesthetist selects the carrier gas composition and dials the flow rate, the desired inspiratory concentrations of both oxygen and the anaesthetic agent as nominal values. According to the actual concentrations, continuously measured in the inspired limb of the patient hose system, the electronic control delivers just these amounts of gases and vapour to precisely establish and maintain the composition of the inspired gas at the desired nominal values. As the gas analyser in this case is an integral part of the control and metering system itself, the machine has to be equipped with a second redundant multi-gas analyser continuously checking the performance of the electronic closed loop feedback control.

The electronic control of the inspired gas composition enables the anaesthetist to set precisely the desired gas composition which shall be delivered to the patient according to the rule 'What you set is what they (the patients) get'. Furthermore, the fresh gas flow rate can be set freely, which may be advantageous if, by intention, a high fresh gas flow is to be used.

An alternative function mode of an electronic gas metering system is the *electronic control of quantitative closed system anaesthesia*: Just those amounts of oxygen, nitrous oxide and volatile anaesthetics taken up by the patient are delivered into the breathing system. The anaesthetist sets the carrier gas composition, the desired inspiratory oxygen and the expiratory anaesthetic concentration as nominal values. The electronic control system delivers just those amounts of gases and vapour needed to quickly establish and maintain the desired gas composition. This mode of electronic control will always deliver only those amounts of gases and vapours that just meet the needs. To quantitatively replace only the gas volumes being consumed by the patient, the electronic control system must be continuously provided with information about the composition and volume of the gas circulating within the system. As the gas analyser again is an integral part of the gas metering system itself, a second gas monitor should supervise its performance.

By this mode of electronic control of the fresh gas supply, quantitative closed system anaesthesia can be performed in routine clinical practice as only the gas and vapour volumes lost via uptake and leakages are replaced. Not only the composition but also the circulating gas volume is kept constant during the course of the anaesthetic procedure.

The gas and vapour consumption is continuously reduced to its utmost minimum, thus rendering it impossible to intentionally work with a certain amount of excess gas as would be advisable, for instance, in cases of smoke and gas intoxication or malignant hyperthermia, or if inhalation anaesthesia is performed using a face mask, which may compromise the exact analysis of the expired gas composition.

7.4.1　PhysioFlex (Dräger Medizintechnik, Lübeck, Germany)

The PhysioFlex anaesthetic machine (Dräger Medizintechnik, Lübeck, Germany) was developed by scientists and engineers of Rotterdam University and the Dutch Physio B.V. under the leadership of W. Erdmann (Figure 7.34a and b). It uses an entirely new technical concept realizing quantitative closed system anaesthesia[65]. The ventilator consists of four membrane chambers connected in parallel, each with a capacity of 625 ml. Depending on the dialled tidal volume, one or several chambers are simultaneously switched into the system. The breathing system itself does not contain any unidirectional valves. Driven by a blower, the anaesthetic gas circulates within the system continuously at a flow of 70 l/min. The membrane chambers are divided into a primary and a secondary compartment by a flexible membrane. If driving gas is fed into the primary compartment of the active membrane chamber, the membrane is pushed towards the other side. The gas contained in the secondary compartment of the membrane chamber is compressed and delivered to the patient. The movement of the metallic membranes is measured capacitively, whereby the ventilation volume is checked. The concentration of oxygen is continuously measured paramagnetically and that of the volatile anaesthetic, of nitrous oxide and carbon dioxide by means of infrared absorption. Oxygen and nitrous oxide are fed into the system via electronically controlled metering systems, whereby the oxygen is proportioned such that the pre-selected oxygen concentration is maintained constant. The volume of nitrous oxide fed into the system is adequate to keep the volume in the breathing system constant. This is verified by capacitive measurement of the expiratory filling of the membrane chambers. The chosen volatile anaesthetic is injected into the system in liquid form by a syringe driven by a stepper motor at such a rate that a desired expiratory concentration is attained rapidly and maintained constant at this level. This mode needs a precise capnographic signal to analyse the expired anaesthetic concentration. Since the anaesthetic gas is circulating continuously within the system, the liquid anaesthetic evaporates quickly so that the gas concentration in the entire system is rapidly equilibrated. A rapid decrease in the anaesthetic concentration is achieved by switching a charcoal filter into the circulating gas (Figure 7.34b: VA filter). If the foreign gas concentration in the system exceeds a value of 10 vol%, a 1-min flushing phase with high fresh gas flow is requested at the monitor.

The time constant of this system is very short due to the technical features mentioned. All data and measured values, including the gas volumes fed into the system, are displayed on a monitor screen and can be transferred for further processing to a computer by means of a communication program via a serial interface. Versichelen and Rolly demonstrated, on the basis of mass spectrometric investigations in clinical use of this anaesthetic machine, that pre-selected anaesthetic gas compositions can reliably be attained and maintained with the aid of the electronically closed loop feedback control[26]. The precise performance of the electronic feedback control system is supervised by a second measurement device, the 'guardian unit'. With the current software version, the anaesthetist is able to switch to a second operation mode. This permits electronic feedback

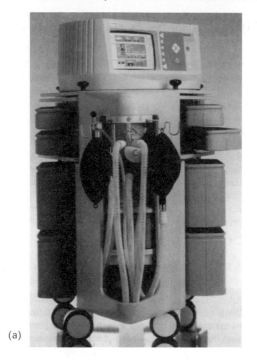

(a)

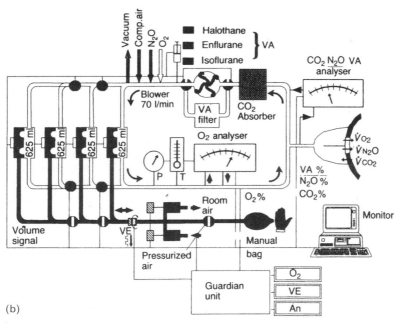

(b)

Figure 7.34   (a) PhysioFlex anaesthetic machine. (b) Flow diagram of the Physio-Flex: anaesthetic machine with closed rebreathing system and electronic closed-loop feedback control of quantitative anaesthetic gas supply. (By courtesy of Dräger Medizintechnik, Lübeck, Germany)

control of the inspired gas composition, in which an excess volume of anaesthetic gas can be supplied to the patient with a flow starting at 1.5 l/min while a pre-selected inspiratory composition of the anaesthetic gas is maintained. This mode is independent of the capnographic signal. In case of gas volume deficiency the flow is automatically increased stepwise to a maximum of 20 l/min. This mode will facilitate the management of all situations in which anaesthetic gas is needed in excess, such as the induction of small children with a face mask, where leakages often are unavoidable.

7.5   Implications for anaesthetic practice. (Table 7.3)

7.5.1   Closed system anaesthesia

Quantitative closed system anaesthesia calls for electronically controlled gas and anaesthetic metering by means of closed loop feedback control.

Until now, this dosage principle is only achieved in the PhysioFlex anaesthetic machine (Dräger Medizintechnik, Lübeck, Germany). Non-quantitative closed system anaesthesia can be performed with all those machines that satisfy the following requirements: the breathing systems must be sufficiently gas tight, flow control systems must permit the accurate adjustment of even the lowest gas flows, vaporizers must work reliably in the low flow range, and comprehensive monitoring of the anaesthetic gas composition must be ensured. These requirements are satisfied, for instance, by the Aestiva 3000, AS/3 ADU, Cato and Cicero EM, Elsa and EAS 9010, Modulus SE and the Megamed anaesthetic machines. Non-quantitative anaesthesia with closed system can be easily performed in routine clinical practice if inhalational anaesthesia without nitrous oxide is performed (see Section 11.3).

7.5.2   Minimal flow anaesthesia

Although the fresh gas flow is reduced to the greatest possible extent in using semi-closed rebreathing systems, minimal flow anaesthesia is performed with a certain excess gas volume and adjustment of standardized fresh gas compositions. This procedure can be adopted in clinical practice without any problems if the following requirements are satisfied: starting with a gas flow of 100 ml/min, oxygen and nitrous oxide must be adjustable in increments of 50 ml, and the flow of already pre-mixed fresh gas to a rate of at least 500 ml/min. Air flow should at least start with a basal flow of 200 ml/min. Furthermore, the vaporizers must work reliably at a flow of 500 ml/min, and the breathing systems must be adequately leakproof. The performance of this technique is considerably facilitated by fresh gas flow compensation of the ventilator and the availability of a gas reservoir, since imbalances in volume can be compensated for and ventilation volume is then independent of the fresh gas flow. These requirements are satisfied by the following anaesthetic machines: Aestiva 3000, AS/3 ADU, Cato, Cicero EM, Elsa, EAS 9010, Fabius, Heyer machines,

Julian, Modulus SE, the Megamed anaesthetic machines, the Siemens Anesthesia Ventilator 711 and the Sulla 909. Besides continuous measurement of inspired oxygen concentration, airway pressure and minute volume, monitoring of the volatile agent concentration within the breathing system should be regarded as indispensable, since accidental overdosage or underdosage of the anaesthetic may be caused by a change from low to high fresh gas flows.

With careful maintenance, the technique can also be adopted for conventional anaesthetic machines like the Sulla 808 V or older type Ohmeda machines. However, this calls for increased vigilance and a sound understanding of the fundamental uptake mechanisms and of the technical function of the anaesthetic machine. Since ventilation is linked to the fresh gas flow by the continuous inflow of fresh gas into the breathing system, and due to the lack of a gas reservoir it needs experience in low flow techniques to safely operate these machines. It is self-evident that the requirements placed on leakproofness must also be satisfied in these machines.

Minimal flow anaesthesia, the low flow technique with the greatest possible flow reduction in the semi-closed use of rebreathing systems, can reliably be performed in clinical practice with the new generation of anaesthetic machines.

7.5.3   Low flow anaesthesia

Low flow anaesthesia, with semi-closed rebreathing systems but with a greater proportion of excess gas volume, should be possible with all appropriately maintained machines, even those of the older generation and conventional technical design.

For the majority of machines, this fresh gas flow corresponds to the range of operation quoted by the manufacturers. The tolerances specified for testing leakproofness during technical inspection and maintenance generally meet the relevant requirements. Continuous measurement of the inspired oxygen concentration, the airway pressure and the minute volume with adjustable alarm limits are indispensable monitoring requirements to guarantee patient safety during the performance of any anaesthetic technique with low fresh gas flow.

Table 7.3   Technical characteristics of anaesthesia machines

	Ventilator	Anaesthetic gas reservoir	Fresh gas flow compensation
Aestiva 3000‡ (Datex–Ohmeda)	Bellows-in-box, ascending and floating bellows arrangement	End-inspiratory volume of the bellows	Ventilator performance adapted to the fresh gas flow
AS/3 ADU‡ (Datex–Engström)	Bellows-in-box, ascending and floating bellows arrangement	End-inspiratory volume of the bellows	Ventilator performance adapted to the fresh gas flow
Cato/Cicero EM‡ (Dräger)	Piston pump ventilator	Manual bag	Fresh gas decoupling valve, discontinuous delivery of the fresh gas
Dogma/Access /Narkomat† (Heyer)	Bellows-in-box, suspended bellows arrangement, actively supported expansion of the bellows[1]	Manual bag	Fresh gas decoupling valve, discontinuous delivery of the fresh gas
Elsa, EAS 9010‡ (Engström)	Bag-in-bottle	End-inspiratory volume of the reservoir bag	Ventilator performance adapted to the fresh gas flow
Fabius†(Dräger)	Piston pump ventilator	Manual bag	Fresh gas decoupling valve, discontinuous delivery of the fresh gas
Julian† (Dräger)	Bellows-in-box, suspended, floating bellows arrangement	End-inspiratory volume of the bellows	Intermittent fresh gas supply only during the expiratory phase
Megamed 700, Mivolan‡ (Megamed)	Bellows-in-box, suspended bellows arrangement, actively supported expansion of the bellows[1]	Manual bag	Fresh gas decoupling valve, discontinuous delivery of the fresh gas
Modulus SE/Excel SE‡ (Ohmeda)	Bellows-in-box, ascending and floating bellows arrangement	End-inspiratory volume of the bellows	Depending on the type of ventilator: 7800: no fresh gas flow compensation 7900: ventilator performance adapted to the fresh gas flow

	Ventilator	Anaesthetic gas reservoir	Fresh gas flow compensation
Narkomed 4* (North American Dräger)	Bellows-in-box, ascending bellows arrangement, expiratory expansion limited to the TV	No	No
SA 2* (Dräger)	Bellows-in-box, suspended bellows arrangement, actively supported expansion of the bellows[1]	Manual bag	Fresh gas decoupling valve, discontinuous delivery of the fresh gas
Servo-Ventilator with circle system* (Siemens)	Bellows-in-box, ascending and floating bellows arrangement	End-inspiratory volume of the bellows	Discontinuous inspiratory delivery of the fresh gas, ventilator performance adapted to the flow
Ventilator 711† (Siemens)	Bag-in-bottle	End-inspiratory volume of the reservoir bag	No
Sulla 800/808* (Dräger)	Bellows-in-box, suspended bellows arrangement, actively supported expansion of the bellows	No	No
Sulla 909† (Dräger)	Bellows-in-box, suspended belows arrangement, actively supported expansion of the bellows[2]	Manual bag	Fresh gas decoupling valve, discontinuous delivery of the fresh gas
Physioflex§ (Dräger)	Membrane chambers	No	Electronically controlled delivery of just that amount of gas needed to maintain the circulating gas volume

[1] Although the expiratory expansion of the suspended bellows is supported by an external force, gas volume deficiency does not result in the development of a negative pressure within the breathing system as the technical concept allows ambient air to entrain the system via an emergency air intake valve.

[2] Although the expiratory expansion of the suspended bellows is supported by an external force, gas volume deficiency does not result in the development of a negative pressure within the breathing system as the technical concept prevents underpressure by corresponding control of the valves.

Suitability of the different machines for low flow anaesthetic techniques: * low flow anaesthesia (1.0 l/min), † low and minimal flow anaesthesia (1.0 and 0.5 l/min), ‡ low-, minimal flow and non-quantitative closed system anaesthesia (1.0, 0.5, 0.2–0.3 l/min), § performance of low flow and quantitative closed system anaesthesia (1.0 l/min, flow equalling total gas uptake).

7.6   References

1. Feigenwinter P, Wallroth CF, Gilly H and Zbinden AM. Normen für Anästhesie, Intensivmedizin und medizinische Versorgungssysteme – Teil 1. *Anästh Intensivmed* 1996; **37**, 587–595.
2. Feigenwinter P, Wallroth CF, Gilly H and Zbinden AM. Normen für Anästhesie, Intensivmedizin und medizinische Versorgungssysteme – Teil 2. *Anästh Intensivmed* 1996; **37**, 644–653.
3. CEN – Comité Européen de Normalisation, ed. Anaesthetic Workstations and their modules – Essential requirements. EN 740. Brussels, 1998.
4. Moyle JTB, Davey A and Ward CS. *Ward's Anaesthetic Equipment*, 4th edn. W. B. Saunders, London, 1998.
5. Ehrenwerth J and Eisenkraft JB. *Anesthesia Equipment. Principles and Applications.* Mosby, St Louis, 1993.
6. Dorsch JA and Dorsch SE. *Understanding Anesthetic Equipment. Construction, Care and Complications*, 3rd. edn. Williams & Wilkins, Baltimore, 1994.
7. Baum J. Technische Voraussetzungen für die Narkoseführung mit reduziertem Frischgasfluß. In Lawin P, van Aken H and Schneider U, eds, *Alternative Methoden der Anästhesie. INA-Schriftenreihe*, Bd. 50. Thieme, Stuttgart, 1985, pp. 43–48.
8. Droh R. Practical application of the closed-circuit system. In Droh R and Spintge R, eds, *Closed-Circuit System and Other Innovations in Anaesthesia.* Springer, Berlin, 1986, pp. 8–12.
9. Götz H and Obermayer A. Wie zuverlässig ist die Narkosegasmessung bei niedrigem Frischgasflow? In Jantzen JPAH and Kleemann PP, eds, *Narkosebeatmung: Low Flow, Minimal Flow, Geschlossenes System.* Schattauer, Stuttgart, 1989, pp. 77–87.
10. Saunders RJ, Calkins JM and Goodin TG. Accuracy of rotameters and linear flowmeters. *Anesthesiology* 1981; **55** (Suppl.), A116.
11. Rügheimer E. Low-flow and closed-circuit anaesthesia. In Dick W, ed., *Kombinationsanästhesie.* Springer, Berlin, 1985, pp. 116–135.
12. Frankenberger H and Wallroth CF. Technische Konzeptionen für ein geschlossenes Narkosesystem. In *Geschlossenes System für Inhalationsnarkosen*, Internationales Symposium, Düsseldorf, 7–8 May 1982 (abstract).
13. Philip JH. Closed circuit anesthesia. In Ehrenwerth J and Eisenkraft JB, eds, *Anesthesia Equipment: Principles and Applications.* Mosby, St Louis 1993, pp. 617–635.
14. Drägerwerk AG, Lübeck: Bedienungsanleitungen (instructions for use).
    - Anästhesie-Ventilator AV 1. GA 5162, May 1989.
    - Cicero, Integrierter Narkose-Arbeitsplatz, GA 5131.001, July 1991.
    - Cicero EM, Integrierter Narkose-Arbeitsplatz, GA 5131.100 d, April, 1994.
    - Julian, Narkosegerät, GA 5132.000 d, October, 1996.
    - Kreissytem 8 ISO. GA 5371, September, 1989.
    - Ergänzung 'Geschlossenes System' zur Gebrauchsanweisung 5371 Kreissystem 8 ISO, October 1989.
    - Narkosemittelverdampfer Vapor 19. GA 5327.0, January 1983.
    - Narkosemittelverdampfer Vapor 19.n. GA 5327.0, April 1986.
    - Narkosemittelverdampfer Vapor 19.n. GA 5327.0, March 1991.
    - Narkosespiromat 650. GA 5161, October 1972.
    - Narkosespiromat 656. GA 5161.1, June 1985.
    - Pulmomat 19 (19.1, 19.3). GA 5323, June 1977.
    - SA 2/RA 2 Inhalation Anaesthetic Machine, GA 5152 e, November 1992.
    - Sulla 808 M/V/MV, Inhalationsnarkosegerät. GA 5191.3, October 1989.
    - Möglichkeit zur Dosierung kleiner Frischgasmengen. Beilage zu den

Gebrauchsanweisungen Sulla 808 V (GA 5191.3) und Sulla 808 V-D (GA 5191.31), May 1988.
- Ventilog und Ventilog 2, Narkosebeatmungsgeräte. GA 5324.0, March 1990.
- Ventilog 3, Narkosebeatmungsgerät, GA 5324.100 d, June 1992.
15. Siemens-Elema AB, Solna: Instructions for Use.
- Servo Anesthesia System (Servo Anesthesia Circle 985)
- Siemens vaporiser 950–952.
16. Rushman GB, Davies NJH and Atkinson RS. *A Short History of Anaesthesia.* Butterworth-Heinemann, Oxford, 1996, pp. 56–57.
17. Frankenberger H, Seidel P and Eichler J. Optimierung eines Narkosemittel-verdunsters für die Inhalationsnarkose. Jahrestagung der DGAW, Lübeck-Travemünde, 7–8 October 1976. Drägerwerk AG, Lübeck 1976.
18. Züchner K, Raffauf EM and Sonntag H. Genauigkeit von Halothanverdampfern unter praxisnahen Betriebsbedingungen. *Anaesthesist* 1983; **32** (Suppl.), 174.
19. Gilly H. Zur Brauchbarkeit herkömmlicher Verdampfer bei Minimal flow. In Jantzen JPAH and Kleemann PP, eds, *Narkosebeatmung: Low Flow, Minimal Flow, Geschlossenes System.* Schattauer, Stuttgart 1989, pp. 67–76.
20. Graham SG. The Desflurane Tec 6 vaporiser. *Br J Anaesth* 1994; **72**, 470–473.
21. Weiskopf RB, Sampson D and Moore MA. The desflurane (Tec 6) vaporiser: design, considerations and performance evaluation. *Br J Anaesth* 1994; **72**, 474–479.
22. Kayser D, Khodja M and Marguerite G. Delivery by a TEC 6 (TM) vaporiser of desflurane vapour above the dialled-in concentration. *Ann Fran Anesth Reanim* 1999; **18**, 691–693.
23. Gambro–Engström AB, Bromma:
- Engström Elsa Anesthesia System, users instructions, May 1988;
- Engström EAS 9020 Ansthesiesystem, Gebrauchsanweisung.
24. Rathgeber J. *Praxis der maschinellen Beatmung*, 2. Aufl. MCN-Verlag, Nürnberg, 1999.
25. Sticher J, Müller M, Zeidler D, Jung HJ and Hempelmann G. Unbeabsichtigte Narkosegasüberdosierung bei den Narkoserespiratoren Servo 900C und D. *Anästhesiol Intensivmed Notfallmed Schmerzther* 1994; **29**, 163–164.
26. Versichelen L and Rolly G. Mass-spectrometric evaluation of some recently introduced low flow, closed circuit systems. *Acta Anaesth Belg* 1990; **41**, 225–237.
27. Hargasser S, Hipp R, Breinbauer B, Mielke L, Entholzner E and Rust M. A lower solubility recommends the use of desflurane more than isoflurane, halothane and enflurane under low-flow conditions. *J Clin Anesth* 1995; **7**, 49–53.
28. Baum J, Berghoff M, Stanke HG, Petermeyer M and Kalff G. Niedrig-flußnarkosen mit Desfluran. *Anaesthesist* 1997; **46**, 287–293.
29. Lockwood GG, Kadim MY, Chakrabarty MK and Whitwam JG. Clinical use of small soda lime canister in a low-flow to-and-fro system. *Anaesthesia* 1992; **47**, 568–573.
30. Megamed AG, Cham. Gebrauchsanweisung Megamed 700. Version AH007, February 1989.
31. Leuenberger M, Feigenwinter P and Zbinden AM. Gas leakage in eight anaesthesia circle systems. *Eur J Anaesthesiol* 1992; **9**, 121–127.
32. Amt für Arbeitsschutz. Merkblatt für den Umgang mit Narkosegasen. Hansestadt Hamburg, August 1990, p. 8.
33. Spintge R and Droh R. The absolutely tight circuit system and the problem of excess humidity. In Droh R, Erdmann W and Spintge R, eds, *Anaesthesia – Innovations in Management.* Springer, Berlin, 1985, pp. 44–45.

34. Baum J. Clinical applications of low flow and closed circuit anaesthesia. *Acta Anaesth Belg* 1990; **41**, 239–247.

35. Oeking R and Weis KH. Zur Sauerstoffkonzentration im Narkosekreissystem. II. Mitteilung: Abhängigkeit vom Typ des Kreissystems. *Anaesthesist* 1973; **22**, 202–206.

36. Zbinden AM, Feigenwinter P and Hutmacher M. Fresh gas utilization of eight circle systems. *Br J Anaesth* 1991; **67**, 492–499.

37. Barth L and Meyer M. CO_2 absorption. In Barth L, Meyer M, eds, *Moderne Narkose* 2nd edn, Fischer, Stuttgart, 1965, pp. 194–209.

38. Gootjes P and Lagerweij E. Quality comparison of different CO_2 absorbents. *Anaesthesist* 1981; **30**, 261–264.

39. Paravicini D, Henning K and Vietor G. Vergleichende Untersuchungen von verschiedenen Atemkalksorten. *Anästh Intensivther Notfallmed* 1982; **17**, 98–101.

40. Wulf R, Siegel E and Wezurek H. Drägersorb 800: Der Indikator-Atemkalk in Pillenform. *Medizintechnik aktuell* 1991; **1**, 10–14.

41. Baum J, Enzenauer J, Krausse Th and Sachs G. Atemkalk – Nutzungsdauer, Verbrauch und Kosten in Abhängigkeit vom Frischgasfluß. *Anaesthesiol Reanimat* 1993; **18**, 108–113.

42. Oehmig H. Atemkalk '85/86'. *Anästh Intensivmed* 1986; **27**, 397–399.

43. Baum J. Atemkalk: Hinweise zu korrektem Umgang und fachgerechter Nutzung. Stellungnahme der Kommission für Normung und technische Sicherheit der DGAI. *Anästh Intensivmed* 1999; **40**, 507–509.

44. Lotz P, Siegel E and Spilker D. *Grundbegriffe der Beatmung*. GIT Verlag Ernst Giebeler, Darmstadt, 1984.

45. Cicman J, Himmelwright H, Skibo V and Yoder J. *Operating Principles of Narkomed Anesthesia Systems*. North American Dräger, Telford, 1993.

46. Baum J and Schneider U. Die Brauchbarkeit verschiedener Narkosebeatmungsgeräte für die Minimal-Flow-Anästhesie. *Anästh Intensivmed* 1983; **24**, 263–269.

47. Baum J. Niedrigflußnarkosen mit dem Beatmungsgerät Ventilog 2. *Anaesthesist* 1998; **47**, 361–364.

48. Klement W and Stühmeier K. Gefahren bei Beatmungsgeräten ohne Reservoir schon bei mittlerem Frischgasflow? *Anaesthesist* 1989; **38** (Suppl. 1), 126.

49. Spieß W. Narkose im geschlossenen System mit kontinuierlicher inspiratorischer Sauerstoffmessung. *Anaesthesist* 1977; **26**, 503–513.

50. Lowe HJ and Ernst EA. *The Quantitative Practice of Anesthesia*. Williams & Wilkins, Baltimore, 1981.

51. Aldrete JA, Adolph AJ, Hanna LM, Farag HA and Ghaemmaghami M. Fresh gas flow rate and I:E ratio affect tidal volume in anaesthesia ventilators. In van Ackern K, Frankenberger H, Konecny E, and Steinbereithner K, eds, *Quantitative Anaesthesia. Anaesthesiology and Intensive Care Medicine*, vol. 204. Springer, Berlin, 1989, pp. 72–80.

52. Baum J and Sachs G. Frischgasflow und Narkosebeatmung – Technische Voraussetzungen für die adäquate Nutzung von Rückatemsystemen. *Anästh Intensivther Notfallmed* 1990; **25**, 72–78.

53. Bund M and Kirchner E. Respiratorbedingte Veränderungen der Beatmungsparameter bei Reduktion des Frischgasflusses. *Anästh Intensivmed* 1991; **32**, 179–183.

54. Rathgeber J. Narkosegeräte und -Respiratoren. *Anaesthesist* 1993; **42**, 885–909.

55. Datex–Ohmeda. Aestiva 3000 Operation Manual, part 1 and 2, Madison, 1999.

56. Peters JWB, Bezstarosti J, Van Eeden J, Erdmann W and Meursing AEE. Safety and efficacy of semi-closed circle ventilation in small infants. *Paediatr Anaesth* 1998; **8**, 299–304.

57. Euliano TY, van Oostrom JH and van der Aa J. Waste gas monitor reduces wasted volatile anesthetic. *J Clin Monit Comput* 1999, **15**, 287–293.

58. Bergmann B. Feldforschung: Anästhesie im Feldlazarett – humanitärer Militäreinsatz im Kosovo. *Medizintechnik aktuell* 1999, 3/99, 6–7.

59. Von dem Hagen T and Kleinschmidt L. Principles of low flow measurement for closed-circuit systems. In Droh R, Erdmann W and Spintge R, eds, *Anaesthesia – Innovations in Management*. Springer, Berlin, 1985, pp. 10–15.

60. Schepp RM, Erdmann W, Westerkamp B and Faithful NS. Automatic ventilation during closed circuit anaesthesia. In Droh R, Erdmann W and Spintge R, eds, *Anaesthesia – Innovations in Management*. Springer, Berlin 1985, pp. 48–53.

61. Spain JA, Jannett TC and Ernst EA. The Alabama automated closed-circuit anesthesia project. In Brown BR, Calkins JL and Saunders RJ, eds, *Future Anesthesia Delivery Systems*. F. A. Davies Company, Philadelphia, 1984, pp. 177–183.

62. Wallroth CF, Jaklitsch R and Wied HA. Technical realisation of quantitative metering and ventilation. In van Ackern K, Frankenberger H, Konecny E and Steinbereithner K, eds, *Quantitative Anaesthesia. Anaesthesiology and Intensive Care Medicine*, vol. 204. Springer, Berlin, 1989, pp. 94–108.

63. Westenskow DR, Jordan WS and Gehmlich DS. Electronic feedback control and measurement of oxygen consumption during closed circuit anaesthesia. In Aldrete JA, Lowe HJ and Virtue RW, eds, *Low Flow and Closed System Anesthesia*. Grune & Stratton, New York, 1979, pp. 135–146.

64. Westenskow DR and Wallroth CF. Closed-loop control for anesthesia breathing systems. *J Clin Monit* 1990; **6**, 249–256.

65. Physio B.V. PhysioFlex, Gesloten Anaesthesie Ventilator. Physio Medical Systems, Hoofddorp, 1990.

66. White D and Royston B. Respiratory feedback effects on vaporisers in circle systems. *Anaesthesia*, 1998; **53**, 555–559.

67. Brosnan S, Royston B and White D. Isoflurane concentrations using uncompensated vaporisers within circle systems. *Anaesthesia*, 1998; **53**, 560–564.

68. Wright D, Brosnan S, Royston B and White D. Controlled ventilation using isoflurane with an in-circle vaporiser. *Anaesthesia*, 1998; **53**, 650–653.

69. Liu EHC and Dhara SS. Sevoflurane anaesthesia with an Oxford Miniature Vaporizer in vaporizer inside circle mode. *Br J Anaesth*, 1999; **82**, 557–560.

70. Stayer SA, Bent ST, Campos CJ, Skjonsby BS and Andropoulos DB. Comparison of NAD 6000 and Servo 900C ventilators in an infant lung model. *Anesth Analg* 2000; **90**, 315–321.

Monitoring

8.1 Technical regulations: safety facilities for inhalation anaesthetic machines

The comments on monitoring will deal primarily with the monitoring of the gas composition in the breathing system. Here, at this interface between patient and anaesthetic machine[1], changes, determined essentially by the fresh gas composition and the patient's uptake, can be observed. While with high flow, the gas composition within the breathing system can be estimated easily from the composition of the fresh gas, this becomes more difficult with lower fresh gas flows[2]. That is why the question arises as to whether additional monitoring devices are required to guarantee patient safety during the performance of low flow anaesthesia.

Independent of the fresh gas flow selection, routine monitoring of the patient and the performance of the machine is obligatory and provided by respective technical regulations, recommendations of scientific and professional organizations and relevant teachings[3-11]. Among other issues, they comprise permanent clinical observation of the electrocardiogram, regular checks on circulation, measurement of the airway pressure and the expired tidal or minute volume (Table 8.1).

According to regulations in the countries of the European Union and in the USA, continuous monitoring of the inspired oxygen concentration is mandatory[3,4,10]. With the new European standard EN 740 monitoring of the anaesthetic agent concentration also became indispensable. In addition, continuous monitoring of the expired carbon dioxide concentration is required. Thus, at least in the countries of the European Union, comprehensive monitoring of the anaesthetic gas composition, as it is already provided for in the modern generation of anaesthetic workstations, has become the obligatory safety standard for inhalation anaesthetic machines[5].

8.2 Main- and side-stream gas analysers

The analysis of gas concentrations by locating the sensor directly in the breathing system or patient hosing is referred to as main-stream

Table 8.1   Safety facilities of inhalation anaesthetic machines

Safety facilities					
Oxygen shortage signal	A	B		D	
Nitrous oxide cut-off	A	B		D	
Oxygen ratio controller		B		D	
Monitoring of equipment function					
Airway pressure with disconnection and obstruction alarm	A	B		D	E
Expired gas volume	(A)	B	C	D	E
Inspired oxygen concentration	A	B	C	D	E
Volatile anaesthetic concentration		B	C	D	E
Carbon dioxide concentration	(A)	B	C	D	(E)
Monitoring of physiological parameters					
Stethoscope			C	D	
ECG	A		C	D	
Blood pressure measurement	A		C	D	
Temperature measurement	(A)		C	(D)	
Pulse oximetry	(A)		C	D	

A: Recommendations given by internationally recognized professional bodies[21].
B: Common European Technical Standard EN 740[5].
C: Recommendations on standard monitoring by Whitcher *et al.*[9]
D: Guidelines by DGAI (German Association for Anaesthesia and Intensive Care Medicine) and BDA (professional organization of the German anaesthetists)[8].
E: Special recommendations on monitoring for safe performance of anaesthesia with a fresh gas flow equal to or less than 1 l/min [12–15].

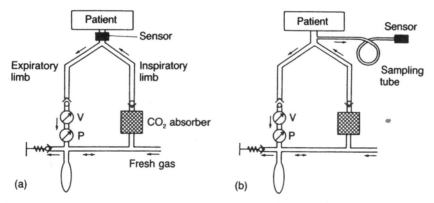

Figure 8.1   Position of sensors for measurement of gas concentrations: (a) measurement directly in the gas stream = main-stream measurement; (b) measurement by withdrawing sampling gas out of the system = side-stream measurement. (From Pockrand[16], by permission)

measurement (Figure 8.1a and b). The advantage of this method is that gas concentrations are measured directly in the stream of the respired gases, and may be displayed without any significant delay if the electronic response time of the device is correspondingly low. However, placement of the sensor directly on to the tube connector is rather involved in daily clinical routine. Due to hygiene regulations, parts of the sensor contaminated by the exhaled gas have to be replaced with each patient, or single use bacterial filters have to be used. In addition, the weight of the mainstream sensor is liable to displace the tube, whereby the free passage of breathing gas may be impaired.

For measurement with the side-stream technique, the gas sample is sucked out of the breathing system and passed to a separate measuring device via a tube. In general, the sample is taken from a point between the tube connector and the Y-piece of the patient hose system. This simple technique can generally be undertaken without any problems during daily clinical practice.

It must be considered on the other hand that, depending on the sampling flow and the dimensions of the sampling hose, alterations of the gas composition in the system may be indicated at the display of the monitor only after a certain time delay. In addition, the amplitude and the characteristics of the measured signal may be subjected to considerable changes by the passage of sampling gas through the hose[16,17].

8.2.1   Return of sampling gas

When a side-stream measuring device is used during low flow anaesthesia, the sampling gas should be returned into the expiratory limb of the breathing system after the measuring procedure is completed. Otherwise, the loss of sampling gas may result in a volume shortage in the system, especially if the sampling gas flow is higher than 100 ml/min and the fresh gas flow about 500 ml/min. If conventional circle absorber systems are used, this can be accomplished by using special connectors. A 30 μm bacterial filter should be connected into the gas return tube to preclude contamination. Within the range of normal airway pressure, the change in pressure at the sampling gas outlet resulting from controlled ventilation has very little influence on the measurement. But even so, some gas analysers are fitted with pressure compensation; for example, the Datex monitors (Datex, Helsinki, Finland) or the PM 8020, 8050 and 8060 monitors (Dräger Medizintechnik, Lübeck, Germany).

Another aspect needs to be considered if sampling gas is returned into the system. If the sampling gas is subject to a measuring technique which alters the molecular structure of the gas, for instance ultraviolet absorption or mass spectrometry, it is self-evident that this gas should not be returned into the breathing system.

Paramagnetic measurement of oxygen concentration calls for simultaneous reference measurement with a gas of known oxygen content. The Datex multi-gas analysers (Datex, Helsinki, Finland), for instance, work with a sampling gas flow of 200 ml/min and, in addition, need approximately 30 ml/min of ambient air as reference gas. Having passed the measurement device, both the sampling and the reference gas are returned together into the breathing system. Using extremely low fresh gas flows, this additional supply of ambient air into the system results in a slow accumulation of nitrogen.

Accumulation of nitrogen within the breathing system can also be

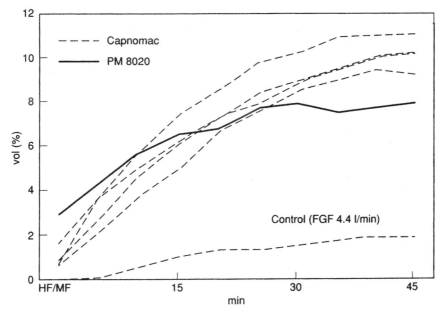

Figure 8.2   Accumulation of foreign gases (nitrogen, water vapour and trace gases) during performance of minimal flow anaesthesia with return of sampling gas. HF/ MF, time of flow reduction. Measurements performed with a Capnomac gas analyser (Datex, Helsinki, Finland) on different groups of patients with the AV 1, Elsa, Megamed 700 and Sulla 800 anaesthetic machines. The measurement with the PM 8020 gas analyser (Dräger Medizintechnik, Lübeck, Germany) was performed at the Cicero anaesthetic workstation. Note: in the control group the high fresh gas flow is maintained during the whole course of anaesthesia

observed with low flow anaesthesia if the measuring system is intermittently calibrated with ambient air. The Dräger monitors 8020, 8050 and 8060 (Dräger Medizintechnik, Lübeck, Germany), for instance, are calibrated with ambient air every 5–10 min during the first 30 min, and thereafter every 30 min at a rate of 150 ml/min (Figure 8.2). The present author cannot agree totally with the recommendation of Bengtson et al.[18], not to return the sampling gas to the breathing system during low flow anaesthesia, in order to avoid nitrogen accumulation. Whereas this recommendation may be acceptable in low flow anaesthesia, in which an excess gas volume of about 600 ml/min is used, in minimal flow anaesthesia the additional loss of the sampling gas into the scavenging system inevitably will result in gas volume deficiency within the breathing system and corresponding alterations of ventilatory patterns. If nitrogen accumulation results in a significant change of the anaesthetic gas composition, a short wash-out phase using high fresh gas flow over a period of about 5 min should be carried out. A sampling gas return device, in general, is a technical feature of most modern anaesthetic workstations, already equipped with multi-gas analysers by the manufacturer.

8.3   Measurement of oxygen concentration

If low flow anaesthesia is performed, it has to be considered that the lower the fresh gas flow, the greater will be the difference between its oxygen concentration and the concentration of oxygen within the breathing system (see Section 3.1). Furthermore, it must be borne in mind that, with the increase of the rebreathing fraction, the inspired oxygen concentration is determined to a considerably greater extent by the patient's individual oxygen consumption than in high flow anaesthesia. These are the reasons why continuous monitoring of oxygen concentration in the breathing system is indispensable to ensure patient safety if anaesthesia is performed with low fresh gas flows[19].

All the various methods of oxygen concentration measurement may be applied. Older types of oxygen monitors fitted with galvanic or polarographic cells, featuring a response time between 5 and 20 s, were essentially slower than newer devices using paramagnetic, magneto-acoustic or mass spectrometric measurement with a response time between 100 and 450 ms. There are now fuel cells available with a response time as low as 500 ms. Nevertheless, extended response times do not impair safety in any way, since concentration changes in the breathing system with low flow anaesthesia only proceed with considerable time delays. Electrochemical methods of oxygen concentration measurement, however, may be affected by humidity, but this problem can be solved by means of humidity condensors and water traps. The measuring accuracy of 1–2% by volume, which is unanimously quoted for all the different methods, is quite adequate to satisfy clinical requirements.

All measuring techniques which feature adequately short response times, for instance the oxygen measurement based on the paramagnetic properties of oxygen molecules, are likely to resolve the measured signal into the inspired and expired values. By the additional measurement of expired oxygen concentration, it is possible to evaluate the efficiency of nitrogen wash-out during pre-oxygenation and to recognize early the development of hypoxia caused by hypoventilation during the emergence phase. Nevertheless, the expired oxygen concentration is not a reliable parameter for evaluating the oxygen consumption, since it is determined to a large extent by the actual nitrous oxide uptake. This is why, following adequate denitrogenation with pure oxygen, the admixture of nitrous oxide results in the following phenomenon: because of the initially high alveolar nitrous oxide uptake, the expired oxygen concentration is higher than the inspired. It takes a period of about 20 min of normoventilation to attain the physiological inspired–expired oxygen difference of 4.5 vol% (Figure 8.3). With a view to patient safety, continuous monitoring of inspired oxygen concentration alone can be regarded as appropriate. In the particular case of anaesthesia with very low fresh gas flow, a reduction in the expired oxygen concentration can clearly be recognized from the distinct simultaneous decrease of the inspired oxygen concentration (see Section 3.1).

Finally, it is emphasized again that continuous monitoring of oxygen concentration is an absolute necessity during anaesthesia with reduced

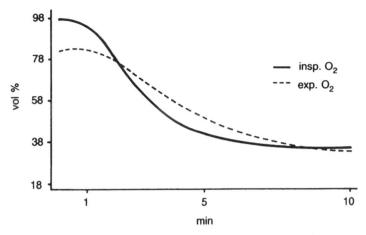

Figure 8.3   Inspired and expired oxygen concentrations during wash-in of nitrous oxide–oxygen mixture (32% O_2, 68% N_2O) after sufficient pre-oxygenation. During the first 10 min the expired oxygen concentration is higher than the inspired due to the initial high nitrous oxide uptake

fresh gas flows. This is already provided by technical standards or recommendations of the scientific societies of several countries, which all demand inhalational anaesthesia machines to be equipped with this safety device.

8.4   Measurement of volatile anaesthetic concentration

The concentration of inhalational anaesthetics can be measured by way of mass spectrometry, crystal oscillometry, infrared absorption, photoacoustic and Raman spectrometry[15,17,20,21]. All these different approaches are employed in clinical practice, but photoacoustic spectrometry and infrared absorption have become the standard clinical methods. Interference by nitrous oxide, carbon dioxide and water vapour can be readily compensated for, and the accuracy of ±0.15% by volume, which is quoted for the majority of measurement devices, is absolutely acceptable for clinical use[14]. However, crystal oscillometry in the main stream (EMMA, Engström, Bromma, Sweden) has not proved to be satisfactory because of its great sensitivity with respect to humidity[22,23]. Where the Servo Gas Monitor 120 (Siemens–Elema, Solna, Sweden) is concerned, a side-stream analyser using the same measurement technique, the cross-sensitivity to water vapour could be considerably reduced. With respect to drift and precision, this unit is also suitable for use in low flow anaesthesia.

The difference between the anaesthetic concentration in the fresh gas and that in the breathing system increases with reduction of the fresh flow (see Section 5.2). With extremely low fresh gas flows, repeated change of anaesthetic fresh gas concentration and repeated flow variation, it is virtually impossible, even for an anaesthetist experienced in low flow techniques, to estimate precisely the anaesthetic concentration in the breathing system. On the other hand, even drastic changes of the anaesthetic concentration in the fresh gas cause only extremely slow changes in the breathing system's gas composition, which can be attributed to the long time constant in low flow anaesthesia. Thus, the risk of accidental over- or underdosage of the inhalational anaesthetic is distinctly lower than with high flow anaesthesia. Anaesthesia with low fresh gas flow in particular allows for an ample period of time to adjust the depth of anaesthesia according to the clinical state of the patient.

An obvious safety problem is encountered in making a change from low to high fresh gas flow. With low fresh gas flow, considerably higher concentrations of volatile anaesthetic in the fresh gas are used than with high fresh gas flow. In changing from low to high flow, the fresh gas concentration of the volatile anaesthetic has to be reduced and thus adapted to the modified condition, since otherwise the concentration of the anaesthetic in the system will increase rapidly and drastically. On the other hand, there is the risk of accidental underdosage if the concentration of the inhalational anaesthetic is not appropriately increased in the case of a reduction of fresh gas flow. Accidental incorrect dosage resulting from changes in the fresh gas flow can only be detected sufficiently early if the anaesthetic concentration in the breathing system is measured and monitored continuously[13,24].

The use of a vaporizer inside the circle (VIC) has always been proscribed during controlled ventilation on account of the potential for drastic rises in vapour concentration. The advent of agent analysers invites the reappraisal of this technique but, as these vaporizers are not (and cannot be) calibrated, it must be accepted that the monitor has to be considered part of the metering system itself. For safety reasons, gas monitoring should be supervised by a second monitoring device. The same statement holds equally for the use of a single analyser during direct injection of liquid agent. This is acknowledged by the inclusion of a guardian unit in the PhysioFlex anaesthetic machine (Dräger Medizintechnik, Lübeck, Germany) as a safety back-up device.

8.4.1   Should anaesthetic agent measurement be performed in the fresh gas or in the breathing system?

There are two alternatives for monitoring inhalational anaesthetics: either the anaesthetic concentration in the breathing system or its fresh gas concentration can be measured. Monitoring the anaesthetic concentration in the breathing system is the only way of precluding false dosage resulting from machine malfunction or handling errors[13]. Measuring in the fresh gas will definitely afford less safety, since only the vaporizer function and adjustment are monitored but not the actual dosage of the inhalational anaesthetic. After all, the technical component by means of which inhalational anaesthetics are really dosed is actually the breathing system. This is where the anaesthetic mixture supplied to the patient is composed in a complex process, determined by the technical design and functional state of the breathing system, the fresh gas flow and the uptake.

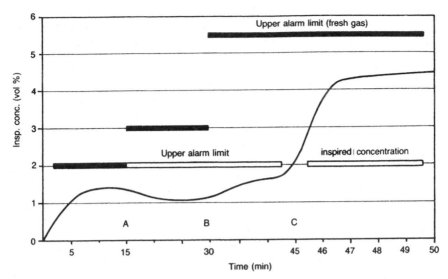

Figure 8.4 Simultaneous monitoring of volatile anaesthetic concentration in the fresh gas and in the breathing system. Only if the concentration within the breathing system is measured will it be possible to adjust the alarm limits independently of the fresh gas flow. Only application of this technique will ensure reliable detection of accidental overdose. (Curve, inspired isoflurane concentration; bars, adjustment of the upper alarm limits). (From Baum[13])

The resultant safety problem shall be explained by an example. A 75 kg patient is anaesthetized with isoflurane via a rebreathing system, whereby the isoflurane concentration is continuously and simultaneously measured and monitored in the fresh gas as well as in the inspiratory limb of the breathing system. At the beginning of anaesthesia, the upper alarm limit of both systems is set to 2% (Figure 8.4).

With a fresh gas flow of 4.4 l/min, the isoflurane concentration is initially set to 1.5 vol%. After 15 min, the flow is reduced to 0.5 l/min, while at the same time the anaesthetic concentration is increased to 2.5 vol% (A). After a period of 30 min, the clinical situation calls for a deeper level of anaesthesia, so that the fresh gas isoflurane concentration is increased to 5 vol% but the flow is left unchanged (B). Due to the long time constant of the system, the changes of the inspired isoflurane concentration proceed very slowly and moderately. The upper alarm limit of 2.0 vol% of the device, monitoring the agent concentration in the breathing system, can be maintained independent of the fresh gas flow selected. On the other hand, the alarm limit of the device, monitoring the fresh gas concentration, has to be adjusted according to the newly dialled fresh gas concentration. This means that at flow reduction the alarm limit has to be increased to 3.0 vol% (A) and at point B to as high as 5.5 vol%.

Emergence from anaesthesia is induced after 45 min by increasing the fresh gas flow to 4.0 l/min (C). Assume that the vaporizer is accidentally left at a setting of 5 vol%. The resulting rapid increase of the inspired anaesthetic concentration to almost 5.0 vol% will only be recognized instantly by continuous monitoring of the inspired concentration. On the other hand, the device monitoring the fresh gas concentration will not warn of the danger of overdosage. This example demonstrates convincingly that only by monitoring the anaesthetic concentration in the breathing system can comprehensive protection against accidental misdosage be achieved. Only if this technique is adopted can the alarm limits be adjusted independently of the fresh gas flow.

As most anaesthetic incidents are based on inappropriate human behaviour and decisions, and not on actual malfunction of the equipment[25,26], misdosage resulting from handling errors should preferably be detected by the monitoring techniques employed. And last but not least, only continuous measurement of the anaesthetic agent concentration in the breathing system significantly facilitates safe and judicious performance of low flow anaesthesia[24].

8.5   Measurement of nitrous oxide concentration

The question of whether the concentration of nitrous oxide should also be monitored continuously is controversial. It is obvious that an overdose of nitrous oxide is precluded by continuous monitoring of the inspired oxygen concentration. Therefore, additional measurement of nitrous oxide concentration seems to be unnecessary. However, misdosage of nitrous oxide cannot always be reliably detected by merely measuring the oxygen concentration. In some anaesthetic machines, featuring active support of the expiratory filling of the ventilator with gas, entrance of ambient air is effected via a special emergency air intake valve (Dräger AS 2 and Fabius, Heyer anaesthesia machines, Megamed anaesthesia machines). In case of gas volume deficiency in the breathing system, the opening of such an emergency air intake valve will make good the gas volume deficit and so prevent possible alterations of the ventilatory patterns in spite of inadequate fresh gas supply. This entrainment of room air may result in significant decrease not only of the nitrous oxide but also the oxygen concentration. In this context, however, a case of considerable decrease of nitrous oxide concentration will be demonstrated which could only be detected by monitoring of the nitrous oxide concentration, as the oxygen concentration remained constant in spite of significant air entrainment (Figure 8.5).

In addition, the accumulation of foreign gas, especially nitrogen, which may be observed in low flow anaesthesia (see Figure 8.2), can only be assessed by additional measurement of the nitrous oxide concentration[15,24]. The proportion of foreign gas can then be calculated from the difference of the sum of all measured inspired gas concentrations (oxygen, nitrous oxide, inhalational anaesthetic) to 100 vol%. The content of water vapour in the inspired gas which, depending on the gas temperature, ranges between 2.3 and 4 vol%[17], is ignored in this calculation. During performance of long-term anaesthesia with extremely low fresh gas flows and return of the sampling gas (see Section 8.2.1), the proportion of foreign gas is liable to rise to values greater than 15 vol%. If the nitrous

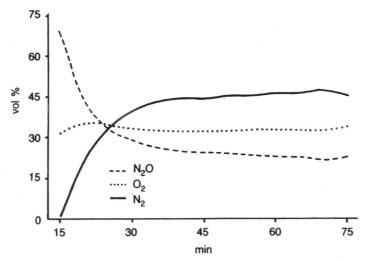

Figure 8.5 Entrainment of room air into the breathing system via an emergency air intake valve during minimal flow anaesthesia due to inappropriate adjustment of the excess gas discharge valve (Megamed 700 anaesthetic machine, Megamed, Cham, Switzerland). In the depicted case, this error in operating the machine can only be detected by means of nitrous oxide concentration measurement, as the oxygen concentration remains stable. (Patient aged 60 years, weight 68 kg, height 1.60 m)

oxide concentration is too low, due to the admixture of foreign gases, the system may be flushed for 2–5 min with a high fresh gas flow. This procedure eliminates the foreign gas from the breathing system and the nitrous oxide concentration can be re-established at the nominal value.

8.6   Measurement of carbon dioxide concentration

In clinical practice, the infrared absorption technique is the most commonly used method for the measurement of carbon dioxide concentration. Both main-stream and side-stream analysers are available. Both capnometry and capnography add considerably to the improvement of patient safety, since this parameter provides considerable information about the patient and the anaesthetic machine[26,27]. However, every alteration of this complex information needs careful and comprehensive analysis[28]. It is self-evident that this analysis also requires detailed knowledge of possible flow-specific artefacts.

8.6.1   Flow-specific artefacts of the capnogram

If gas taken directly from the Y-piece is analysed, the reduction of the fresh gas flow is liable to cause contamination of the expired gas with inspiratory gas. This phenomenon may be observed if controlled ventilation is performed with conventional anaesthetic machines featuring constant flow of fresh gas into the system and hanging bellows, which

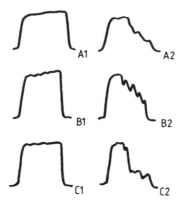

Figure 8.6 Artificial changes in configuration of capnographic curves due to fresh gas flow reduction: with high flow of 4.4 l/min, typical waveform with ascending plateau (A1, B1, C1); after flow reduction to 0.5 l/min, descending curve during exhalation without a plateau (A2, B2, C2). Records taken during the use of a conventional anaesthetic machine with continuous supply of fresh gas into the breathing system and hanging bellows

are actively expanded during expiration[27,29]. The capnograph curves may not show the typical waveform with a slightly ascending expiratory plateau. On the contrary, the curves tend to descend during the course of exhalation without having formed a distinct plateau. Mostly the capnograph curves then show superimposed cardiogenic oscillations (Figure 8.6). These artificial changes of the capnograms result from the fact that the reduction of the fresh gas flow results in an increase of initial negative expiratory pressure, generated by the descending bellows, with corresponding changes in the gas flow at the Y-piece. The changes may be accentuated by a high sampling gas flow in case of side-stream anaesthetic gas measurement, but they may also occur in main-stream capnography.

Correspondingly, the arterial–end-expiratory partial pressure difference of carbon dioxide ($aeDCO_2$) increases in both side- and main-stream measurement. The $aeDCO_2$ is the difference between the arterial carbon dioxide partial pressure ($PaCO_2$), obtained by blood gas analysis, and the end-expiratory carbon dioxide partial pressure ($PeCO_2$), calculated from the expired carbon dioxide concentration. In patients who are not suffering from pulmonary disease, this value increases by about 3 mmHg (Figure 8.7). The $aeDCO_2$ is a measure of the alveolar dead space ventilation and under normal physiological conditions amounts to about 4 mmHg[30]. In a considerable number of diseases causing imbalances of the lung's ventilation perfusion ratio[30,31], this value is increased, which also applies if gas free from carbon dioxide is admixed to the expired gas[32,33]. On the contrary, the $aeDCO_2$ decreases with forced ventilation[30]. If, during performance of low flow anaesthesia, a defined arterial carbon dioxide partial pressure shall be adjusted precisely by capnometry, the $PaCO_2$ should be established by blood gas analysis only if the flow has already been reduced. The $PeCO_2$ should be measured at the same time and the $aeDCO_2$, specific to the given low flow condition, can then be calculated

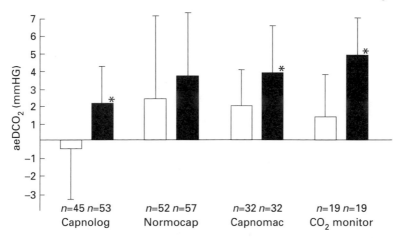

Figure 8.7 Increase of the arterial–end-expiratory carbon dioxide partial pressure difference (aeDCO$_2$) due to changing from high to low fresh gas flow. Identical changes of readings in both main-stream (Capnolog) and side-stream monitors (Normocap, Capnomac, CO$_2$ monitor). White columns, aeDCO$_2$ with high fresh gas flow (4.2–4.4 l/min); black columns, aeDCO$_2$ with low fresh gas flow (0.5 l/ min). (*Statistical significance of difference (Student's *t*-test): p <0.001)

from these two values. This is the only way of estimating an actual PaCO$_2$ correctly during the following course of anaesthesia by using the formula:

$$PaCO_2 = PeCO_2 + aeDCO_2$$

The aforementioned procedure-specific alterations in carbon dioxide measurement are relevant for anaesthetic practice in so far as misinterpretations of capnometric values and capnogram configuration can only be prevented if these facts are known[29]. However, these artificial alterations of the carbon dioxide signal and resultant increase of aeDCO$_2$ are not observed if low flow anaesthesia is performed with anaesthetic machines of the new generation (see Section 7.2.6) featuring a gas reservoir and discontinuous fresh gas supply.

8.6.2 Zero calibration

Main-stream and side-stream analysers may differ greatly in respect of the technique of zero calibration. While in most side-stream analysers, zero calibration is effected by reference measurement with carbon dioxide free gas, in some of the main-stream analysers zero calibration is performed during the inspiratory phase. This calibration technique can only be correct under the proviso that the inspired gas is definitely free from carbon dioxide. If carbon dioxide absorption is insufficient due to soda lime exhaustion, this will not cause any serious problem with high fresh gas flows due to the low rebreathing fraction and the resultant high wash-out effect[34]. But in the case of low flow anaesthesia, a considerable increase of the carbon dioxide concentration in the inspiratory limb of

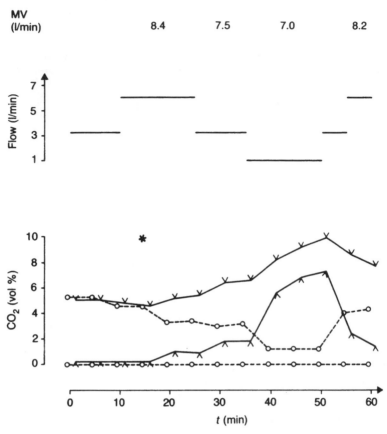

Figure 8.8   Simulation of soda lime exhaustion: at *, removal of the carbon dioxide absorber from the breathing system; ——, measurement with Normocap (side-stream analyser); – –, measurement with Capnolog D (main-stream analyser). The inspired and expired carbon dioxide concentration increase considerably with reduction of the fresh gas flow, but decrease only with the increase of flow. Contrary to that, the readings displayed by the Capnolog D are lower the higher the inspired carbon dioxide concentration. Zero calibration is effected with inspired gas during each ventilation stroke. (Patient aged 16 years, weight 70 kg, height 1.83 m)

the breathing system will result from exhaustion of the absorbent. This equipment failure, which is especially serious with low flow anaesthesia, and which is not reliably indicated by a colour change of the indicator (see Section 7.2.5.2), cannot be detected by means of such main-stream analysers. On the contrary, these devices indicate paradoxically low figures in the event of soda lime exhaustion (Figure 8.8). Both expired and inspired carbon dioxide concentration can be reliably measured by means of side-stream analysers, in which the zero calibration is effected with carbon dioxide free reference gas, or by main-stream analysers, working with a chopper wheel and different filters. Only by these techniques of zero calibration is it possible to detect exhaustion of soda lime reliably, which is essential in low flow anaesthesia.

If, however, carbon dioxide absorption is ensured by using two 1-litre canisters in tandem arrangement or Jumbo absorbers, and if in addition the soda lime is regularly exchanged after each working day, monitoring of absorber function by continuous carbon dioxide measurement must not be assumed to be necessary for safe performance of low flow anaesthesia[2,35].

8.6.3   Implications for anaesthetic practice

With capnometry and capnography the anaesthetist has two monitoring parameters available, which, independent of the fresh gas flow selected, provide essential information on the clinical condition of the patient and the function of the anaesthetic machine[27]. This monitoring adds considerably to the safety of the anaesthetized patient[10,36]. It should be available at each anaesthetic workplace, irrespective of the anaesthetic technique applied. The common European norm EN 740 demands carbon dioxide monitoring as a standard safety device for all inhalation anaesthetic machines[5].

It is for these reasons of safety that in low flow anaesthesia only monitoring equipment which ensures reliable measurement of the carbon dioxide concentration should be used. Main-stream analysers whose zero point is calibrated by the use of inspired gas are not suitable for this anaesthetic technique. However, if continuous monitoring of inspired and expired carbon dioxide concentration is available, for reasons of economy and ecology, the soda lime should only be discarded if exhausted or, routinely, once a week[35] (see Sections 6.2.2, 7.2.5 and 9.1.2.2.4).

8.7   Multi-gas analysers

Complex analysis of gas composition in the breathing system is made possible by using a mass spectrometer or a multi-gas analyser. To date, only a few clinical centres are making significant use of mass spectrometry in routine anaesthetic practice[37–39].

However, several different multi-gas analysers are now available for clinical use. These devices either work on the principle of infrared absorption spectrometry (Datex, Dräger, Hellige, Nellcor), photoacoustic spectrometry (Brüel & Kjaer, Hewlett Packard) or Raman scattering (Ohmeda)[21]. All these different measurement techniques facilitate simultaneous measurement of carbon dioxide, nitrous oxide and volatile anaesthetic concentration. Oxygen concentration is determined by the paramagnetic technique or with the aid of electrochemical devices with fast response time. All these techniques permit measurement not only of the inspired but also the expired oxygen concentration. Nearly all multi-gas analysers are side-stream monitors which can be easily handled. They work reliably and are barely susceptible to malfunction, assisting the anaesthetist in analysing the gas composition in the system and its changes during the course of anaesthesia. The previously mentioned measurement techniques do not modify the gas molecules, so that the sampling gas can be returned to the breathing system once it has passed the device[16]. Accumulation of foreign gas has to be expected to a certain degree as, in addition to the sampling gas, gas for reference measurement and calibration routines may also be drawn into the system. However, foreign gas accumulation takes place very slowly and can reliably be detected by the simultaneous measurement of oxygen and nitrous oxide. If required, this gas can be eliminated by briefly flushing the system with a high fresh gas flow.

Automatic gas identification is a great advantage in concentration measurement of volatile anaesthetics. Setting errors in devices without this facility may result in the display of wrong readings with clinically relevant deviation from real concentrations[14,40]. Due to the delayed wash-out effect, however, if the agent was changed in low flow anaesthesia an alarm will indicate the presence an anaesthetic mixture within the breathing system over a longer period of time.

Without any doubt, the use of multi-gas analysers will considerably increase the acceptance of adequate routine reduction of the fresh gas flow. Significantly, it facilitates the performance of the different techniques of low flow anaesthesia. In addition, it has to be emphasized that the use of multi-gas analysers, which is required for safe performance of minimal flow anaesthesia is already established as an integral part of the safety facilities of inhalation anaesthetic machines in the technical norm EN 740. Together with capnometry, continuous analysis of anaesthetic gas composition allows the comprehensive monitoring of both the patient's physical status and the functions of the anaesthetic machine, so that virtually all potential complications can be detected sufficiently early (Figure 8.9).

	Disconnection	Hypoventilation	Oesophageal intubation	Hypoxic gas mixture	Overdose by anaesthetics	Hypovolaemia	Pneumothorax	Air embolism	Hyperthermia	Aspiration	Arrhythmia	Acid-base disbalance	Overdose i.v. drug
Pulse oximetry	●	●	●	●			●	●	■	■	■		●
Capnometry	▲	●	▲			■	■	●	▲	■		●	■
Spirometry	▲	▲	■				■		■				■
Blood pressure					●	▲	■	●					●
Conc. of vol. anaesthetics	■				▲								
Insp. O₂ concentration				▲									
ECG							■				▲		
Temperature									●				
Auscultation	●	■	●		■		■	■		■	●		■

Figure 8.9 Value of different monitoring parameters for early detection of complications. ▲, maximum value; ●, medium value, ■, low value. (From Whitcher *et al.*[9], by permission)

8.8 References

1. Frankenberger H. Monitoring während Narkosen mit reduziertem Frischgasfluß. In Lawin P, van Aken H and Schneider U, eds, *Alternative Methoden der Anästhesie*, INA-Schriftenreihe, Bd. 50. Thieme, Stuttgart 1985, pp. 19–32.
2. Nunn J F. Monitoring of totally closed systems. In Aldrete JA, Lowe HJ and Virtue RW, eds, *Low Flow and Closed System Anesthesia*. Grune & Stratton, New York, 1979, pp. 199–209.
3. American Society of Anesthesiologists (ASA). Standards for basic anesthetic monitoring. In Miller RD, ed., *Anesthesia*, 5th edn. Churchill Livingstone, Philadelphia, 1999, pp. 1468–1469.
4. American Society for Testing and Materials, ed. ASTM designation: F 1161–88: Standard Specification for Minimum Performance and Safety Requirements for Components and Systems of Anesthesia Gas Machines. ASTM Standards, 1988, pp. 509–532.
5. CEN – Comité Européen de Normalisation, ed. Anaesthetic Workstations and their modules – Particular requirements. EN 740. Brussels, 1998.
6. International Organization for Standardization: ISO 5358 – Anaesthetic machines for use with humans, 2nd edn. Geneva, 1992.
7. Pasch T. Basismonitoring: Empfehlungen und Standards. *Anaesthesist* 1991; **40**, (Suppl. 2), S126.
8. Schmucker P. Qualitätssicherung in der Anästhesiologie. Fortschreibung der Richtlinien der Deutschen Gesellschaft für Anästhesiologie und Intensivmedizin und des Berufsverbandes Deutscher Anästhesisten (*Anästh Intensivmed* 1989; **30**, 307–314). *Anästh Intensivmed* 1995; **36**, 250–254.
9. Whitcher C, Ream AK, Parsons D, Rubsamen D, Scott J, Champeau M, Sterman W and Siegel L. Anesthetic mishaps and the cost of monitoring: a proposed standard for monitoring equipment. *J Clin Monit* 1988; **4**, 5–15.
10. Winter A and Spence AA. An International Consensus on Monitoring? *Br J Anaesth* 1990; **64**, 263–266.
11. WFSA (World Federation of Societies of Anaesthesiologists). International standards for a safe practice of anaesthesia. *Eur J Anaesth* 1993; **10** (Suppl. 7), 12–15.
12. Baum J. Technische Voraussetzungen für die Narkoseführung mit reduziertem Frischgasfluß. In Lawin P, van Aken H and Schneider U, eds, *Alternative Methoden der Anästhesie*, INA-Band 50. Thieme, Stuttgart, 1985, pp. 43–48.
13. Baum J. Die Messung der Anästhesiemittelkonzentration. *Anästh Intensivmed* 1991, **32**, 284–286.
14. Gilly H. Muß die Konzentration volatiler Anästhetika überwacht werden? *Anaesthesist* 1991; **40** (Suppl. 2), S128.
15. Jantzen JPAH. Monitoring der Narkosebeatmung. In Jantzen JPAH and Kleemann PP, eds, *Narkosebeatmung: Low Flow, Minimal Flow, Geschlossenes System*. Schattauer, Stuttgart, 1989, pp. 25–47.
16. Pockrand I. Optische Gasanalyse in der Medizin. *Techn Messen* 1985; **52**, 247–252.
17. Gravenstein JS. *Gas Monitoring and Pulse Oximetry*. Butterworth-Heinemann, Boston, 1990.
18. Bengtson JP, Bengtsson J, Bengtsson A and Stenqvist O. Sampled gas need not be returned during low-flow anesthesia. *J Clin Monit* 1993; **9**, 330–334.
19. Spieß W. Narkose im geschlossenem System mit kontinuierlicher inspiratorischer Sauerstoffmessung. *Anaesthesist* 1977; **26**, 503–513.

20. Block FE. Monitoring the end-tidal concentration of inhalation agents. In Torri G and Damia G, eds, *Update on Modern Inhalation Anaesthetics*. Worldwide Medical Communications, New York, 1989, pp. 125–129.
21. Moyle JTB, Davey A and Ward CS. *Ward's Anaesthetic Equipment*, 4th edn. W. B. Saunders, London, 1998.
22. Hayes JK, Westenskow DR and Jordan WS. Continuous monitoring of inspiratory and end-tidal anesthetic vapor using a piezoelectric detector. *Anesthesiology* 1982; **57**, A180.
23. Linstromberg JW and Muir JJ: Cross-sensitivity in water vapor in the Engström EMMA. *Anesth Analg* 1987; **63**, 75–78.
24. Whitcher C. Monitoring of anesthetic halocarbons: self-contained ('standalone') equipment. *Sem Anesth* 1986; **5**, 213–223.
25. Cooper JB, Newborner RS and Kitz RJ. An analysis of major errors and equipment failures in anesthesia management: considerations for prevention and detection. *Anesthesiology* 1984; **60**, 34–42.
26. Lotz P. Sicherheitstechnische Aspekte bei der Anwendung medizinisch-technischer Geräte im Krankenhaus. *mt-Medizintechnik* 1984; **104**, 133–137.
27. Baum J. Kapnometrie und Kapnographie als Sicherheitsfaktoren in der Anästhesie. *Anaesthesiol Reanimat* 1991; **16**, 12–22.
28. Kalenda Z. *Mastering Infrared Capnography*. Kerkebosch BV, Zeist, 1989.
29. Baum J and Sachs G. Frischgasflow und Narkosebeatmung – Technische Voraussetzungen für die adquate Nutzung von Rückatemsystemen. *Anästh Intensivther Notfallmed* 1990; **25**, 72–78.
30. Lenz G, Klöss Th and Schorer R. Grundlagen und Anwendung der Kapnometrie. *Anästh Intensivmed* 1985; **26**, 133–141.
31. Lindahl SGE, Yates AP and Hatch DJ. Relationship between invasive and noninvasive measurements of gas exchange in anesthetized infants and children. *Anesthesiology* 1987; **66**, 168–175.
32. Badgwell JM, Heavner JE, May WS, Goldthorn JF and Lerman J. End-tidal PCO_2 monitoring in infants and children ventilated with either a partial rebreathing or a non-rebreathing circuit. *Anesthesiology* 1987; **66**, 405–410.
33. Lenz G, Heipertz W, Leidig E and Madee S. Intraoperatives Monitoring der Beatmung bei Früh- und Neugeborenen. *Anästh Intensivther Notfallmed* 1986; **21**, 122–126.
34. Spoerel WE. 1st Atemkalk überflüssig? *Anaesthesist* 1977; **26**, 518–524.
35. Baum J, Enzenauer J, Krausse Th and Sachs G. Atemkalk – Nutzungsdauer, Kosten und Verbrauch in Abhängigkeit vom Frischgasfluß. *Anaesthesiol Reanimat* 1993; **18**, 108–113.
36. Tinker JH, Dull DL, Caplan RA, Ward RJ and Cheney FW. Role of monitoring devices in prevention of anesthetic mishaps: a closed claims analysis. *Anesthesiology* 1989; **71**, 541–546.
37. Gravenstein JS and Paulus DA. *Praxis der Patientenüberwachung*. Gustav Fischer, Stuttgart, 1985.
38. Sodal IE and Swanson GD. Mass spectrometry: current technology and implications for anesthesia. In Aldrete JA, Lowe HJ and Virtue RW, eds. *Low Flow and Closed System Anesthesia*. Grune & Stratton, New York, 1979, pp. 167–182.
39. Weingarten M. Synopsis of the application of the mass spectrometer to the practice of anesthesia. In Aldrete JA, Lowe HJ and Virtue RW, eds, *Low Flow and Closed System Anesthesia*. Grune & Stratton, New York 1979, pp. 183–191.
40. Walder B, Lauber R and Zbinden AM. Genauigkeit und Kreuzempfindlichkeit von volatilen Anästhetika-Analysatoren. *Anaesthesist* 1991; **40** (Suppl. 2), S151.

9

Patient safety aspects of low flow anaesthesia

In this chapter the prejudices against low flow anaesthesia will be discussed comprehensively. They are the main obstacles against a judicious use of technically advanced rebreathing systems by adequate flow reduction. To illustrate the problem, reference will primarily be made to minimal flow anaesthesia, which is a low flow technique practicable in clinical routine, wherein the flow is virtually reduced to the minimum possible.

9.1 Specific risks of anaesthetic techniques with reduced fresh gas flow

9.1.1 Risks attributable to inadequate technical equipment

The requirements concerning technical equipment have already been subject to extensive discussion (see Chapters 7 and 8). Once more it should be pointed out that the extent of safety facilities for anaesthetic machines is specified by different national and international standards such as the common European Norm EN 740. Thus, only those potential risks directly resulting from the reduction of fresh gas flow and the corresponding increase of the rebreathing fraction will be discussed.

9.1.1.1 Hypoxia

It cannot be denied that the preconditions for performance of low flow anaesthesia are not ideal if the flow control systems of older anaesthesia machines do not meet the specifications quoted by the manufacturer in the low flow range (see Section 7.2.2). For anaesthesia management with reduced fresh gas flow, some manufacturers of anaesthesia machines offer to optionally replace old unsuitable flowmeters by special low flow tubes (see Figure 7.1). Furthermore, non-precise adjustment of the flow controls, due to bad performance of the fine needle valves, is liable to cause unexpected alterations of the inspired oxygen concentration and hence possibly hypoxia. In older anaesthetic machines, insufficient gas tightness with corresponding higher loss of gas via leaks, as well as poor fresh gas utilization of older type breathing systems, may be the cause of unexpected decrease of the inspired oxygen concentration.

However, under the provisions of most of the national and international safety standards, continuous monitoring of the oxygen concentration is mandatory during performance of inhalational anaesthesia. With correct setting of the lower alarm limit, there is no procedure-specific risk involved for the patient. If required, the fresh gas flow and its composition have to be adapted to the specific properties of the available equipment.

9.1.1.2   Hypoventilation and alterations in ventilation patterns

Gas volume deficiency in the breathing system resulting from significant leakage losses will cause a reduction of the ventilatory minute volume and possibly even a change in the ventilation pattern. This is the reason why all anaesthetic machines, breathing systems and ventilators should be subjected to a leak test before minimal flow anaesthesia is implemented. It should be guaranteed at the least that the leakage tolerances quoted by the manufacturer are not exceeded. In the common European standard, maximum tolerances of leakage gas loss at a defined pressure are established: $\leq 150\,ml/min$ at $3\,kPa$ ($30\,cmH_2O$).

An important shortcoming of conventional anaesthetic machines is the aforementioned linkage between tidal and fresh gas volume (see Section 7.2.6.1) if the machines does not feature fresh gas flow compensation. When the fresh gas flow is reduced the tidal volume is diminished likewise, since the gas volume which is additionally fed into the system during inspiration decreases. In clinical routine, reduction of the fresh gas flow from 4.4 to $0.5\,l/min$ decreases the minute volume of a normal-weight adult patient by an average of 0.6–1.2 litres. From a clinical point of view, this merely results in a normalization of ventilation for most of the patients, as common routine pre-adjustment of ventilation causes a more or less significant hyperventilation. On the other hand, the reduction of the respired gas volume can be recognized immediately by means of the mandatory continuous monitoring of the expired minute volume, and corrected by increasing the tidal volume. Using low fresh gas flows, additional gas loss via leakages results in a further decrease of gas volume circulating in the system, thus prompting hypoventilation and possibly alternating pressure ventilation. This in turn can be detected sufficiently early by the mandatory airway pressure monitoring. Provided that the disconnection alarm is adjusted correctly to $5\,mbar$ below the peak pressure, hypoventilation resulting from gas volume deficiency will cause an immediate alarm.

Basically, high leakage gas losses involve the risk of alterations in the ventilatory patterns in addition to the corresponding hypoventilation. However, this can be rapidly recognized and corrected when monitoring standards are followed. Anaesthetic machines with an anaesthetic gas reservoir are far better suited for use with low fresh gas flows, and the problems described will not arise as long as the reservoir is filled sufficiently. Essentially, all problems resulting from leakage gas loss can be minimized by appropriate maintenance of the anaesthetic machines.

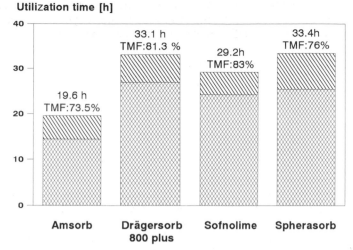

Figure 9.1 Utilization times (mean values) of different brands of carbon dioxide absorbents (1.5 litre canister). Potassium-free soda lime: Spherasorb™ (Intersurgical), Sofnolime™ (Molecular Products), Drägersorb 800 plus™ (Dräger Medizintechnik) versus calcium hydroxide lime: Amsorb™ (Armstrong Medical). Utilization time: time during which a patient was connected to the breathing system, from the filling date until exhaustion, marked by an increase of the inspired CO_2 concentration to 1.0 vol%. TMF: Percentage of time during which a low fresh gas flow between 0.5 and 0.25 l/min was used[100]

9.1.1.3 Carbon dioxide accumulation in the breathing system

In contrast to high flow anaesthesia, efficient carbon dioxide elimination is essential in the performance of anaesthesia with low fresh gas flow since, with the increase in rebreathing volume, the carbon dioxide concentration in the breathing system may rise considerably if the absorbers are exhausted (see Figure 8.8).

According to the author's own investigations, the usage period of absorbers (Figure 9.1) is considerably longer than previously quoted in relevant textbooks (see Section 7.2.5.1). If suitable carbon dioxide monitoring is available (see Section 8.6.2), the soda lime should be used until it is completely exhausted and only changed routinely once a week. But if an anaesthetic machine is used which does not permit constant carbon dioxide measurement, use should be made of double canisters in tandem arrangement or Jumbo absorbers and the soda lime should be discarded routinely at shorter intervals, at least whenever a colour change of the indicator signals the beginning of exhaustion. Proceeding in this way, the patient is reliably protected from carbon dioxide rebreathing[1,2].

9.1.1.4 Accidental increase of the airway pressure

It had been recommended to increase the gas tightness of some older type anaesthesia ventilators, having no gas reservoir and featuring active support of the expiratory expansion of the bellows, by switching on the

PEEP function if the fresh gas flow is reduced (see Section 7.2.6.1.1). When the PEEP valve is fitted to the exhaust port of the ventilator this manoeuvre improves the gas tightness of the system. If the leakage loss is small, a positive end-expiratory pressure may be established requiring adequate readjustment of the PEEP valve. In case of accidental inattentiveness this may not be carried out, resulting in an unexpected increase of the pressure within the breathing system. However, this will not really threaten the patient as this problem will be recognized early if the occlusion alarm is set correctly and activated, and the PEEP in older type ventilators is in any case limited to a maximum of 15 mbar.

In some anaesthetic ventilators, such as the Megamed 700 (Megamed, Cham, Switzerland), the excess gas is not discharged via an automatically opening excess gas valve but via an overflow valve, which is operated manually. Working with extremely low flows, this valve needs to be closed virtually completely. If this valve is not appropriately adjusted to the fresh gas flow and the loss of gas volume resulting from uptake and leaks, this may cause either gas volume deficiency or the development of an increasing positive pressure within the breathing system. This fault in operating the machine will also soon be detected if occlusion and disconnection alarms are set appropriately. Another safety feature to prevent an accidental barotrauma is the airway pressure limit valve (APL valve), which opens automatically if a pre-adjusted positive pressure within the breathing system is reached.

9.1.1.5   Accidental overdose of volatile anaesthetics

Even with severe maladjustment of plenum vaporizers outside the circle, it is virtually impossible that this will result in a rapidly occurring overdose during low flow anaesthesia. On the one hand, this can be attributed to the link between the vaporizer output and the fresh gas flow; on the other hand, to the fact that, due to different safety regulations, the output of nearly all vaporizers is limited. In low flow anaesthesia, alterations of the anaesthetic concentration proceed very slowly due to the long time constant of the breathing system (Figure 9.2a and b). In the event of accidental maladjustment, changes in volatile agent concentration can always be recognized sufficiently early by means of careful clinical observation of the patient. Increase in rebreathing volume just does not involve a higher risk of overdose of inhalational anaesthetics.

From this point of view, this technique is evidently safer than anaesthesia with high fresh gas flow where accidental adjustment errors at the vaporizer result in immediate drastic, possibly dangerous, changes of the anaesthetic concentration in the breathing system.

It has been pointed out before (see Section 8.4.1) that it is just the change from low back to high fresh gas flow which may result in serious overdose if the setting at the vaporizer is not readjusted appropriately to the higher flow with its shorter time constant. This is the reason why anaesthesia using a flow lower than 1 l/min should not be carried out without continuously monitoring the anaesthetic concentration in the breathing system. Once more it must be pointed out that continuous monitoring of inhalation anaesthetic concentration is obligatory under

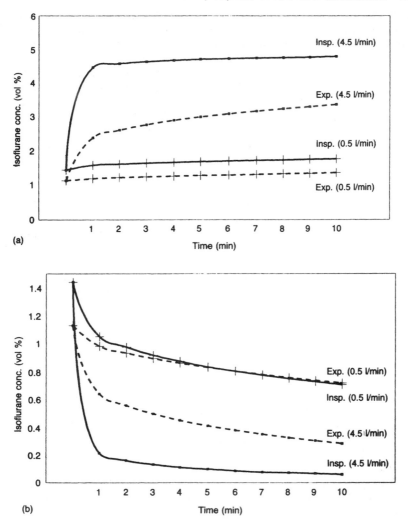

Figure 9.2 Course of inspired and expired isoflurane concentration in case of accidental adjustment error of the vaporizer: (a) vaporizer accidentally set to its maximum output; (b) vaporizer accidentally closed. (Patient 75 kg, MV 5.6 l/min (Gas uptake simulation))

the European standard EN 740 demanding all inhalation anaesthetic machines to be equipped with this safety facility.

9.1.2   Risks which are directly caused by reduction of the fresh gas flow

9.1.2.1   The long time constant

The assumption that the long time constant poses a specific risk due to the inability to rapidly change the anaesthetic gas composition if required

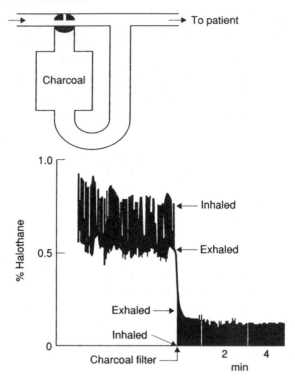

Figure 9.3 Charcoal filter, switched by bypass into the breathing system, for rapid elimination of inhalational anaesthetics in low flow anaesthetic techniques. (From Ernst and Spain[5], by permission)

during low flow anaesthesia is absolutely unfounded. A desired gas composition can be immediately attained at any time with short time constant simply by switching back from low to high fresh gas flow. This approach is especially recommended to those anaesthetists who are gaining their initial experience with minimal flow anaesthesia. Once familiar with the technique, rapid increase of anaesthetic depth can be achieved by intravenous injection of supplementary drugs. Rapid lightening of the anaesthetic, on the other hand, can only be achieved by increasing the fresh gas flow.

It will only be possible to rapidly reduce the concentration of volatile anaesthetic while maintaining a low fresh gas flow rate if the anaesthetic machine is equipped with a charcoal filter (see Section 7.4.1). The anaesthetic concentration will drop instantly whenever the filter is switched into the breathing system (Figure 9.3)[3,4].

9.1.2.2   Accumulation of foreign gas

9.1.2.2.1   Nitrogen
For a patient of normal weight, the nitrogen volume stored in the body and in the lungs can be assumed to be 2.7 litres. If denitrogenation is

performed over a period of 15–20 min with high fresh gas flow, a volume of about 2 litres nitrogen is washed out of all compartments during this period. The remaining 0.7 litres is only slowly released from the less perfused tissues[5,6]. If the fresh gas flow is reduced to extremely low values after such an apparently sufficient denitrogenation, the nitrogen concentration in the breathing system will rise to about 3–10% within the next hour[6–14]. Nitrogen accumulation in the breathing system may increase even more if side-stream gas analysers are used, since considerable volumes of ambient air, which serves as calibration or reference gas, may be returned into the system together with the sampling gas. Depending on the volume of ambient air admixed to the sampling gas and the degree of flow reduction, nitrogen concentrations of 15% or even higher can be observed in the case of long-term minimal flow anaesthesia (see Sections 8.2.1, 8.5 and 8.7). Should undesirable nitrogen concentrations be reached in the breathing system, nitrogen can be washed out by a 2–5 min flushing phase with a high fresh gas flow[9–11,15]. During anaesthesia, accumulation of nitrogen in the system can only be detected by means of a mass spectrometer or a multi-gas analyser. It must be emphasized, however, that nitrogen accumulation does not involve any risk for the patient as long as hypoxia can be definitely excluded. However, the nitrous oxide concentration may be reduced considerably by nitrogen accumulation, thus lessening its anaesthetic effects. To overcome this problem intermittent flushing with an appropriate gas mixture at a high fresh gas flow rate may be carried out, or anaesthesia can be supplemented by the administration of intravenous or volatile anaesthetics.

9.1.2.2.2   Acetone

Acetone is generated by oxidative metabolism of free fatty acids. Increased formation may be observed in the state of starvation, in decompensated diabetes mellitus, and in the case of an increased release of anti-insulin hormones. If isoflurane anaesthesia with closed system is performed over a period of 6 h, average acetone blood concentrations of about 50 mg/l, but in individual cases as high as 200 mg/l, were observed[16]. The increase in acetone concentration during closed system anaesthesia depends on its preoperative value and on the duration of the anaesthetic procedure[17,18]. A blood concentration higher than 50 mg/l is said to extend the emergence period and to be liable to increase postoperative vomiting[17]. In performing anaesthesia with closed system over a period of 4 h, Morita et al.[11] found an average increase of acetone concentration from 1.3 to 5.9 ppm in the breathing gas. The MAK value (German list of maximum workplace concentrations) assessed for acetone is 1000 ppm, the normal value for blood concentration less than 5 mg/l, the limit value tolerated with respect to industrial hygiene is 20 mg/l. However, the US Navy concentration limit for acetone in ambient air in submarines is established at 2000 ppm over a period of 24 h[19]!

Furthermore, it has to be emphasized that even with the use of semi-open breathing systems, considerable increase of blood acetone concentration cannot be prevented. During the first 5 h of anaesthesia, Strauß et al. could not establish a significant difference when comparing the use of

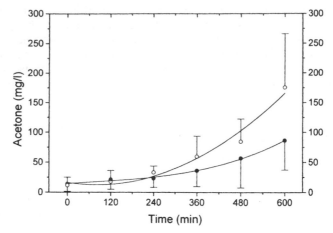

Figure 9.4   Acetone blood concentrations during the course of anaesthesia: • semi-open rebreathing system, ○, closed rebreathing system. Regression curves. (From Strauß et al.[17], by permission)

closed and semi-open breathing systems[18]. Differences only became clinically relevant after 6 h of anaesthesia (Figure 9.4).

Because of its high solubility in water and fat, the acetone concentration cannot be lowered by means of intermittent short-term high flow flushing phases[11]. For safety reasons it is recommended, in patients suffering from decompensated diabetes mellitus and patients with otherwise raised blood acetone concentration, not to use fresh gas flows lower than 1 l/min during long-term anaesthesia. By the resulting continuous wash-out effect, undesired trace gas accumulation can be prevented. The most simple and best way to decrease the metabolism of free fatty acids, and hence acetone generation, would be the infusion of low concentration solutions of glucose. Intra-operative stress, which also promotes endogenous acetone production, should be prevented in long-term anaesthesia by the additional administration of opioids, in accordance with the concept of balanced anaesthesia.

9.1.2.2.3   Ethanol
Ethanol, with a gas–water solubility coefficient of 1200, may accumulate in the closed system similarly to acetone, and its concentration in the breathing gas can barely be decreased by short-term intermittent wash-out phases[11]. However, high ethanol concentrations result exclusively from exogenous intoxication. If a surgical intervention has to be performed urgently on an alcoholized patient, elimination of ethanol by exhalation would be made impossible by anaesthesia with a closed system. Again it seems prudent in these cases not to reduce the fresh gas flow to below 1 l/min in order to provide an adequate wash-out effect.

9.1.2.2.4   Carbon monoxide
During performance of anaesthesia with a closed system over a period of

2 h, the carbon monoxide concentration in the breathing system was found to increase to an average of 80 ppm within the range of 20–210 ppm[20]. After 6 h anaesthesia with closed system carbon monoxide haemoglobin concentrations (COHb) of non-smokers amounted to 0.5–1.5%, while for smokers the values reached 3% COHb. The average increase for both groups amounted to 0.4% COHb, but in an individual case an increase of up to 3.5% COHb was observed[21].

The physiological value of COHb amounts to 0.4–0.8%, but with habitual smokers this value may even reach 10%. Concentrations of 100 ppm over an exposure period of 8 h, and 400 ppm over a period of 1 h, are considered harmful. The toxicity of carbon monoxide can be estimated with the Henderson and Haggard toxicity index I_{tox}[22]:

$$I_{tox} = C_{CO} \times t$$

where C_{CO} = carbon monoxide concentration (ppm) and t = exposure period (h).

No effects were observed with an I_{tox} of 300 ppm/h, symptoms of beginning intoxication with 600 ppm/h, vomiting and headache with 900 ppm/h; a value of 1500 ppm/h is life-threatening. Middleton et al.[20] point out that, in the case of closed system anaesthesia, a toxicity index of about 200–300 ppm/h may be reached.

Only a very small volume of carbon monoxide (0.42 ± 0.07 ml/h) is endogenously produced under normal conditions. However, in the closed system, the concentration may rise to values of clinical relevance in the case of heavy smokers, haemolysis, anaemia, porphyria and blood transfusions, particularly when blood donated by smokers is given. Where high risk patients are concerned, such as heavy smokers suffering from severe anaemia with considerable regional perfusion restriction, low flow anaesthesia should be performed in preference to closed system anaesthesia to ensure continuous wash-out of carbon monoxide. Due to its high affinity for haemoglobin, intermittent short flushing with high fresh gas flow will be insufficient as only the amount of carbon monoxide within the gas-containing space (lung and breathing system) is washed-out. As soon as the flow is reduced again, the carbon monoxide concentration will be re-established, balancing the partial pressure difference.

About 10 years ago isolated cases of accidental intra-operative carbon monoxide poisoning with COHb concentrations up to 30% were observed[23,24]. According to the classification given by Pankow these cases represent subacute carbon monoxide poisoning in which the COHb concentration can amount to 20–50%[25]. Slow generation of carbon monoxide in the carbon dioxide absorbent following exposure to fluorinated agents was assumed to be the cause for this intoxication[23,24]. Canisters which had been in place for longer periods of time were more likely to contain high carbon monoxide concentrations. To avoid accidental carbon monoxide intoxication, Moon recommended the consistent use of fresh gas flows as high or even higher than 5 l/min, to flush the system with pure oxygen before starting the list, and to frequently change the absorbent[26]. Fang et al. analysed the preconditions facilitating the generation of carbon monoxide: absolutely dry absorbents react eagerly with all volatile anaesthetics containing the CHF_2 moiety, with the reactivity decreasing in the order desflurane > enflurane > isoflurane. Halothane, like sevoflurane, hardly generates carbon monoxide with carbon dioxide absorbents[27,28]. Baralyme reacts more eagerly with volatile agents than does soda lime. Only partial wetting of the absorbent, however, results in a significant decrease in carbon monoxide generation. If the water content in soda lime amounts to more than 4.8%, or in Baralyme to more than 9.5%, carbon monoxide generation ceases completely. Fresh carbon dioxide absorbents contain about 15–16% of water. Although up to now only one single case of significant accidental intra-operative carbon monoxide poisoning has been reported[29], all measures should be taken to prevent desiccation of the absorbent[2,30]:

- All needle valves at the flowmeter block should be turned off after each anaesthetic. In addition, when the daily list is finished, the pipeline connectors should be disconnected from the sockets of the central gas piping system.
- A breathing system equipped with an absorber canister must never be dried out by switching on a continuous gas flow at the flow control system, or by opening the Y-piece and switching on the ventilator, while the machine is idle during the night or at the weekend.
- Whenever the canister is newly filled with absorbent it should be labelled with the filling date written on an adhesive strip. The absorbent should be changed at least once a week. This, however, only can be recommended if the anaesthetic machine is equipped with a gas monitor reliably measuring the inspired carbon dioxide concentration.
- The absorber canisters of anaesthetic machines left idle for a longer period of time should not be filled with absorbent. To safely protect the absorbent from desiccation it should be stored in the unopened original packaging near to the machine. The canister should then be filled only in case of use. However, if the machine has to be used urgently, leaving no time for filling of the canister, a fresh gas flow rate equalling the minute volume will provide adequate elimination of expired carbon dioxide out of the breathing system via the exhaust port.
- As recommended by the manufacturers, opened original packaging containing carbon dioxide absorbents should be closed carefully again after use.

A sufficient water content of the carbon dioxide absorbent is one of the essential factors to prevent carbon monoxide generation. Thus, quite contrary to Moon, Fang et al. recommend the consistent use of fresh gas flow rates not higher than 2–3 l/min to prevent accidental desiccation of the absorbent[27]. The preservation of humidity contained in the absorbent is one of the specific advantages of low flow anaesthetic techniques. In addition, the increase in rebreathing will improve water generation resulting from the chemical reaction of the exhaled carbon dioxide with the absorbent. Consistent performance of low flow anaesthetic techniques, thus, significantly decreases the danger of accidental carbon monoxide intoxication.

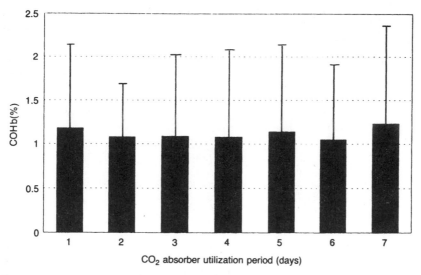

Figure 9.5 Concentration of carbon monoxide haemoglobin as a function of the carbon dioxide absorber's utilization period. All blood samples were taken about 30 min after fresh gas flow reduction from 4.4 to 0.5 l/min.

Another factor essentially favouring the chemical reaction of anaesthetic agents, characterized by a difluoromethoxy moiety, with the carbon dioxide absorbent, is the sodium and potassium hydroxide content. Murray *et al.* found that calcium hydroxide lime, containing predominantly calcium hydroxide together with small amounts of calcium chloride and sulphate but neither potassium nor sodium hydroxide, does not degrade anaesthetic agents to carbon monoxide, even when desiccated[31,32]. The consistent use of absorbents containing preferably no sodium hydroxide but certainly no potassium hydroxide is a further measure to reduce the danger of carbon monoxide generation.

In a clinical trial of 1258 unselected patients 45 min after induction, i.e. 30 min after fresh gas flow reduction from 4.4 to 0.5 l/min, COHb concentration was measured: the mean COHb concentration was 1.22%, the standard deviation 0.98%, the range 0.0–7.6%[33]. The same values were found independently of the utilization period of the absorbent, although the soda lime was only changed once a week (Figure 9.5). Compared with the reference concentration of 2.14 ± 0.93% COHb, taken before starting the anaesthetic, the COHb concentration decreased by about 0.8% to 1.38 ± 0.86% after 60 min minimal flow anaesthesia. Even after 2 h of minimal flow anaesthesia the COHb concentration amounted to not more than 1.42 ± 0.79% (Figure 9.6). A significant decrease of COHb concentration can already be found in the initial high flow phase, just 5 min after connecting the patient to the breathing system (Figure 9.7). This is based on the fact that, starting with pre-oxygenation, gas mixtures containing significantly higher oxygen partial pressures are applied to the lung of the patient[34]. Based on extensive clinical experience, the following conclusions can be made. In a trial of 1800 patients, in not a single case

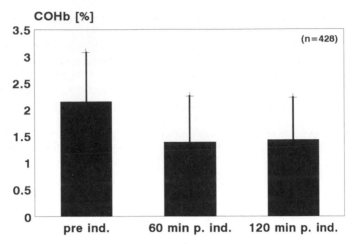

Figure 9.6 COHb concentration (paired values, mean and standard deviation) during the course of minimal flow anaesthesia. The blood samples were taken directly prior ('pre ind.') and 60 and 120 min after induction ('p. ind.')

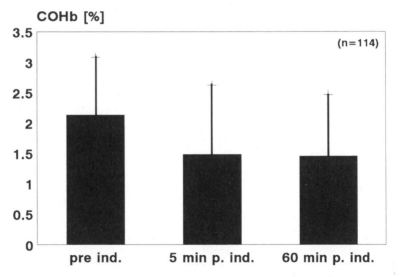

Figure 9.7 COHb concentration (paired values, mean and standard deviation) during the course of minimal flow anaesthesia. The blood samples were taken directly prior ('pre ind.') and 5 and 60 min after induction ('p. ind.')

was significant or even dangerous increase of COHb concentration observed although extremely low fresh gas flow rates were consistently used and the absorbent was changed only once a week. The small mean increase by 0.4% in COHb during long duration closed system anaesthesia is negligible if compared with its decrease during the initial high flow phase. There is absolutely no increased procedure-specific risk for accidental carbon monoxide intoxication resulting from the performance of low

flow anaesthetic techniques[35]. On the contrary, the consistent use of low fresh
gas flow rates is an essential measure to prevent carbon monoxide generation[30]. This equally holds for minimal flow anaesthesia using desflurane: $n = 112$, COHb concentration before induction, $2.13 \pm 1.05\%$; COHb concentration 45 min after flow reduction from 4.4 to 0.5 l/min, $1.42 \pm 1.01\%$; COHb concentration 105 min after flow reduction, $1.41 \pm 0.78\%$.

If the carbon dioxide absorbent contains a sufficient amount of water there is absolutely no increased risk for accidental carbon monoxide intoxication even when an extremely low fresh gas flow rate and desflurane are used[36].

9.1.2.2.5 Argon

Oxygen concentrators separate nitrogen contained in ambient air by an adsorption process using molecular sieves. At the outlet respirable oxygen-enriched gas is supplied consisting of a maximum of about 95% oxygen, the remnant being mainly the noble gas argon[37,38]. The concentration of oxygen essentially depends on the gas flow demanded from the device and amounts to more than 90% at flows lower than 5 l/min, but decreases to about 50% at a flow of 15 l/min. If oxygen is supplied by an oxygen concentrator to the anaesthetic machine, in longer-lasting low flow anaesthesia argon may accumulate within the breathing system. At a fresh gas flow rate of 1.0 l/min in long-lasting procedures the argon concentration may amount to 5–6%, at a flow rate of 0.5 l/min – depending on the oxygen concentration desired – the concentration may increase from 8% to more than 15%. The anaesthetic gas monitoring is not influenced in any way by the argon accumulation[37], which furthermore is harmless from a medical aspect[39]. The accumulation of argon can be opposed by brief intermittent wash-out with a high fresh gas flow every 90 min[38].

9.1.2.2.6 Methane

Methane, which is generated in the intestines by bacterial decomposition processes, is a physiological constituent of intestinal gases. It may accumulate in the anaesthetic gas during anaesthesia with a closed system[6]. The average methane concentration measured after 2 h of anaesthesia amounted to 11.2 ppm. The maximum value measured in an individual case was 229 ppm. Methane concentrations of up to 100 ppm are found in the expired air of healthy test persons. Being a non-toxic foreign gas, methane is of significance only in so far as it is flammable if mixed with oxygen (5–60% in oxygen) or nitrous oxide (4–40% in nitrous oxide). However, such methane concentrations are not attained even in long-term closed system anaesthesia[35,40].

Rolly and co-workers, however, recently published observations gained during performance of total intravenous anaesthesia on patients being ventilated with an oxygen–air mixture with the aid of the closed circuit PhysioFlex apparatus (Dräger Medizintechnik, Lübeck, Germany). Although a volatile agent was not used, the in-built infrared analyser indicated unexpected values for halothane in patients undergoing gynaecological laparoscopies with carbon dioxide insufflation[41,42]. The mean concentration of methane was 861 ppm, ranging from 139 to even 4130 ppm, in closed system anaesthesia lasting from 45 to 150 min. Thus, the methane concentrations were much higher than mentioned previously. Such high methane concentrations, however, are only liable to influence halothane measurement by non-dispersive infrared absorption, with 800 ppm methane being misinterpreted as 1% halothane by the measuring device. Especially if halothane is metered electronically gas analysers have to be used, guaranteeing no cross-sensitivity to methane.

9.1.2.2.7   Hydrogen

Hydrogen, which is discharged via the lungs in a volume of up to 0.6 ml/min, also may accumulate in the anaesthetic gas during anaesthesia with a closed system. On average, the concentration rises by 200 ppm/h[43]. However, flammable hydrogen concentrations (4.6–94% in oxygen, 5.8–86% in nitrous oxide) are likewise not reached in long-term anaesthesia with closed systems.

9.1.2.2.8   Haloalkenes

Some of the volatile anaesthetics react chemically with the carbon dioxide absorbents by generating volatile haloalkenes which may accumulate as foreign trace gases within the breathing system during performance of low flow anaesthesia. Thus, 2-bromo-2-chloro-1,1-difluoroethylene, CF_2CBrCl (BCDFE), a gaseous decomposition product of halothane, may reach concentrations of 4–5 ppm with a closed system[44]. Experiments with model rebreathing systems indicate that 0.02% of the halothane is transformed into BCDFE within 4 h. Although the levels of BCDFE, gained during closed system anaesthesia, are significantly less than the toxic concentration, quoted as 250 ppm according to Sharp et al.[44], these findings do raise concern regarding the use of closed circuit halothane administration.

Sevoflurane reacts with carbon dioxide absorbents by formation of several degradation products, named compounds A–E[45]. Only one of these compounds, compound A, fluoromethyl-2,2-difluoro-1-trifluoro-methyl-vinylether, reaches clinically significant concentrations. The concentration of compound A in rebreathing systems increases with the sevoflurane concentration of the anaesthetic gas, the temperature of the carbon dioxide absorbent, with decreasing water content of the absorbent, and with decreasing fresh gas flow rate. The latter results from the increased carbon dioxide load of the absorbent, which on its part leads to an increase of the temperature in the absorbent canister, and a diminished wash-out effect. If the absorbent is desiccated a complex equilibrium is established resulting from compound A generation and decomposition[46–48]. Baralyme is more liable to degrade sevoflurane to compound A than soda lime due to its higher potassium hydroxide content and a higher temperature during carbon dioxide absorption[31,49].

In animal experiments with rats the lethal concentration, LD_{50}, of compound A was about 1000 ppm at an exposure time of 1 h, about 400 ppm at 3 h, about 200 ppm at 6 h, and about 130 ppm at an exposition time of $12\,h^{45,50,51}$. After an exposure lasting 3h at a compound A concentration between 50 and 100 ppm, early mild and reversible injuries of the renal tubular epithelium with corresponding minor disturbances of renal function were found in rats[52,53].

Compound A itself is not known to be nephrotoxic, but there remain some concerns about its metabolites. After coupling to glutathione in the liver, extrahepatic formation of cysteine S-conjugates and N-acetylation to mercapturic acids, compound A is excreted via the kidneys – the detoxification pathway. By an alternative metabolic process, however, the cysteine S-conjugates are metabolized by renal β-lyase to reactive nephrotoxic intermediates – the toxification pathway[54]. The β-lyase activity in the renal tissue of rats, however, is at least 10 times higher than in humans[54-56]. This justifies the conclusion that the nephrotoxicity of compound A in rats can not be assumed to apply in humans. According to their own experimental findings Eger and co-workers, for their part, strongly call this conclusion into question[57]. The experimentally induced decrease of glutathione S- and cysteine S-conjugates and the inhibition of the renal β-lyase activity did not result in decreased nephrotoxicity but, in some animals, even to a higher degree of renal damage. The Eger group even argues that the β-lyase metabolism of compound A conjugates may be the detoxificating pathway.

Thus, some authors already regard a compound A load of 150–240 ppm/h as potentially nephrotoxic in humans[58-60] and recommend that sevoflurane is not used with flows lower than 2.0 l/min. In contrast, other authors estimate low flow anaesthesia with sevoflurane to be safe, arguing that mean peak concentrations in different studies did not exceed 25 ppm and emphasize that no signs of renal impairment were observed in any patient[61-63]. Mazze et al. recently reported the results of an investigation on nephrotoxicity of compound A in primates, demonstrating that only at a load of at least 800 ppm did nephrotoxic effects occur[64]. Accepting this threshold for nephrotoxic load with compound A absolutely no flow restriction would be justified. Even long-lasting minimal flow anaesthesia with sevoflurane could be performed safely, although compound A peak concentrations were found to reach 50–60 ppm with this technique[65]. Unlike in the USA, sevoflurane has been approved for clinical use without any fresh gas flow restriction in all countries of the European Community. Nevertheless, whenever in clinical practice there might be assumed the possibility of accumulation of potentially harmful trace gases, for safety reasons, a low flow technique using a flow of at least 1 l/min should be performed, guaranteeing a sufficient continuous wash-out effect[66].

Haloalkene generation from chemical reaction of the volatile anaesthetics with carbon dioxide absorbents seems to be bound to the sodium and especially the potassium hydroxide contained in the different absorbents. The removal of just the potassium hydroxide from the absorbent leads to a significant reduction of haloalkene formation[67,68]. Murray and co-workers even demonstrated that the use of calcium hydroxide lime, which is absolutely free from these strong alkaline hydroxides, prevents haloalkene generation totally[32]. Thus, the simplest way to avoid any risk for the patient will be the consistent use of absorbents containing no alkali metal hydroxides, but especially no potassium hydroxide[2,31].

The following conclusions on haloalkene formation in rebreathing systems seem to be justified:

- The compound A problem has been the focus of a vast number of scientific publications, however the scientific discussion is not yet over.
- Clinical trials have failed to show clinically relevant harmful effects on renal or hepatic function in humans after longer duration sevoflurane anaesthesia. This also holds for prolonged use of sevoflurane with low flow anaesthetic techniques or even for performance of sevoflurane anaesthesia in patients suffering from chronic renal insufficiency[69]. Only mild disturbances of the renal and hepatic function were observed in some of the trials[70-75]. Thus, it seems justified to conclude that neither sevoflurane metabolism itself nor the compound A generated in breathing systems and its metabolism, in normal clinical use, will actually result in significant harmful disturbance of renal or hepatic function in humans.
- During low flow anaesthesia mean maximum compound A concentration of about 25 ppm has been observed. Thus, even in cases lasting up to 5 h, the compound A load will not reach the nephrotoxic threshold, even if the low limit of 150–200 ppm/h given by Eger and co-workers is accepted.
- In 1998 even the American FDA stated that fresh gas flow rates of 1.0 l/min were acceptable but should not exceed 2 MACh, and flow rates less than 1.0 l/min were not recommended[31]. In the countries of the European Community sevoflurane was approved without any flow restriction.
- As long as the scientific discussion concerning potential nephrotoxic, hepatotoxic or even neurotoxic effects of compound A in humans is not concluded, anaesthetists should follow the recommendations of the FDA. If extremely low fresh gas flow rates are used consistently, then potassium-free soda lime or, what seems to be the best alternative, calcium hydroxide lime should be used[31,32,67,100]. Baralyme should not be used at all in low flow sevoflurane anaesthesia.

It seems unlikely that cooling of the absorber canister[76] or the admixture of chemical compound A scavengers[77] as measures to reduce compound A generation will win through against the simple technique of increasing the fresh gas flow rate. Driven by a fan, in the PhysioFlex anaesthetic machine (Dräger Medizintechnik, Lübeck, Germany) the breathing gas circulates continuously at a flow of 70 l/min, resulting in a cooling effect guaranteeing comparatively low absorbent temperatures. Thus, the mean compound A concentration was found to be lower than 10 ppm, even though this device may realize quantitative closed system anaesthesia[78,79].

9.1.2.2.9   Implications for anaesthetic practice

Foreign gases may accumulate in the breathing system if anaesthesia is performed with extremely low fresh gas flows. These are gases which

- may be formed in the body itself, such as acetone, carbon monoxide, methane and hydrogen;

Table 9.1   Contaminants of medical gases*

	Oxygen for medical use (ppm)	Nitrous oxide for anaesthesia (ppm)
$Ar + N_2$	≈ 5000	< 10
CO	< 5	< 10
CO_2	< 50	< 300
Halogens		< 1
H_2S		< 5
NH_3	< 1	< 5
NO/NO_2	< 1	< 5
Cl_2	< 0.5	
SO_2	< 1	
$N_2 + O_2$		≈ 4600

*The low concentrations of O_2 contaminants meet the requirements of the German and European Pharmacopoeias, the levels of N_2O contaminants the requirements of the European, US and German Pharmacopoeias (Source: Messer Griesheim, Frankfurt a. Main, Germany)

- may be absorbed by the body, stored in the tissues and discharged via the lungs, such as ethanol, carbon monoxide and nitrogen; and
- may either be generated in the system, or fed into the breathing system as contaminants together with the fresh or the sampling gas, such as argon, carbon monoxide, haloalkenes and nitrogen (Table 9.1).

Sparingly soluble gases, such as nitrogen, methane and hydrogen, can be washed out from the system, if required, by brief intermittent flushing with a high fresh gas flow. However, gases readily soluble in water and fat or featuring high affinity to the tissues – such as acetone, alcohol or carbon monoxide – cannot be washed out by intermittent short increase of the fresh gas flow. Accumulation within the breathing system can be avoided by performance of low flow anaesthesia, because a flow rate of 1.0 l/min already guarantees a sufficient continuous wash-out of trace gases by the discharge of excess gas.

For safety reasons it seems wise to follow these recommendations whenever trace or foreign gases are liable to accumulate in considerable and possibly harmful concentrations. Nevertheless, although foreign gas accumulation needs to be considered thoroughly, the author agrees with Baumgarten and Reynolds[19] that the trace gas issue cannot '... justify the continued waste and pollution resulting from high flow anaesthesia'.

9.2   Specific safety features of anaesthetic techniques with reduced fresh gas flow

9.2.1   Improved equipment maintenance

The increased demands placed on the technical equipment call for more painstaking care, maintenance and testing of anaesthetic machines. When technical inspections are carried out, particular interest should be focused upon testing the equipment in the lower flow ranges to ensure that it at least meets the technical specifications of the manufacturer. The equipment should be carefully tested and readjusted if required over the entire specified operation range as given in the service manuals. There cannot be any doubt that the high demands placed on equipment care and maintenance are an essential factor in terms of patient safety. It must be emphasized that it is the anaesthetist himself who is ultimately responsible for careful handling and maintenance of anaesthetic equipment[80], to avoid technical complications like those described in detail by Good et al.[81], Johnstone[82] and Müchler[83].

9.2.2   The long time constant

The long time constant of the breathing system is an extraordinary safety factor in low flow anaesthesia. Schreiber[84,85] analyses a potentially hazardous situation threatening the patient's safety as consisting of different periods (Figure 9.8):

- Pre-alarm period: the time from occurrence of an adverse condition to the generation of the alarm (A–B).

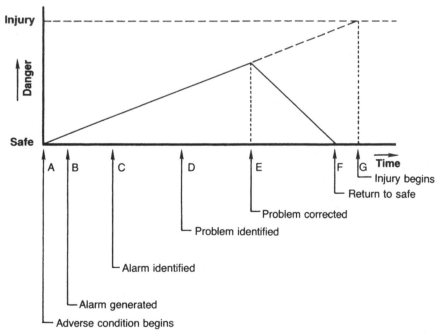

Figure 9.8   Analysis of a critical incident: A–B, pre-alarm period; B–D, identification period; D–E, correction period; E–F, restitution period; B–G, reaction period – the time from onset of the alarm to definite injury. (From Schreiber and Schreiber[85], by permission)

- Identification period: the time it takes on the part of the anaesthetist to identify the origin of the alarm (B–C); it takes some further time for the anaesthetist to identify exactly the cause of the alarm (C–D).
- Correction period: after having analysed the particular cause of the problem, it takes some time for the corrective action to be carried out and the system starts with its corresponding reaction (D–E).
- Restitution period: the time which elapses until the system returns to its safe starting condition (E–F).

If any of these phases of a critical incident is prolonged, the danger to the patient may escalate to that point where injury cannot be prevented by correcting measures (G). The time from the generation of an alarm to the actual occurrence of an injury is referred to as the reaction period (B–G). This is the maximum period that the anaesthetist has available to protect the patient from being injured.

When these different phases are very short, the period available for adequate corrective measures preventing the patient from a life-threatening hazard may quickly be exceeded.

The increase in safety achieved by the long time constants, especially in minimal flow anaesthesia, can be impressively demonstrated by a clinical example. The following situation was simulated on a young healthy male patient in the presence of two anaesthetists (Figure 9.9).

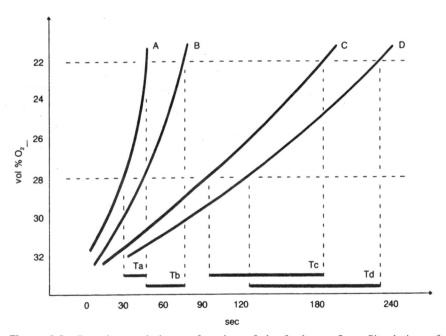

Figure 9.9 Reaction period as a function of the fresh gas flow. Simulation of accidental interruption of oxygen flow on an anaesthetic machine without oxygen ratio controller. With low fresh gas flows (Tc and Td), the reaction period takes considerably longer than with high fresh gas flows (Ta and Tb). Fresh gas flow: A = 6 l/min, B = 3 l/min, C = 1 l/min, D = 0.5 l/min

During anaesthesia using an older type anaesthetic machine, and starting each time with an inspired oxygen concentration of 32% at steady-state conditions, the oxygen supply was interrupted while the nitrous oxide supply remained unchanged. This test was performed with different fresh gas flows of 6, 3, 1 and 0.5 l/min. The lower alarm limit of the oxygen monitor was set to 28%. The test was interrupted immediately if an inspired oxygen concentration of 22% was reached, and the breathing system flushed with pure oxygen. In this test, the oxygen concentration of 22% will represent the critical limit at which potential injury may endanger the patient.

It can clearly be recognized from the illustration that, with a fresh gas flow of 1.0 or 0.5 l/min, the reaction period (Tc and Td) is considerably longer than with a high fresh gas flow of 6 or 3 l/min (Ta and Tb). This in turn means that with low fresh gas flow considerably more time is left for identification and correction of an operating error at the flow controls than with high fresh gas flow. The long time constants of low flow anaesthesia are a specific safety factor which is directly based on the reduction of the fresh gas flow. It prevents sudden accidental hypoxia or anaesthetic agent misdosage in case of inadvertent errors in operating the anaesthetic machine. As regards this point, low flow anaesthetic techniques definitely involve less risks than anaesthesia with high fresh gas flow.

9.2.3 Improved knowledge of the theory and practice of inhalation anaesthesia

An essential safety factor will be improved knowledge about inhalation anaesthesia gained by dealing with the theoretical basis and clinical characteristics of low flow anaesthetic techniques. Prior to performance of such methods, the anaesthetist has to be committed to many specific aspects of anaesthesia. This in turn enhances the understanding of kinetic uptake processes during the course of anaesthesia and of the technical details and features of the anaesthetic machines.

It is self-evident that the early period of training, when first experiences are gained with this technique, requires increased attention to the observation of both the patient and the machine. But in no way can it be claimed that such increased care and attention during anaesthesia should be considered a disadvantage of the method[86]. On the contrary, increased care and attention reduces the risk involved for the patient. Whenever the anaesthetist feels overstrained in a certain clinical situation, he or she is free at any time to switch back to high fresh gas flow and to continue anaesthesia using a more familiar method.

It can be emphasized from the author's own experience that, in dealing with low flow techniques, the anaesthetist learns much about both the patients and the anaesthetic machine[87,88]. This corresponds with the observation published by Deshane and Edsall[89]: the incidence of hypoxaemia with the use of nitrous oxide and varying fresh gas flows during general anaesthetic maintenance were retrospectively studied using computerized patient records on 1064 patients. No hypoxaemia occurred with fresh gas flow less than 3 l/min and the incidence of expired oxygen concentration lower than 26% was significantly ($p < 0.20$) greater with fresh gas flows higher than 3 l/min. The reported results support the thesis that perform-ance of low flow techniques results in increased appreciation of problems and correspondingly careful management of anaesthesia.

9.3   Implications for anaesthetic practice

The potential risks involved in reduction of the fresh gas flow nowadays can always be detected early due to the safety features (Table 9.2) specified by the different technical standards and regulations. The performance of low flow anaesthetic techniques, thus, does not specifically increase the risk for the patient, and, if anaesthetic machines of the new generation are available, generally will not require additional monitoring.

It must be pointed out, however, that conventional anaesthetic machines may be inadequate in terms both of guaranteeing a constant gas volume during mechanical ventilation and with respect to the precision of the flow control systems. Only the anaesthetic machines of the new generation satisfy completely all the technical requirements which facilitate anaesthe-sia with maximally reduced fresh gas flows. Essential technical features are the fresh gas flow compensation of the ventilators and the existence of anaesthetic gas reservoirs. These technical details compensate for the minor volume imbalances, which typically may occur with minimal flow anaesthesia. Anaesthetic machines specifically designed for the use of low fresh gas flows and for judicious use of rebreathing technique do not present any problems in the routine performance even of minimal flow anaesthesia. If, however, use is made of the older conventional machines mentioned above, performance of this anaesthetic method calls for careful observation of ventilation parameters and may need more readjustments in machine settings.

Essentially, the risk involved for the patient during anaesthesia depends on the anaesthetist's familiarity with the anaesthetic method selected and his knowledge regarding the potential for procedure-specific complications[90].

Table 9.2   Safety features of inhalation anaesthetic machines (as required by the common European standard EN 740)

Power failure alarm
Oxygen supply failure alarm
Nitrous oxide cut-off
Oxygen bypass
Oxygen ratio controller
Device for guaranteeing single vaporizer operation
Monitoring of inspired oxygen concentration
Airway pressure monitoring with disconnection and occlusion alarm
Monitoring of expired gas volume
Monitoring of respired carbon dioxide concentration
Monitoring of volatile anaesthetic concentration

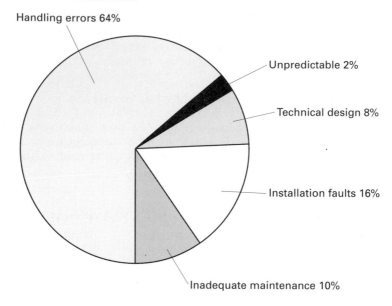

Figure 9.10   Causes of incidents with technical equipment used in medicine. (From Lotz[91], by permission)

It has been demonstrated that only about 4–11% of anaesthetic incidents are definitely caused by malfunction of equipment[80,85,91,92], while 70–80% must be attributed to human error[85,93–95]. Complications are frequently correlated with inadequate equipment testing and maintenance, insufficient knowledge and familiarity with the machine and the anaesthetic method plus incorrect operation of the controls (Figure 9.10). Calkins[93] points out that complications may arise, in particular, if the interactions between breathing system and anaesthetic machine are misjudged.

The following conclusions may be drawn from these points of discussion:

- Dealing with low flow anaesthetic methods should be made a rule in the training of all young anaesthetists. Improved understanding of technical and physiological processes during inhalation anaesthesia provides an essential safety factor for the patient.
- Young anaesthetists who are still in the training phase should perform low flow techniques only under the supervision of an experienced consultant. This is even more important if the technical equipment does not perfectly satisfy all the ideal technical requirements of this method.
- In the management of critical situations and patients, the anaesthetists should adhere to that method in which they are best trained and familiarized. To proceed in this manner always reduces the risk to the patient.
- Selection of the fresh gas flow should be flexibly adapted to the

respective conditions which are a function of the surgical procedure, the equipment and the anaesthetist's state of training.

- The safety of the patient must always assume first priority in the anaesthetist's decision concerning the anaesthetic method[86,96].

If these self-evident rules are borne in mind when a decision is made in favour of an anaesthetic method, low flow anaesthesia can be understood as an alternative technique just as safe as anaesthesia with high fresh gas flow[87,97–99]. But it is only with minimal and low flow anaesthesia that the advantages of rebreathing rendered by the sophisticated technical standards of present-day anaesthetic machines can be used to their best potential.

9.4   Contraindications for low flow anaesthetic techniques

9.4.1   Relative contraindications

In inhalation anaesthesia lasting less than 10–15 min, fresh gas flow reduction is unsuitable because – especially if nitrous oxide is used – there is an increased risk of:

- insufficient denitrogenation;
- inadequate depth of anaesthesia; and
- gas volume deficiency.

If using equipment which does not meet the required technical preconditions, fresh gas flow reduction may become difficult or even impossible:

- due to insufficient gas tightness of the breathing system or the ventilator;
- due to imprecise performance of the gas flow controls in the low flow range;
- during anaesthesia with a face mask;
- in case of rigid bronchoscopy;
- possibly, when using uncuffed endotracheal tubes;
- when using non-rebreathing systems, for instance during magnetic resonance imaging;
- if anaesthetic machines are used featuring no gas reservoir and a ventilator in which the expiratory expansion of the bellows is supported by an additional force, especially in patients suffering from acute bronchospasm.

If there is an increased risk of accumulation of potentially dangerous trace gases, the fresh gas flow should be at least 1 l/min so as to guarantee a continuous wash-out effect. Such contraindications for the use of extremely low fresh gas flow rates – minimal flow or closed system anaesthesia – include:

- decompensated diabetes mellitus;
- the state of long-term starvation;
- anaesthesia performed on chronic alcoholics;

- anaesthesia performed on patients with acute alcohol intoxication;
- heavy smokers suffering from severe restriction of regional perfusion undergoing mass transfusion;
- the use of halothane or sevoflurane in cases lasting longer than 3 h, unless calcium hydroxide lime is used, or with the exception of fan-driven machines such as the PhysioFlex anaesthetic machine.

9.4.2 Absolute contraindications

Whenever a continuous wash-out of dangerous or toxic gases is required or extremely high gas uptake has to be expected, low flow anaesthetic techniques must not be performed. Thus, in case of:

- smoke or gas intoxication;
- malignant hyperthermia; and
- septicaemia.

Furthermore, all conditions in which the equipment does not meet essential requirements to ensure patient safety are generally absolute contraindications of the rebreathing techniques. These include:

- soda lime exhaustion;
- failure of the oxygen monitor (unless pure oxygen is used as carrier gas); and
- failure of the anaesthetic agent monitor (if it is part of the dosing system itself).

9.5 References

1. Baum J, Enzenauer J, Krausse Th and Sachs G. Atemkalk, Nutzungsdauer, Verbrauch und Kosten in Abhängigkeit vom Frischgasfluß. *Anaesthesiol Reanimat* 1993; **18**, 108–113.
2. Baum J. Atemkalk: Hinweise zu korrektem Umgang und fachgerechter Nutzung. Stellungnahme der Kommission für Normung und technische Sicherheit der DGAI. *Anästh Intensivmed* 1999; **40**, 507–509.
3. Ernst EA. Use of charcoal to rapidly decrease depth of anesthesia while maintaining a closed circuit. *Anesthesiology* 1982; **57**, 343.
4. Romano E, Pegoraro M, Vacri A, Pecchiari C and Auci E. Low-flow anaesthesia systems, charcoal and isoflurane kinetics. *Anaesthesia* 1992; **47**, 1098–1099.
5. Ernst EA and Spain JA. Closed-circuit and high-flow systems: examining alternatives. In Brown BR, Calkins JM and Saunders RJ, eds, *Future Anesthesia Delivery Systems. Contemporary Anesthesia Practice*, vol VIII. F. A. Davies, Philadelphia, 1984, pp. 11–38.
6. Barton F and Nunn JF. Totally closed circuit nitrous oxide/oxygen anaesthesia. *Br J Anaesth* 1975; **47**, 350–357.
7. Nunn JF. Techniques for induction of closed circuit anaesthesia. In Aldrete JA, Lowe HJ and Virtue RW, eds, *Low Flow and Closed System Anesthesia*. Grune & Stratton, New York, 1979, pp. 3–10.
8. Barton F and Nunn JF. Use of refractometry to determine nitrogen accumulation in closed circuits. *Br J Anaesth* 1975; **47**, 346–348.

9. Bengtson JP, Bengtsson J, Bengtsson A and Stenqvist O. Sampled gas need not be returned during low-flow anesthesia. *J Clin Monit* 1993; **9**, 330–334.
10. Lin CY, Mostert JW and Benson DW. Closed circle systems. A new direction in the practice of anesthesia. *Acta Anaesth Scand* 1980; **24**, 354–361.
11. Morita S, Latta W, Hambro K and Snider MT. Accumulation of methane, acetone, and nitrogen in the inspired gas during closed-circuit anesthesia. *Anesth Analg* 1985; **64**, 343–347.
12. Versichelen L and Rolly G. Nitrogen accumulation during closed circuit anaesthesia. *Circular* 1989; **6**, 10.
13. Versichelen L and Rolly G. Mass-spectrometric evaluation of some recently introduced low flow, closed circuit systems. *Acta Anaesth Belg* 1990; **41**, 225–237.
14. Westenskow DR, Jordan WS and Gehmlich DS. Electronic feedback control and measurement of oxygen consumption during closed circuit anesthesia. In Aldrete JA, Lowe HJ and Virtue RW, eds, *Low Flow and Closed System Anesthesia*. Grune & Stratton, New York, 1979, pp. 135–146.
15. Spieß W. Narkose im geschlossenen System mit kontinuierlicher inspiratorischer Sauerstoffmessung. *Anaesthesist*, 1977; **26**, 503–513.
16. Strauß J, Hausdörfer J, Bannasch W and Bang S. Akkumulation von Aceton während Langzeitnarkosen in halboffenen und geschlossenen Kreissystemen. *Anaesthesist*, 1991; **40** (Suppl. 2), S260.
17. Strauß JM and Hausdörfer J. Accumulation of acetone in blood during long-term anaesthesia with closed system. *Br J Anaesth* 1993; **70**, 363–364.
18. Strauß JM, Krohn S and Sümpelmann R. Pulmonale Elimination von Azeton und Beatmung im geschlossenen System. *Anaesthesist* 1993; **42** (Suppl. 1), S290.
19. Baumgarten RK and Reynolds WJ. Much ado about nothing: trace gaseous metabolites in the closed circuit. *Anesth Analg* 1985; **64**, 1029–1030.
20. Middleton V, van Poznak A, Artusio JF and Smith SM. Carbon monoxide accumulation in closed circle anesthesia systems. *Anesthesiology* 1965; **26**, 715–719.
21. Strauß JM, Bannasch W, Hausdörfer J and Bang S. Die Entwicklung von Carboxyhmoglobin während Langzeitnarkosen im geschlossenen Kreissystem. *Anaesthesist* 1991; **40**, 324–327.
22. Henderson M and Haggard HW. The treatment of carbon monoxide asphyxia by means of oxygen and CO_2 inhalation. A method for the rapid elimination of carbon monoxide from the blood. *JAMA* 1922; **79**, 1137.
23. Moon RE, Meyer AF, Scott DL, Fox E, Millington DS and Norwood DM. Intraoperative carbon monoxide toxicity. *Anesthesiology* 1990; **73**, A1049.
24. Moon RE, Ingram C, Brunner EA and Meyer AF. Spontaneous generation of carbon monoxide within anaesthetic circuits. *Anesthesiology* 1991; **75**, A873.
25. Pankow D. *Toxikologie des Kohlenmonoxids*. VEB Verlag Volk und Gesundheit, Berlin, 1981, S.55 u.87.
26. Moon RE. Carbon monoxide gas may be linked to CO_2 absorbent. *Anesthesia Patient Safety Foundation Newsletter* 1991; **6**, 8.
27. Fang ZX, Eger II EI, Laster MJ, Chortkoff BS, Kandel L and Ionescu P. Carbon monoxide production from degradation of desflurane, enflurane, isoflurane, halothane and sevoflurane by soda lime and baralyme. *Anesth Analg* 1995; **80**, 1187–1193.
28. Strauß JM, Baum J, Sümpelmann R, Krohn S and Callies A. Zersetzung von Halothan, Enfluran und Isofluran an trockenem Atemkalk zu Kohlenmonoxid. *Anaesthesist* 1996; **45**, 798–801.
29. Berry PD, Sessler DI and Larson MD. Severe carbon monoxide poisoning during desflurane anesthesia. *Anesthesiology* 1999; **90**, 613–616.

30. Baum J and Strauß JM. Kohlenmonoxidbildung am Atemkalk. *Anästh Intensivmed* 1995; **36**, 237–240.
31. Kharasch ED. Putting the brakes on anesthetic breakdown. *Anesthesiology* 1999; **91**, 1192–1194.
32. Murray JM, Renfrew CW, Bedi A, McCrystal CB, Jones DS and Fee JPH. Amsorb: a new carbon dioxide absorbent for use in anaesthetic breathing systems. *Anesthesiology* 1999; **91**, 1342–1348.
33. Baum J, Sachs G, v. d. Driesch C and Stanke HG. Carbon monoxide generation in carbon dioxide absorbents. *Anesth Analg* 1995; **81**, 144–146.
34. Zacharowski K. Die unblutige und präzise Bestimmung von Carboxyhämoglobin und Blutvolumen. Inauguraldissertation der Johannes Gutenberg-Universität Mainz, Fachbereich Medizin, 1995.
35. Morita S. Inspired gas contamination by non-anesthetic gases during closed circuit anesthesia. *Circular* 1985; **2**, 24–25.
36. Baum J, v. Legat M and Leier M. The carbon monoxide story. *Eur J Anaesth* 1997; **14**, 57–58.
37. Rathgeber J, Züchner K, Kietzmann D and Kraus E. Leistungsfähigkeit eines mobilen Sauerstoffkonzentrators für die Narkosebeatmung. *Anästhesist* 1995; **44**, 643–650.
38. Parker CJR and Snowdon SL. Predicted and measured oxygen concentrations in the circle system using low fresh gas flows with oxygen supplied by an oxygen concentrator. *Br J Anaesth* 1988; **61**, 397–402.
39. Aldrete JA and Virtue RW. Prolonged inhalation of inert gases by rats. *Anesth Analg* 1967; **46**, 562–565.
40. Morita S, Latta W and Snider M. Accumulation of methane, acetone and nitrogen in the inspired gas during closed-circuit anesthesia. *Anesth Analg* 1985; **64**, 343–347.
41. Rolly G, Versichelen LF and Mortier E. Methane accumulation during closed-circuit anesthesia. *Anesth Analg* 1994; **79**, 545–547.
42. Versichelen L, Rolly G and Vermeulen H. Accumulation of foreign gases during closed-system anaesthesia. *Br J Anaesth* 1996; **76**, 668–672.
43. Morita S, Toyooka H and Nagase M. Hydrogen accumulation in closed circuit. *Jpn J Anesth* 1985; **34**, 468–472.
44. Sharp HJ, Trudell JR and Cohen EN. Volatile metabolites and decomposition products of halothane in man. *Anesthesiology* 1979; **50**, 2–8.
45. Kenna JG and Jones RM. The organ toxicity of inhaled anesthetics. *Anesth Analg* 1995; **81**, S51–S66.
46. Fang ZX and Eger II EI. Factors affecting the concentration of compound A resulting from degradation of sevoflurane by soda lime and Baralyme® in a standard anesthetic circuit. *Anesth Analg* 1995; **81**, 564–568.
47. Fang ZX, Kandel L, Laster MJ, Ionescu P and Eger II EI. Factors affecting production of compound A from the interaction of sevoflurane with Baralyme® and soda lime. *Anesth Analg* 1996; **82**, 775–781.
48. Bito H and Ikeda K. Effect of total flow rate on the concentration of degradation products generated by the reaction between sevoflurane and soda lime. *Br J Anaesth* 1995; **74**, 667–669.
49. Bito H and Ikeda K. Long-duration, low-flow sevoflurane anesthesia using two carbon dioxide absorbents. *Anesthesiology* 1994; **81**, 340–345.
50. Morio M, Fujii K, Satoh N, Imai M, Kawakami U, Mizuno T, Kawai Y, Ogasawara Y, Tamura T, Negishi A, Kumagai Y and Kawai T. Reaction of sevoflurane and its degradation products with soda lime. Toxicity of the byproducts. *Anesthesiology* 1992; **77**, 1155–1164.
51. Smith I, Nathanson M and White PF. Sevoflurane – a long-awaited volatile anaesthetic. *Br J Anaesth* 1996; **76**, 435–445.

52. Gonsowski CT, Laster MJ, Eger II EI, Ferrell LD and Kerschmann RL. Toxicity of compound A in rats. Effect of a 3-hour administration. *Anesthesiology* 1994; **80**, 556–565.
53. Keller KA, Callan C, Prokocimer P, Delgado-Herrera L, Friedman MB, Hoffman GM, Wooding WL, Cusick PK and Krasula RW. Inhalation toxicity study of a haloalkene degradant of sevoflurane, compound A (PIFE), in Sprague–Dawley rats. *Anesthesiology* 1995; **83**, 1220–1232.
54. Kharasch ED and Jubert C. Compound A uptake and metabolism to mercapturic acids and 3,3-trifluoro-2-fluoromethoxypropanoic acid during low flow sevoflurane anesthesia. *Anesthesiology* 1999; **91**, 1267–1278.
55. Jin L, Baillie TA, Davis MR and Kharasch ED. Nephrotoxicity of sevoflurane compound A in rats: evidence for glutathione and cysteine conjugate formation and the role of renal cysteine conjugate β-lyase. *Biochem Biophys Res Commun* 1995; **210**, 498–506.
56. Ramaswamy AI and Anders MW. Cysteine conjugate β-lyase-dependent biotransformation of the cysteine S-conjugates of the sevoflurane degradation product compound A in human, nonhuman primate, and rat kidney cytosol and mitochondria. *Anesthesiology* 1996; **85**, 454–461.
57. Martin JL, Laster MJ, Kandel L, Kerschmann RL, Reed GF and Eger II EI. Metabolism of compound A by renal cysteine-S-conjugate beta-lyase is not the mechanism of compound A-induced renal injury in the rat. *Anesth Analg* 1996; **82**, 770–774.
58. Eger EI, Gong D, Koblin DD, Bowland T, Ionescu P, Laster MJ and Weiskopf RB. Dose-related biochemical markers of renal injury after sevoflurane versus desflurane anesthesia in volunteers. *Anesth Analg* 1997; **85**, 1154–1163.
59. Eger EI, Gong D, Koblin DD, Bowland T, Ionescu P, Laster MJ and Weiskopf RB. The effect of anesthetic duration on kinetic and recovery characteristics of desflurane versus sevoflurane, and on the kinetic characteristics of compound A in volunteers. *Anesth Analg* 1998; **86**, 414–421.
60. Goldberg ME, Cantillo J, Gratz I, Deal E, Vekeman D, McDougall R, Afshar M, Zafeiridis A and Larijani G. Dose of compound A, not sevoflurane, determines changes in the biochemical markers of renal injury in healthy volunteers. *Anesth Analg* 1999; **88**, 437–445.
61. Mazze RI and Jamison RL. Low-flow (1 l/min) sevoflurane – is it safe? *Anesthesiology* 1997; **86**, 1225–1227.
62. Bito H, Ikeuchi Y and Ikeda K. Effects of low-flow sevoflurane anesthesia on renal function. Comparison with high-flow sevoflurane and low-flow isoflurane anesthesia. *Anesthesiology* 1997; **86**, 1231–1237.
63. Kharash ED, Frink EJ, Zager R, Bowdle TA, Artru A and Nogami WM. Assessment of low-flow sevoflurane and isoflurane effects on renal function using sensitive markers of tubular toxicity. *Anesthesiology* 1997; **86** 1238–1253.
64. Mazze RI, Friedman M, Delgado-Herrera L, Galvez ST and Mayer DB. Renal toxicity of compound A plus sevoflurane compared with isoflurane in non-human primates. *Anesthesiology* 1998; **89**: A490.
65. Reinhardt C, Gronau E, Wüsten R, Goeters C, Vrana S, Baum J and van Aken H. Compound A in minimal flow sevoflurane. *Anesthesiology* 1998, **89**, A142.
66. Baum JA. Low-flow anesthesia: theory, practice, technical preconditions, advantages, and foreign gas accumulation. *J Anesth* 1999; **13**, 166–174.
67. Neumann MA, Laster MJ, Weiskopf RB, Gong DH, Dudziak R, Forster H and Eger EI. The elimination of sodium and potassium hydroxides from

desiccated soda lime diminishes degradation of desflurane to carbon monoxide and sevoflurane to compound A but does not compromise carbon dioxide absorption. *Anesth Analg* 1999; **89**, 768–773.

68. Funk W, Gruber M, Wild K and Hobbhahn J. Dry soda lime markedly degrades sevoflurane during simulated inhalation induction. *Br J Anaesth* 1999; **82**, 193–198.

69. Conzen PF, Nuscheler M, Melotte A, Verhaegen M, Leupolt T, van Aken H and Peter K. Renal function and serum fluoride concentrations in patients with stable renal insufficiency after anaesthesia with sevoflurane or enflurane. *Anesth Analg* 1995; **81**, 569–575.

70. Frink EJ, Malan TP, Isner RJ, Brown EA, Morgan SE and Brown BR. Renal concentration function with prolonged sevoflurane or enflurane anesthesia in volunteers. *Anesthesiology* 1994; **80**, 1019–1025.

71. Goldberg ME, Cantillo J, Larijani GE, Torjman M, Vekeman D and Schieren H. Sevoflurane versus isoflurane for maintenance of anesthesia: are serum inorganic fluoride ion concentrations of concern? *Anesth Analg* 1996; **82**, 1268–1272.

72. Eger EI, Koblin DD, Bowland T, Ionescu P, Laster MJ, Fang Z, Gong D, Sonner J and Weiskopf RB. Nephrotoxicity of sevoflurane versus desflurane anesthesia in volunteers. *Anesth Analg* 1997; **84**, 160–168.

73. Higuchi H, Sumita S, Wada H, Ura T, Ikemoto T, Nakai T, Kanno M and Satoh T. Effects of sevoflurane and isoflurane on renal function and on possible markers of nephrotoxicity. *Anesthesiology* 1998; **89**, 307–322.

74. Nishiyama T and Hanaoka K. Inorganic fluoride kinetics and renal and hepatic function after repeated sevoflurane anaesthesia. *Anesth Analg* 1998; **87** 468–473.

75. Bito H and Ikeda K. Renal and hepatic function in surgical patients after low-flow sevoflurane or isoflurane anesthesia. *Anesth Analg* 1996; **82**, 173–176.

76. Ruzicka JA, Hidalgo JC, Tinker JH and Baker MT. Inhibition of volatile sevoflurane degradation product formation in an anesthetic circuit by a reduction in soda lime temperature. *Anesthesiology* 1994; **81**, 238–244.

77. Cunnigham DD, Huang S, Webster J, Mayoral J and Grabenkort RW. Sevoflurane degradation to compound A in anaesthesia breathing systems. *Br J Anaesth* 1996; **77**, 537–543.

78. Wissing H, Kuhn I and Kessler P. Das Wärme-Feuchte-Profil des Physioflex. Untersuchungen am Modell. *Anaesthesist* 1997; **46**, 201–206.

79. Funk W, Gruber M, Jakob W and Hobbhahn J. Compound A does not accumulate during closed circuit sevoflurane anaesthesia with the Physioflex. *Br J Anaesth* 1999; **83**, 571–575.

80. Ahnefeld FW, Kilian J and Friesdorf W. Sicherheit und Instandhaltung medizinisch-technischer Geräte. *Anästh Intensivmed* 1981; **22**, 291–308.

81. Good ML and Paulus DA. Equipment. In Gravenstein N., ed., *Manual of Complications During Anesthesia*. J. B. Lippincott, Philadelphia, 1991, pp. 83–120.

82. Johnstone RE. Equipment malfunction. In Orkin FK, Cooperman LH, eds, *Complications in Anesthesiology*. J. B. Lippincott, Philadelphia, 1983, pp. 639–645.

83. Müchler HC. Das technische Narkoserisiko. *Prakt Anästh* 1978; **13**, 368–378.

84. Schreiber P. Anesthesia systems. In North American Draeger Safety Guidelines. Merchants Press, Boston, 1985.

85. Schreiber P and Schreiber JM. Electronic surveillance during anesthesia. North American Draeger, Telford, 1986.

86. Opderbecke HW. Ärztliche Sorgfaltspflicht bei der Narkoseführung mit reduziertem Frischgasflow. In Lawin P, van Aken H and Schneider U. *Alternative*

Methoden in der Anästhesie, INA-Schriftenreihe, Bd. 50. Thieme, Stuttgart, 1985, pp. 49–52.

87. Cullen SC. Who is watching the patient? *Anesthesiology* 1972; **37**, 361–362.
88. Edsall DW. Economy is not the major benefit of closed-system anesthesia. *Anesthesiology* 1981; **54**, 258.
89. Deshane PD and Edsall DW. Incidence of hypoxemia due to a hypoxic mixture in low flow anesthesia when using nitrous oxide. Abstracts of the Annual Meeting of The Society for Technology in Anesthesia 1993 'Human Performance and Anesthesia Technology', New Orleans, p. 49.
90. Eyrich K. Sorgfalt bei der Prämedikation und Wahl des Anästhesieverfahrens. *Anästh Intensivmed* 1979; **20**, 39–43.
91. Lotz P. Sicherheitstechnische Aspekte bei der Anwendung medizinisch-technischer Geräte im Krankenhaus. *mt-Medizintechnik* 1984; **104**, 133–137.
92. Lunn JN and Mushin WW. *Mortality Associated with Anaesthesia*. Nuffield Provincial Hospitals Trust, London, 1982.
93. Calkins JM. Why new delivery systems? In Brown BR, ed., *Future Anesthesia Delivery Systems. Contemporary Anesthesia Practice*, vol. VIII. Davies, Philadelphia, 1984, pp. 3–9.
94. Cooper JB, Newborner RS and Kitz RJ. An analysis of major errors and equipment failures in anesthesia management: considerations for prevention and detection. *Anesthesiology* 1984; **60**, 34–42.
95. Keats AS. What do we know about anesthetic mortality? *Anesthesiology* 1979; **50**, 387–392.
96. Opderbecke HW. Sorgfalt bei der Durchführung und Überwachung der Anästhesie. *Anästh Intensivmed* 1979; **20**, 59–62.
97. Mazzia VDB and Simon AH. Low flow and close system anesthesia: legal liability and some specific cases. In Aldrete JA, Lowe HJ and Virtue RW, eds, *Low Flow and Closed System Anesthesia*. Grune & Stratton, New York, 1979, pp. 315–321.
98. Spieß W. Minimal-flow Anästhesie – eine zeitgemäße Alternative für die Klinikroutine. *Anaesth Reanim* 1980; **5**, 145–159.
99. Virtue RW. Toward closed system anesthesia. *Anaesthesist* 1977; **26**, 545–546.
100. Baum J and van Aken H. Calcium hydroxide lime – a new carbon dioxide absorbent. A rationale for judicious use of different absorbents. *Eur J Anaesth* 2000; **17**, 597–600.

10

Low flow anaesthesia in clinical practice

Chapters 10 and 11 will focus exclusively on all practical aspects of low flow anaesthesia, minimal flow anaesthesia and closed system anaesthesia. During low flow anaesthesia a considerable amount of excess gas is still used, rendering the clinical performance of this technique especially simple. If nitrous oxide is used, minimal flow anaesthesia is the low flow technique in which the fresh gas flow is reduced to the greatest possible extent assuming that modern anaesthetic equipment is available. Both techniques are extreme variants of the semi-closed use of rebreathing systems, which is the designed use for most anaesthetic machines. Thus, minimal flow anaesthesia still corresponds well to the defined range of operation of the apparatus. The safety facilities provided by different American and European standards and regulations comprehensively meet the requirements, being specific preconditions for safe performance of low flow techniques. If, however, nitrous oxide as a carrier gas is omitted, even non-quantitative anaesthesia may become an anaesthetic technique in clinical routine practice.

At first, low flow anaesthetic techniques should only be applied in uncomplicated surgical procedures and on patients not suffering from critical disease. Thus, full attention can be paid to both the patient and the anaesthetic machine while gaining early experience with the new technique. It ought to go without saying, yet it should be emphasized once more, that, in the case of high risk patients or surgical interventions, the anaesthetist must only employ a suitable anaesthetic method he is best acquainted with. From the medicolegal aspect, however, all the different low flow anaesthetic techniques are anaesthetic methods appropriate for routine clinical use. Much scientific investigation has been dedicated to these methods which thus are nowadays widely accepted and approved anaesthetic techniques. As early as 1986, Bergmann[1] pointed out that performance of anaesthesia with high fresh gas flow rates, as it was still widely employed at that time, is in marked contrast to the high technical standards of modern anaesthetic machines.

10.1 Maintenance of the equipment

Following daily use, the breathing system, including all valves, is completely disassembled, cleaned, sterilized or disinfected according to the respective instructions for use. It must be ensured that all sealing rings are removed from their grooves to be carefully cleaned. Thereafter, all components are dried and laid out for cooling. If a conventional breathing system is still equipped with a switch to operate the excess gas discharge valve, prior to re-assembly of the cleaned components, the stopcock has to be lubricated with an oxygen-safe grease (e.g. Oxygenoex S4, Dräger Medizintechnik, Lübeck, Germany). The leakproofness required for minimal flow or closed system anaesthesia can only be achieved if brittle and hard seals are removed and all screw connections of the circle system are tightened carefully but not excessively. Plastic components of the system such as absorber canisters and valve domes have to be thoroughly checked for hairline cracks and replaced if necessary. Metal tapers have to be checked for damage, and cleanliness and the correct fit of all metal-to-metal connections must be verified. This approach ensures that the required gas tightness of the breathing system with a leakage loss less than $100\,ml/min$ at a pressure of $2\,kPa$ ($\approx 20\,cmH_2O$) can always be achieved in routine clinical use. It is good practice to keep a small number of seals and plastic components available as spare parts.

Where the use of two absorbers in tandem arrangement is concerned, the contents of the absorber adjacent to the circle system should be discarded whenever the soda lime is exhausted, but routinely at least it should be replaced after 1 week's use. The same procedure should be adopted if single absorbers are used, provided continuous carbon dioxide monitoring is in use. Bacteriological investigations in the author's own department confirmed that this procedure can be considered to be very safe in terms of hygiene[2,3]. When the absorbent is discarded, the absorber canister should be disassembled as far as possible, and care should be taken again that rubber seals are removed from their grooves. The disassembled absorber has to be disinfected or sterilized in accordance with the manufacturer's instructions for use. After cleaning, the sealing rings and components are re-assembled when they have cooled down to room temperature. When the clean absorber has been refilled, a label indicating the filling date must be attached to the canister. Care must be taken not to risk accidental desiccation of the carbon dioxide absorbent (see Section 7.2.5).

A patient hose system is attached to the circle system immediately after re-assembly and the breathing system carefully tested for leaks. The APL valve at the circle absorber system has to be closed and the hoses attached to the Y-piece as shown in Figure 10.1. A high oxygen flow is then supplied to the system in order to build up a pressure of $2\,kPa$ ($20\,cmH_2O$) within the system. Then the oxygen flow is reduced to $100\,ml/min$: under these conditions, the pressure of $2\,kPa$ must not fall over a period of 1 min. In the author's department, the leak test is performed routinely at a pressure of $3\,kPa$ ($\approx 30\,cmH_2O$), a tightness which can be achieved even in routine use of the anaesthetic machines if maintenance is conducted in the described manner.

The gas tightness of modern anaesthetic machines like AS/3 ADU (Datex, Helsinki, Finland), Cato, Cicero EM and Julian (Dräger Medizintechnik, Lübeck, Germany), or Elsa and EAS 9010 (Gambro-Engström, Bromma, Sweden) is tested in test sequences which run

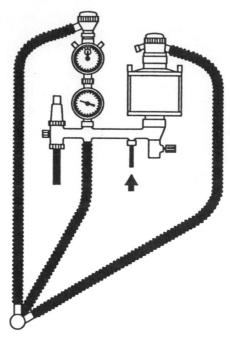

Figure 10.1 Connections of hose assembly for performance of leak test: circle absorption system 8 ISO (Dräger Medizintechnik, Lübeck, Germany)

automatically (see Section 7.2.4.1). After having passed the check success-fully, the gas tightness of the breathing system and the ventilator will always meet the requirements for the performance of each kind of low flow technique.

Testing of the other modules of the cleaned machine is carried out in line with the respective instructions for use.

Proper function of all monitoring systems has to be checked at the beginning of each working day. This includes, if required, calibration and zero adjustment of the gas analyser and calibration of the oxygen monitor to 21% O_2 with ambient air. Furthermore, readiness for use of the anaesthetic machine and gas tightness of the breathing system must be tested again every day prior to the start of the daily list.

10.1.1   Are there greater demands on disinfection or sterilization of the equipment resulting from fresh gas flow reduction?

In low flow anaesthetic techniques the temperature and the humidity of the anaesthetic gases increase significantly. As increased warmth and humidity facilitates bacterial growth in the event of contamination, the question may be raised of whether routine performance of low flow anaesthesia increases the risk of bacterial contamination of the breathing system.

In the author's own investigation on this topic, 546 bacteriological

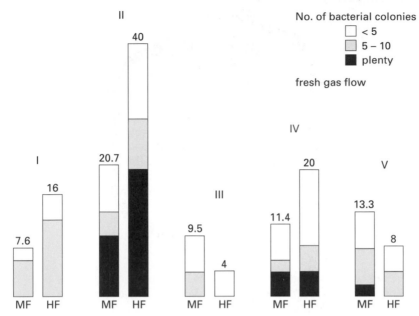

Figure 10.2 Percentage of positive bacteriological samples, related to the total number of samples taken at the corresponding sample site I–V. Comparison between the high flow (HF) and the minimal flow (MF) group. I, connection between expired hose and expired valve; II, connection between manual bag and breathing system; III, taper at the expired side of the CO_2 absorber; IV, taper at the inspired side of the CO_2 absorber; V, connection between inspired hose and inspired valve. (From Baum[2])

samples were taken with the aid of cotton-tipped swabs at different sites in the breathing system 55 (about 10%) of them showed bacterial contamination. Twenty-one (38%) of the 55 positive results were found at the point where the manual bag is attached to the anaesthetic circuit with a rubber hose (Figure 10.2: sampling site II). At the other sampling sites, only minor bacterial contamination was found. Even if the results were differentiated according to the number of bacterial colonies, the highest incidence of plentiful colonies could be found at this particular sampling site II.

With two anaesthetic machines, minimal flow anaesthesia was performed routinely, while with another anaesthetic apparatus, anaesthesia with high fresh gas flow was carried out exclusively. If the results were differentiated according to the fresh gas flow used, a statistical difference could not be established between the two groups (Figure 10.2). There is, therefore, no evidence of increased bacterial contamination caused by flow reduction. These results correspond with the findings of Bengtson et al.[4].

The investigation was performed under the conditions of routine daily maintenance: according to the recommendations given by the German Society of Anaesthesiology and Intensive Care Medicine, DGAI,[5] the face masks, the Y-pieces and the patient hosing were changed with every patient. If, however, a bacterial filter is inserted between the tube connector and the Y-piece, as became routine practice about 2 years ago, the hosing is only changed once after finishing the daily list. All parts of the breathing system which can be disassembled were disinfected on a daily schedule, and all breathing gas containing parts of the complete circle system and the ventilator were sterilized weekly. As, at the time of the investigation, the manual bag with its connecting tube was considered to be a part of the circuit itself, it was only changed and disinfected weekly. The results of the investigation, however, suggest that the manual bag and the connecting rubber tube should also preferably be changed on a daily basis. The site where the rubber hose is connected to the circuit seems to be a favoured location for bacterial growth. Generally, this is the lowest point of the breathing circle, where accumulation of condensed water is likely, facilitating the growth of microbes like *Pseudomonas* which prefer a warm and humid environment.

The results of our investigations justify the following statements and recommendations:

- The routine performance of low flow anaesthetic techniques does not increase the risk of bacterial contamination of the breathing system if cleaning and sterilizing procedures are accomplished properly.
- Bacterial contamination, however, seems to increase if a previously used breathing system is left idle without cleaning for a longer period of time.
- There is absolutely no evidence that there is an aerogenic spread of bacterial contamination by the gas flow, neither in the high flow nor the low flow group. This corresponds well to the results of comprehensive investigations in this field by Stober *et al.*[6,7].
- Care should be taken to change the manual bag with its connecting hose on a daily schedule. It is recommended not to attach the new connecting hose to the circuit prior to its use the next working day, but preferably to leave the adapter open in the night, thus allowing adequate drying of the metal-to-rubber connection.
- As most of the identified bacterial strains are common skin commensals, the hands should be disinfected before re-assembling the circuit after cleaning and sterilizing; furthermore, disinfection of the hands should be obligatory whenever the patient hoses are changed after use.

Whether the use of bacterial filters offers real advantages in preventing cross-contamination by anaesthetic equipment has long been controversial[8]. According to the author's experiences the use of bacterial filters saves time and money, resulting from a significant reduction of parts needing daily disinfection. Furthermore, bacterial filters reduce contamination of the equipment[9], but Luttropp and Berntman also admit that their absence does not increase contamination either of the circle or the ventilator. Nevertheless, if the hosing is used over the period of one whole operating list a new bacterial filter must be used with each patient to exclude any risk for the patients from Y-piece contamination. Whether the use of bacterial filters, or even heat and moisture exchangers (HMEs), reduces the water condensation within the breathing system and hosing during low flow anaesthesia has not yet been verified. The use of HMEs to ensure adequate humidification and warming of the anaesthetic gases is judged to be unnecessary if anaesthesia is performed with low flow techniques[10] (see Section 6.4).

10.2   Practice of low flow anaesthesia with halothane, enflurane and isoflurane

Please note that all details about metering of the anaesthetic agent and controlling of the gas flows are clinically proven guidelines for the safe performance of low flow anaesthesia in adult patients of normal body weight.

10.2.1   Pre-medication and induction

The pre-medication can follow the usual scheme; there are absolutely no method-specific requirements with respect to the low flow techniques.

The induction of low flow anaesthesia also follows the normal routine: after pre-oxygenation, i.v. injection of a hypnotic and (if necessary) neuromuscular relaxation, an endotracheal tube or a laryngeal mask is inserted. The patient is then connected to a rebreathing system.

Low flow anaesthetic techniques must only be performed if the monitoring essential for safe performance of these methods is available and working reliably, the alarm limits are carefully adjusted and the alarms activated as soon as the patient is connected to the breathing system. The lower alarm limit of the inspired oxygen concentration should be set to 28–30 vol%, the disconnect alarm to 5 cmH$_2$O below the respective peak pressure, the occlusion alarm to 30 cmH$_2$O, and the lower alarm of the expired gas volume monitoring to 500 ml less than the desired minute volume. The upper alarm limit for the anaesthetic agent monitoring should be set to a threshold of 2.0–2.5 vol% for halothane, enflurane and isoflurane.

10.2.2   Initial phase of low flow inhalation anaesthesia

An initial phase in which a high fresh gas flow of about 4 l/min is used (in the author's department 1.4 l/min O$_2$, 3.0 l/min N$_2$O) has to precede the reduction of the fresh gas flow rate. During this initial phase, a sufficient denitrogenation will be gained, the desired gas composition must be washed-in into the breathing system, and the desired concentration of the chosen anaesthetic agent has to be established, guaranteeing a sufficient anaesthetic level. The comparatively high excess gas volume, furthermore, prevents accidental gas volume deficiency which especially might occur in the initial phase which is characterized by high nitrous oxide uptake. The duration of this initial high flow phase depends on the extent of the flow reduction and the individual's total gas uptake.

Using a fresh gas flow rate between 4 and 5 l/min (fresh gas composition: 32% O$_2$, 68% N$_2$O) denitrogenation will be finished after about

6–8 min. After 10 min an oxygen concentration of about 30 vol% and a nitrous oxide concentration of about 65 vol% will be established within the breathing system. When the vaporizer is set to 1.5% isoflurane, 2.5% enflurane or 1.3% halothane, respectively, after 10–15 min an expired agent concentration will be gained, being about $0.8 \times MAC$ of the chosen anaesthetic agent. This concentration, together with a nitrous oxide concentration between 50 and 65%, will result in an additive effect which equals the AD_{95}, the agent concentration needed to guarantee that 95% of patients will tolerate the initial skin incision without any motor response.

10.2.3   The change from high to low fresh gas flow rate

10.2.3.1   Low flow anaesthesia

Ten minutes after connecting the patient to the rebreathing system the total gas uptake can be assumed to be still about 600 ml/min. In low flow anaesthesia at that time the fresh gas flow rate is reduced to 1.0 l/min. The fresh gas volume exceeds the individual uptake; thus, a sufficient amount of excess gas is available to balance an additive loss of gas volume.

The reduction of the fresh gas flow rate results in a significant increase of the rebreathing fraction and, correspondingly, the share of oxygen-depleted gas. The inspired oxygen concentration of 30 vol% can only be maintained if at the moment of flow reduction the oxygen concentration of the fresh gas is raised to at least 40%, and preferably 50%.

Using a vaporizer outside the circle, the reduction of the flow rate will result in a corresponding decrease of the amount of anaesthetic vapour supplied into the breathing system. To maintain the nominal anaesthetic concentration of $0.8 \times MAC$ its fresh gas concentration has to be increased: isoflurane to 2.0 vol%, enflurane to 3.0 vol%, and halothane to 2.0 vol% (Figure 10.3a–c).

10.2.3.2   Minimal flow anaesthesia

If minimal flow anaesthesia is performed, the fresh gas flow rate is reduced to 0.5 l/min. An initial phase lasting at least 15 min, in very strong patients as long as 20 min, must precede the flow reduction. Early reduction of the fresh gas flow will increase the risk of gas volume deficiency, as a gas volume as low as 0.5 l/min might not meet the gas loss via high initial uptake and leakages. Gas volume deficiency will lead to insufficient ventilation.

As, compared to low flow anaesthesia, the rebreathing fraction is still increasing, the oxygen content of the fresh gas has to be raised, probably to 60 vol%, but at least to 50 vol%. The target nominal anaesthetic concentration of $0.8 \times MAC$ can only be maintained by increasing the fresh gas volatile agent concentration: isoflurane to 2.5 vol%, enflurane to 3.5 vol%, and halothane to 3.0 vol% (Figure 10.3a–c).

10.2.3.3   Anaesthetic gas composition

During performance of inhalation anaesthesia with a fresh gas flow rate close to the minute volume the rebreathing fraction becomes negligible. Irrespective of the use of a rebreathing system the exhaled gases are discharged out of the system almost completely. The composition of the anaesthetic gas is similar to that of the fresh gas, and remains unchanged during the course of the anaesthetic.

However, in minimal flow anaesthesia the composition of the gases exhaled by the patient to a large extent determines the composition of the gas within the breathing system. The composition of the exhaled gases, for its part, is mainly determined by the individual's uptake of oxygen, nitrous oxide and anaesthetic agent, the latter both of which are changing continuously and independently during the course of the anaesthetic. Initially these alterations of the uptake of the different gas components are rapid and extensive, whereas after a certain period of time they become small and insignificant. Thus, after the initial phase is finished, a constant fresh gas composition can be used according to a standardized scheme over a longer period of time. This can be clinically realized in low and minimal flow anaesthesia and significantly facilitates routine clinical performance of these low flow techniques. However, when using a fixed fresh gas composition, due to the continuous alterations of uptake, very slow but continuous alterations of the anaesthetic gas composition have to be accepted[11].

10.2.3.3.1   Inspired oxygen concentration
In the first 30–45 min after flow reduction an increase of the inspired oxygen concentration can be observed. During this period the nitrous oxide uptake is still significant. As, however, the nitrous oxide uptake continuously declines, in longer anaesthetics this gas begins to accumulate within the breathing system, causing a slow but continuous decrease of the oxygen concentration. Whenever the inspired oxygen concentration falls below the lower alarm limit of 30 vol%, the oxygen flow should be increased by 10% of the total fresh gas flow rate and the nitrous oxide flow reduced by the same amount. Thus, in low flow anaesthesia the oxygen flow is increased by 100 ml/min, i.e. from 500 to 600 ml/min, and the nitrous oxide flow reduced by the same amount, i.e. from 500 to 400 ml/min. Accordingly, in minimal flow anaesthesia the flow of both carrier gas components is changed by 50 ml/min. After these corrections the inspired oxygen concentration will increase but after a certain period of time will tend to decrease again. Whenever the lower alarm threshold is reached again, appropriate corrections of the gas flows have to be made (Figure 10.4).

If, in order to more efficiently use the analgesic and amnesic effects of nitrous oxide[12–14], minimal flow anaesthesia is performed with a fresh gas oxygen concentration of only 50 vol%, the inspired oxygen concentration in 30% of all cases decreases to 28 vol% in the first 60 min following flow reduction (Figure 10.5a and b). The lower the oxygen content of the fresh

Exp. halothane concentration (vol %)

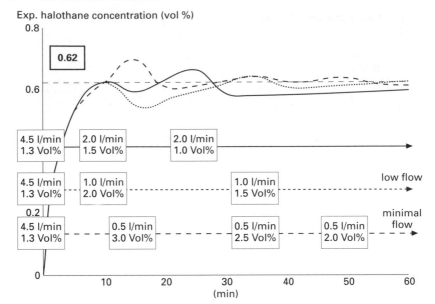

Figure 10.3a

Exp. enflurane concentration (vol %)

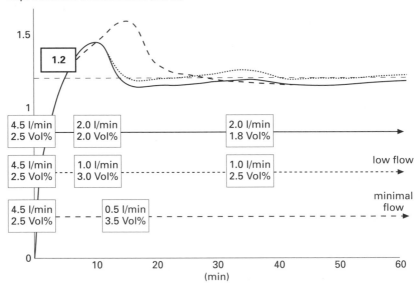

Figure 10.3b

gas after flow reduction, the more frequently will the fresh gas composition have to be changed in favour of oxygen.

During low flow anaesthetic techniques, the inspired oxygen concentration is determined mainly by the individual's oxygen consumption. The

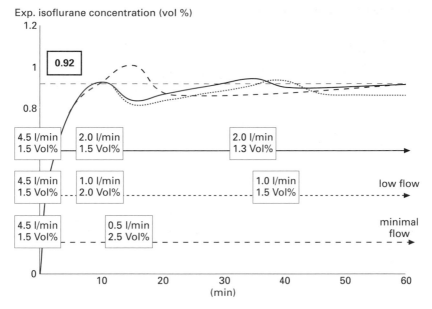

Figure 10.3c

Figure 10.3 Inhalation anaesthetic concentrations to be selected at different fresh gas flow rates to establish and maintain a desired expiratory concentration of about 0.8 MAC of the respective agent (assumed body weight of the patient = 75 kg). (a) Halothane, desired expired concentration 0.62 vol%; (b) enflurane, desired expired concentration 1.2 vol%; (c) isoflurane, desired expired concentration 0.92 vol%

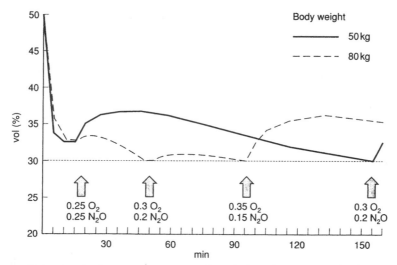

Figure 10.4 Inspired oxygen concentration during the course of minimal flow anaesthesia as a function of body weight (correlates to the oxygen uptake). At flow reduction, oxygen and nitrous oxide flow are set to 0.25 l/min each. Whenever the concentration drops to 30%, oxygen flow is increased by 0.05 l/min and nitrous oxide flow decreased by the same value

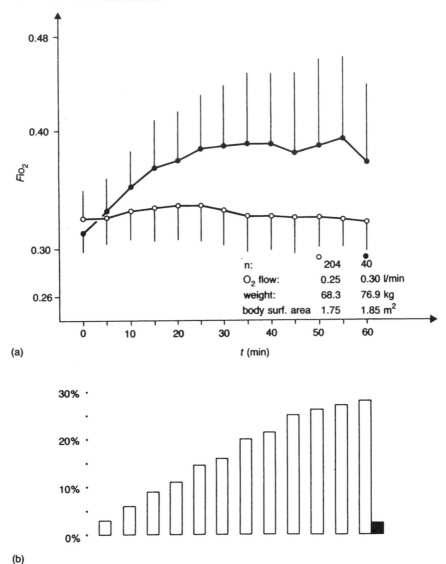

Figure 10.5   (a) Alterations of the inspired oxygen concentration (F_{iO_2}) during the course of minimal flow anaesthesia as a function of fresh gas composition: fresh gas flow 0.5 l/min–0.25 l/min O_2 and 0.25 l/min N_2O versus fresh gas flow 0.5 l/min–0.3 l/min O_2 and 0.2 l/min N_2O. Ordinate: F_{iO_2}, mean values and standard deviation; abscissa: time, starting with flow reduction. (b) Cumulative presentation of the relative frequency at which F_{iO_2} drops below the value of 0.28

inspired oxygen concentration is significantly lower in young, strong and athletic patients than in old, small and asthenic patients with less muscle tissue (Figure 10.6). If the oxygen consumption and the resulting oxygen uptake is high, due to the high oxygen extraction from the alveolar gas,

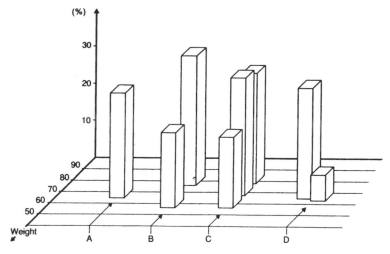

Figure 10.6 Percentage of patients in whom the inspired oxygen concentration drops to a value of 28%, as a function of patient weight, constitution and age: *y*-axis, percentage of patients (%); *z*-axis, body weight (kg). A, Whole group of patients: average weight 69 kg, average age 41.5 years. Differentiated according to: B, Body weight: average weight 59 kg versus average weight 78 kg; C, Constitution in accordance with the Broca index: underweight (average weight 58 kg) versus normal weight (average weight 67 kg) versus overweight patients (average weight 79 kg); D, Age: average age 38 years versus average age 62 years (with virtually identical weight and stature)

the oxygen content of the exhaled gases is correspondingly low[15]. The rebreathing fraction which, mixed with the fresh gas, is supplied back to the patient contains less oxygen the higher is the individual oxygen consumption of the patient.

10.2.3.3.2   Metering inhalation anaesthetics

10.2.3.3.2.1   Isoflurane   Due to its specific pharmacokinetic and pharmacodynamic properties, isoflurane is the most suitable of the group of the older conventional anaesthetic agents to be used in low flow anaesthesia (Table 10.1). Its low blood solubility gives a sufficiently quick wash-in and wash-out of the agent, and its low MAC value results in the quick establishment of an adequate anaesthetic level[16,17]. Only 0.2% of an inhaled dose of isoflurane is biotransformed[23] so the uptake is not at all influenced by its metabolism. The amount of isoflurane, calculated in accordance with Lowe's formula (see Section 3.3.1.2), which has to be supplied to the breathing system to maintain a desired expiratory concentration is lower than the equi-anaesthetic dose of halothane or enflurane. The dosing scheme is correspondingly simple: during an initial phase using a high fresh gas flow of 4.4 l/min the vaporizer is set to 1.5%. Performing low flow anaesthesia, after 10 min the fresh gas flow is reduced to 1.0 l/min and the vaporizer setting increased to 2.0%. Performing minimal flow

Table 10.1   Physicochemical and pharmacological properties of inhalation anaesthetics

	MAC	$\lambda_{B/G}$	$\lambda_{oil/gas}$	VAP	MR
Nitrous oxide	101	0.47	1.4	$\varnothing$	0.004
Halothane	0.77	2.3	224	228	15–30
Enflurane	1.68	1.78	96.5	199	2–7
Isoflurane	1.15	1.41	90.8	196	0.2–1
Sevoflurane	2.0	0.65	42	183	3–7
Desflurane	~4–6	0.42	18	209	0.02
Xenon	71	0.14	1.9	$\varnothing$	$\varnothing$

MAC: minimum alveolar concentration [vol%]; $\lambda_{B/G}$: blood/gas partition coefficient; $\lambda_{oil/gas}$: oil/gas partition coefficient; VAP: ml vapour per ml fluid of the volatile anaesthetic at 20°C [ml]; MR: metabolic rate [%] (after references 16–22)

anaesthesia, the initial high flow phase, assuming a similar fresh gas composition as above, should last about 15–20 min. After reduction of the fresh gas flow to 0.5 l/min, the vaporizer is set to a standard value of 2.5 vol%[24]. It goes without saying that modifications of this scheme have to be made in accordance with the requirements of the surgical intervention or the individual reaction of the patient, as, indeed, would be the case during high flow isoflurane anaesthesia.

Applying this standardized dosage scheme results in an average expired and, thus, approximately alveolar isoflurane concentration of 0.8–0.9 vol%, i.e. about 0.7–0.8 × MAC (Figure 10.7). If, corresponding to a nitrous oxide concentration of 55–65 vol%, the MAC_{N_2O} share of 0.6 is added to this value[25], a common MAC value of 1.3 is achieved. This is the alveolar anaesthetic concentration at which 95% of all patients do not react to the skin incision (AD_{95}). The expired isoflurane concentration of 0.8% is achieved virtually independent of patient characteristics such as weight, constitution and age (Figure 10.8).

It must be pointed out, however, that the MAC varies with a number of individual factors such as age, body temperature and, furthermore, with variations of anaesthetic management, such as supplementary analgesics and pre-medication[23,26]. Furthermore, the pharmacokinetics of a volatile anaesthetic vary as a function of individual parameters such as age and cardiac output[23,25,26]. Although, applying this dosage scheme, quotations for patients' average values can be made with sufficient accuracy with respect to inspired and expired isoflurane concentrations, in the individual case the concentration may differ considerably from the predicted values. In addition, it must be emphasized that only a certain gas concentration is predictable by applying this dosage scheme. It is not possible, however, to predict precisely whether the anaesthetic depth achieved with this concentration will meet the demands of the specific surgical intervention or the individual status of the patient. Based on the standard scheme of the anaesthetic fresh gas concentration, further adjustment of the agent concentration has to be made in the light of current clinical requirements, as is the case with high flow anaesthesia. Nevertheless, the standardized dosage

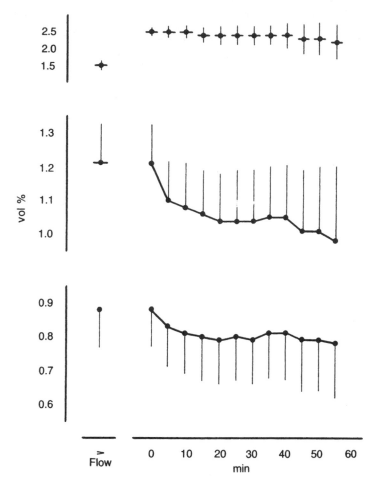

Figure 10.7 Inspired and expired isoflurane concentration immediately prior to, and during the course of 60 min after flow reduction to 0.5 l/min (mean values and standard deviation). Group of patients: average weight 74 kg, average age 51 years. Upper ordinate: vaporizer setting = fresh gas concentration; centre ordinate: inspired isoflurane concentration; bottom ordinate: expired isoflurane concentration. Measuring device: Normac (Datex, Helsinki, Finland)

scheme for isoflurane has proved its worth outstandingly in clinical practice. This confirms Lin's thesis (see Section 3.3.1.4) that, following an initial phase of anaesthesia during which the gas concentrations within the whole system are brought to equilibrium, the uptake of volatile anaesthetics remains relatively constant. Assuming stable cardiac output and unaltered ventilation, it is essentially a function of the alveolar–capillary partial pressure difference. Lin therefore recommends replacing the low uptake loss by administering only correspondingly low amounts of the anaesthetic, which, furthermore, can be kept constant over a longer period of time: involved calculations and frequent changes of the

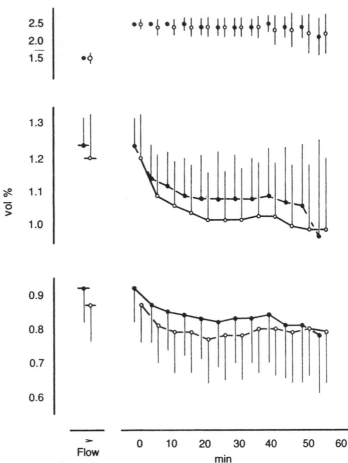

Figure 10.8 Inspired and expired isoflurane concentration immediately prior to, and during the course of 60 min after flow reduction to 0.5 l/min (mean values and standard deviation). Differentiation of the whole group (see Figure 10.7) according to body weight: ● average weight 62 kg (average age 49 years) versus ○ average weight 81 kg (average age 52 years). Upper ordinate: vaporizer setting = fresh gas concentration; centre ordinate: inspired isoflurane concentration; bottom ordinate: expired isoflurane concentration

vaporizer's settings in accordance with a complex exponential function would be absolutely unnecessary. Following on from Lin's quotations on halothane and enflurane, the following formula can be used for calculation of isoflurane dosage. After an initial equilibrium phase, the uptake for the following 60 min can be estimated by means of the formula

$$\dot{V}_{ISO} = 10\text{--}15 \, ml/min \text{ vapour per } \% \text{ desired expiratory concentration.}$$

With reference to a recently published investigation on uptake of isoflurane and desflurane[27] Eger also emphasizes that, contrary to earlier findings, the uptake of volatile agents was found to change only slightly during the course of inhalation anaesthesia[28]. The demand for greater amounts of anaesthetic vapour during the initial phase of an anaesthetic results from the fact that a great vapour volume is needed for washing-in and establishing the desired anaesthetic concentration within the whole gas-containing space, i.e. the machine's volume and the volume contained in the lung of the patient. Thus, the anaesthetist need not be engaged in applying involved mathematical calculations of the individual uptake and frequent adaptation of the settings of the gas flow controls, but instead may use very simple dosing schemes. Similar considerations, however, were equally the basis of the standardized schemes for low and minimal flow anaesthesia recommended here.

Anyhow, the practising anaesthetist has to deal with the fact that initially a large amount of agent vapour has to be supplied into the breathing system, followed by a decline to significantly lower amounts. For the practitioner it makes no difference whether the initial high demand for the inhalation anaesthetic results from individual uptake or from wash-in processes, which both follow exponential characteristics.

10.2.3.3.2.2 Enflurane The dosage schemes for enflurane are equally simple. During an initial phase lasting 10 min or 15–20 min, respectively, during which a high fresh gas flow of 4.4 l/min is used, the fresh gas concentration of 2.5 vol% enflurane results in an average expired concentration between 1.1 and 1.35 vol%. In low flow anaesthesia the flow is reduced to 1.0 l/min and the vaporizer set to 3.0 vol% after 10 min, whereas in minimal flow anaesthesia the flow is reduced to 0.5 l/min and the vaporizer set to 3.5 vol% after 15–20 min. These standardized settings will result in an average expired enflurane concentration of about 1.0 vol% (0.65 × MAC). Together with an additive MAC_{N_2O} of about 0.60–0.65 the corresponding anaesthetic level will be sufficient to start most of all surgical interventions (Figure 10.9). The individual uptake of enflurane, much more than that of isoflurane, determines the concentration which finally builds up within the breathing system. Thus, standardized settings of the fresh gas concentration assumed, the enflurane concentration is higher in slim patients with low body weight than in strong and athletic ones (Figure 10.10).

The following conclusion can be drawn from clinical experience with this standardized scheme for enflurane dosage in low flow anaesthesia. It is perfectly possible to obtain good clinical results by standardization of enflurane dosage without involved calculations according to a time-dependent scheme. However, equilibrium processes after flow reduction proceed slower than those with isoflurane. The inspired and expired concentrations depend to a distinctly greater extent on patient characteristics such as weight and constitution.

10.2.3.3.2.3 Halothane The first experiences gained in the performance of low flow anaesthesia with halothane and guidelines for its use in anaesthesia with extensive flow reduction were published as early as 1959 by Robson *et al.*[29] and in 1969 by Zinganell[30]. A dosage concept for halothane will only be mentioned in order to complete the discussion. At least where adults are concerned, its use is viewed rather critically

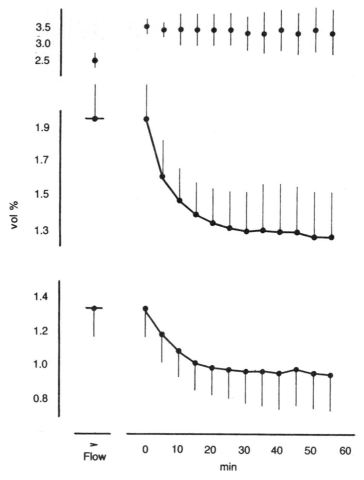

Figure 10.9 Inspired and expired enflurane concentration immediately prior to, and during the course of 60 min after flow reduction to 0.5 l/min (mean values and standard deviation). Group of patients: average weight 71 kg, average age 42 years. Upper ordinate: vaporizer setting = fresh gas concentration; centre ordinate: inspired enflurane concentration; bottom ordinate: expired enflurane concentration

because of the potential hepatotoxic side-effects, the aforementioned degradation of this agent with soda lime (see Section 9.1.2.2.8), and the alternative universal availability of other volatile agents[31–33]. As this volatile anaesthetic has not been used for more than 18 years in the author's department, the following dosing scheme for halothane is not based on personal clinical experience and has to be applied very carefully. In the initial high flow phase of anaesthesia, lasting 15–20 min, a fresh gas halothane concentration of about 1.0–1.3 vol% with a flow of 4.4 l/min seems reasonable. After flow reduction in low flow anaesthesia (1.0 l/min) the vaporizer may be set to 2.0 vol%, in minimal flow

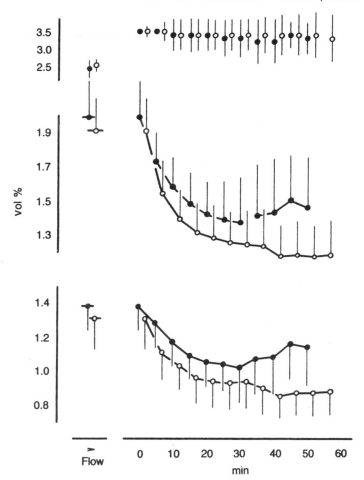

vol %

Flow

0   10   20   30   40   50   60
min

Figure 10.10   Inspired and expired enflurane concentration immediately prior to, and during the course of 60 min after flow reduction to 0.5 l/min (mean values and standard deviation). Differentiation of the group (see Figure 10.9) according to body weight: ● average weight 62 kg (average age 39 years) versus ○ average weight 79 kg (average age 44 years). Upper ordinate: vaporizer setting = fresh gas concentration; centre ordinate: inspired enflurane concentration; bottom ordinate: expired enflurane concentration

anaesthesia (0.5 l/min) to 3.0 vol%. According to the author's extremely limited experience with halothane minimal flow anaesthesia, initially an expired concentration of about 0.6 vol% is gained and will be maintained after flow reduction during the following course of the anaesthetic. Pronounced individual differences in the halothane concentration, building up in the breathing system, have to be expected. If, in spite of the problems mentioned above, halothane is to be used with a standardized dosage concept, the values obtained in clinical practice may differ considerably from the quoted average values.

10.2.3.3.3   Control of the concentration of inhalation anaesthetics

Low flow anaesthetic techniques are specifically characterized by the great delay in which alterations of the anaesthetic agent's fresh gas concentration will result in corresponding alterations of its concentration in the breathing system. This characteristic can be described precisely by the time constant (see Section 5.2.3), which for its part is proportional to the circulating gas volume and (assuming a nearly constant individual uptake) inversely proportional to the amount of agent supplied into the breathing system, thus it is also inversely proportional to the fresh gas flow rate.

The long time constants of low flow techniques are of considerable clinical significance. If the anaesthetic level has to be changed this can be achieved by corresponding alterations of the vaporizer setting. Using extremely low fresh gas flow rates, however, even drastic alterations of the dial setting will result in only very delayed corresponding alterations of the agent concentration within the breathing system. It is nearly impossible to rapidly change the concentrations of the gases supplied to the patients (Figure 10.11).

If the situation requires a rapid change of the anaesthetic agent concentration, the fresh gas flow rate must be increased to 4–5 l/min and the dialled concentration has to exceed or fall below the desired concentration by 0.5 vol% accordingly. The change from long to short time constant is essential to rapidly change the agent concentration within the breathing system (Figure 10.12). Generally, after about 5 min the desired concentration is established. The fresh gas flow can be reduced again, the vaporizer

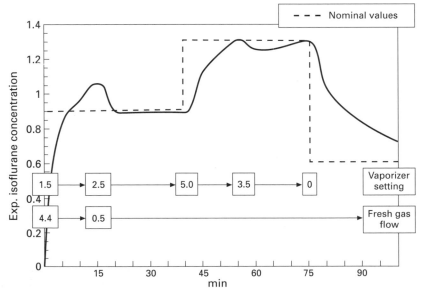

Figure 10.11   Minimal flow anaesthesia: alteration of the expired isoflurane concentration to new desired nominal values only by variation of the vaporizer setting. Anaesthesia management maintaining long time constant

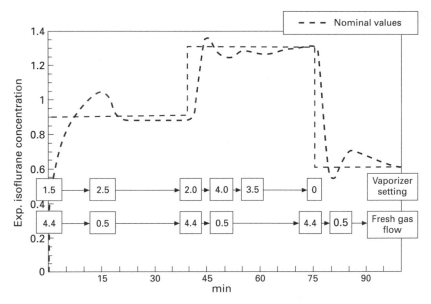

Figure 10.12 Minimal flow anaesthesia: alteration of the expired isoflurane concentration to new desired nominal values by variation of fresh gas flow and vaporizer setting. Anaesthesia management with changing time constants

has to be adjusted to maintain the new nominal value, and the system again performs with long time constants. An alternative way to rapidly increase the anaesthetic depth while maintaining the low fresh gas flow rate is the intravenous application of supplementary doses of hypnotics or opioids.

It must always be kept in mind, however, that metering of volatile anaesthetics is not aimed to a distinct concentration but always to a sufficient anaesthetic depth. Thus, all the simple dosing schemes are only rough guidelines which, in the individual case, have to be adapted carefully according to the respective needs. If, for instance, a lower concentration shall be used consistently during the course of the anaesthetic, the standard settings of the vaporizer have to be given up in favour of lower fresh gas concentrations, not only in the initial high flow phase but also after flow reduction (Figures 10.13 and 10.14).

10.2.4 Emergence phase

Due to the long time constant and depending on the duration of anaesthesia, the admixture of the volatile agent to the fresh gas can be stopped about 15–30 min before the end of the surgical intervention, provided the low fresh gas flow rate is maintained. The lower is the flow, the slower is the decrease in the anaesthetic concentration. The patient is then subjected to assisted manual ventilation until spontaneous breathing is restored. Approximately 5–10 min prior to extubation, the anaesthetic gases are washed out of the system completely with an oxygen flow of 4–6 l/min

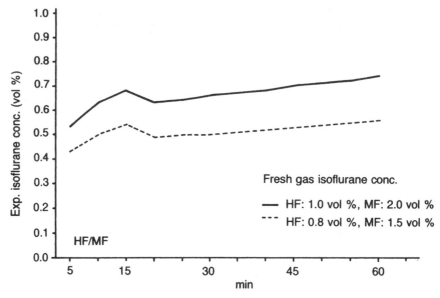

Figure 10.13   Expired isoflurane concentration during the course of minimal flow anaesthesia with lower standard settings of the vaporizer. (Simulation using the Gas Uptake Simulation computer program, assuming an adult patient with normal body weight; HF/MF, flow reduction from 4.4 to 0.5 l/min)

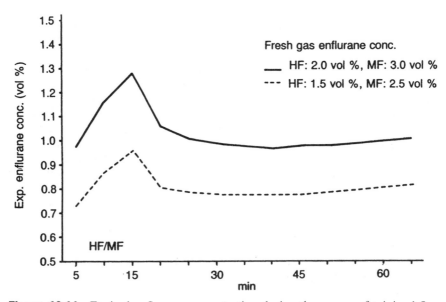

Figure 10.14   Expired enflurane concentration during the course of minimal flow anaesthesia with lower standard settings of the vaporizer. (Simulation using the Gas Uptake Simulation computer program, assuming an adult patient with normal body weight; HF/MF, flow reduction from 4.4 to 0.5 l/min)

after the APL valve has been opened and nitrous oxide administration ceased. The immediate postoperative care of the patient takes place in the usual manner.

✕ 10.3   Practice of low flow anaesthesia with desflurane and sevoflurane

With respect to their low solubility, the new inhalation anaesthetics desflurane and sevoflurane are quite different from the conventional volatile agents halothane, enflurane and isoflurane. The blood–gas partition coefficient is 0.65 for sevoflurane and 0.42 for desflurane, hence the solubility of both agents is in the order of that of nitrous oxide. All wash-in and wash-out processes are correspondingly short, and clinical experience verifies induction and emergence to be rapid, and control of the concentration of agents to be performed quickly and easily. At room temperature desflurane has a vapour pressure of 669 mmHg, thus to use this agent a special electronically controlled vaporizer is needed (see Section 7.3.2.4). The vapour pressure of sevoflurane, however, is very similar to that of enflurane and this agent can be administered using a plenum vaporizer featuring conventional technology. Compared to the other inhalation agents, the anaesthetic potency of desflurane is low, its MAC value being 4–8 vol%, depending on the age of the patient. Thus, a comparatively high alveolar concentration has to be established and maintained to guarantee a sufficient anaesthetic level. The anaesthetic potency of sevoflurane, however, is only slightly less than that of enflurane, the MAC value being about 2.0–2.5 vol%. With respect to their biotransformation, both new agents differ considerably, as the desflurane metabolism of 0.02% is absolutely negligible whereas some 3–7% of an inhaled dose of sevoflurane is metabolized, this rate being somewhat higher than for enflurane. The increase of serum fluoride concentration by hepatic sevoflurane metabolism, contrary to the increase of serum fluoride resulting from renal decomposition of methoxyflurane, does not impair renal function, which corresponds to clinical experience in a vast number of cases. While during sevoflurane anaesthesia all cardiovascular parameters are quite stable, a rapid increase of the desflurane concentration to values higher than 1.5 MAC will result in significant sympathetic reactions with an increase of heart beat rate and blood pressure. The desflurane vapour is pungent, making it unsuitable for induction by inhalation via a face mask, as is done frequently in paediatric anaesthesia. In contrast, sevoflurane is especially suitable to be used in paediatric anaesthesia[34–37]. Both new inhalation anaesthetics are degraded by absorbent limes; desflurane reacts to generate carbon monoxide and sevoflurane is broken down to produce compound A (see Section 9.1.2.2).

10.3.1   Desflurane

The initial wash-in of desflurane is so rapid that 10 min after induction an inspired desflurane concentration is achieved being about 85% of the fresh

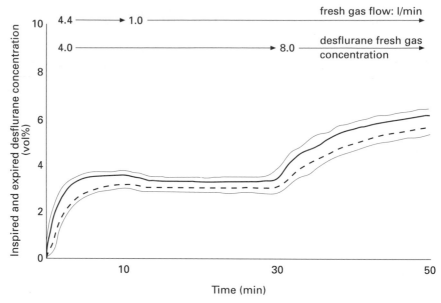

Figure 10.15 Inspired (——) and expired (– –) desflurane concentration (mean values) during the course of low flow anaesthesia. In spite of its low solubility, one has to expect delayed increase of inspired and expired desflurane concentration with considerably prolonged time constant when the fresh gas concentration only is increased moderately. Enveloping curves: standard deviation. (From Baum et al.[38])

gas concentration. At that time the quotient ($Q_{i/f}$) resulting from the division of the inspired (C_i) by the fresh gas concentration (C_f), $Q_{i/f} = C_i/C_f$, amounts to about 0.85. Ten minutes after induction, nitrogen is nearly completely washed out of all gas-containing compartments and the desired anaesthetic gas composition is already established within the breathing system. Thus, using desflurane the fresh gas flow rate can be reduced at that time, not only in low flow but also in minimal flow anaesthesia. To proceed in this way, however, can only be recommended if anaesthetic ventilators featuring a gas reservoir are used, as 10 min after induction in some cases the nitrous oxide uptake might still be high, increasing the risk of accidental gas volume deficiency.

If low flow anaesthesia with a flow rate of 1.0 l/min is performed, the vaporizer setting can be maintained at flow reduction. The concentration gained during the initial high flow phase remains stable, and during the following 60 min the quotient $Q_{i/f}$ again reaches 0.85 (Figure 10.15). In minimal flow anaesthesia, using a fresh gas flow rate of 0.5 l/min, an increase of the fresh gas desflurane concentration by 1 vol% at flow reduction is sufficient to maintain the agent concentration in the breathing system gained during the initial high flow phase. If, at flow reduction, the fresh gas concentration is increased by 2 vol%, a delayed but continuous rise of the desflurane concentration within the breathing system can be observed (Figure 10.16). Corresponding to the respective

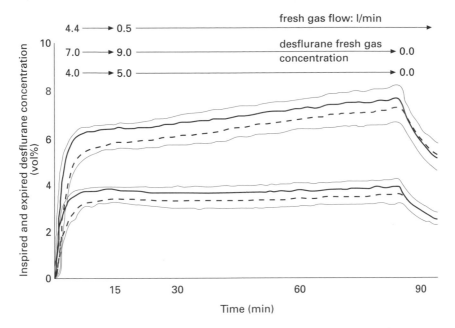

Figure 10.16 Inspired (——) and expired (– –) desflurane concentrations (mean values) during the course of minimal flow anaesthesia. Inspired and expired desflurane concentrations remain constant if the fresh gas concentration is increased by 1.0 vol% at flow reduction. Inspired and expired desflurane concentrations increase slowly but continuously if the fresh gas concentration is increased by 2.0 vol% at flow reduction. Enveloping curves: standard deviation (From Baum *et al.*[38]).

flow rate and the fresh gas concentration, the inspired desflurane concentration amounts to about 65–85% of the fresh gas concentration.

Due to the low anaesthetic potency of desflurane, the maximum output of 18 vol% of the agent-specific vaporizer is comparatively high. This enables the delivery of quite high amounts of desflurane vapour into the breathing system, even if extremely low fresh gas flow rates are used. Provided the vaporizer dial is set to its maximum, 110 ml desflurane vapour per minute will be supplied at a flow as low as 0.5 l/min. Due to the fact that, at the same time, the individual uptake is comparatively low, the concentration of desflurane can be increased in a considerably short time despite the fresh gas flow being maintained at a low rate. When a concentration is dialled being 2 times the desired nominal value the anaesthetic level can be increased rapidly, even in minimal flow anaesthesia (Figure 10.17). The use of desflurane shortens the time constant of low flow anaesthesia if use is made of the wide range of the agent-specific vaporizer. If, however, only the newly desired concentration is dialled as the fresh gas concentration in low flow anaesthesia (Figure 10.15), irrespective of the use of desflurane, a considerably prolonged time constant must be expected.

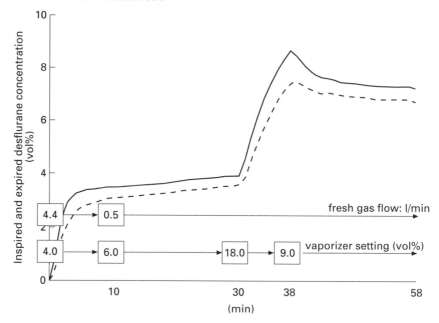

Figure 10.17   Inspired (——) and expired (– –) desflurane concentrations (mean values) during the course of minimal flow anaesthesia. Inspired and expired desflurane concentrations increase rapidly if use is made of the maximum output of the agent-specific vaporizer, although the fresh gas flow is maintained at the low rate of 0.5 l/min. Enveloping curves: standard deviation. (From Baum *et al.*[38])

Even if the fresh gas flow is maintained at a rate of 0.5 l/min, the desflurane concentration declines considerably by 35% during the 10 min after switching the vaporizer off.

Desflurane much more vigorously than enflurane or isoflurane reacts with completely desiccated soda lime, generating carbon monoxide (see Section 9.1.2.2.4). Nevertheless, even during long-lasting minimal flow anaesthetics, in not a single case was any accidental increase of carbon monoxide haemoglobin observed in the author's department, proper maintenance of the absorbent provided. In this context, it should again be emphasized that preservation of a sufficient water content of the absorbent is of great clinical importance. All measures have to be observed to prevent any accidental desiccation of the absorbent. Proper maintenance of the absorbent will, therefore, safely prevent the degradation of desflurane to carbon monoxide.

The characteristics of low flow anaesthesia with desflurane can be summarized as follows[38]:

- Due to its low solubility, the initial high flow phase can be shortened to 10 min even in minimal flow anaesthesia[39]. As there might be the risk of gas volume imbalances, this can only be recommended if anaesthetic ventilators featuring a gas reservoir are used.

● The desired inspiratory desflurane concentration in low flow anaesthesia can be maintained without any increase of its fresh gas concentration at flow reduction. In minimal flow anaesthesia the fresh gas concentration of desflurane has to be increased by 1–2 vol% at that time. Even with extremely low fresh gas flow rates, the difference between inspired and fresh gas concentration is comparatively small. If use is made of the wide dosage range of the desflurane vaporizer, the desflurane concentration of the respired gases can be increased with short time constants while maintaining the fresh gas flow at low rates. Due to its low solubility and the wide range of the vaporizer, desflurane is especially suitable for use with low flow anaesthetic techniques[38–40].

10.3.2   Sevoflurane

Sevoflurane is also characterized by low solubility. Thus, the initial wash-in is achieved rapidly and after a 10-min initial phase, using a fresh gas flow of 4.4 l/min and a fresh gas sevoflurane concentration of 2.5 vol%, an inspired concentration is attained of about 85% of the fresh gas concentration[41]. The mean expired concentration at that time amounts to 1.7 vol%, which is equal to $0.8 \times MAC$ of sevoflurane. As with desflurane, it is possible to make an early reduction in flow after this short period of time, provided the anaesthetic ventilator is equipped with a gas reservoir.

If low flow anaesthesia is performed, the flow is reduced to 1.0 l/min and the fresh gas concentration of sevoflurane raised to 3.0 vol%. The expired concentration decreases slightly to 1.5–1.6 vol%, a concentration guaranteeing a sufficient anaesthetic level in most cases. During the following 60 min the quotient $Q_{i/f}$ will attain a value of about 0.6 (Figure 10.18). If minimal flow anaesthesia is performed, using a fresh gas flow of 0.5 l/min, the fresh gas concentration has to be increased to 3.5 vol% to maintain an expired concentration of 1.6–1.7 vol%. Under these conditions of minimal flow anaesthesia the quotient $Q_{i/f}$ will achieve a value of about 0.5–0.55 (Figure 10.19).

The short time constant of sevoflurane low flow anaesthesia depends on its low tissue solubility and also on the relatively high output of the agent-specific vaporizer. The maximum output of the sevoflurane vaporizer is limited to 8.0 vol%. At a fresh gas flow as low as 0.5 l/min, 43.5 ml of sevoflurane vapour per minute can be supplied into the breathing system, at a flow of 1.0 l/min the amount of vapour increases to 87 ml/min. This permits increasing the anaesthetic level in a sufficiently short period of time while maintaining the low flow technique (Figure 10.18).

Carbon dioxide absorbents degrade sevoflurane to compound A, which is potentially nephro- and neurotoxic (see Section 9.1.2.2.8). Using anaesthetic machines equipped with heated breathing systems during minimal flow anaesthesia, peak concentrations up to 60 ppm were observed, whereas during low flow anaesthesia mean peak concentrations rarely exceeded 25 ppm. Thus, the American FDA recommends not to use fresh gas flows lower than 1 l/min and not to exceed a maximum load of 2 MAC·h sevoflurane with low flow techniques[42]. This limitation may be unnecessary if the new carbon dioxide absorbent calcium

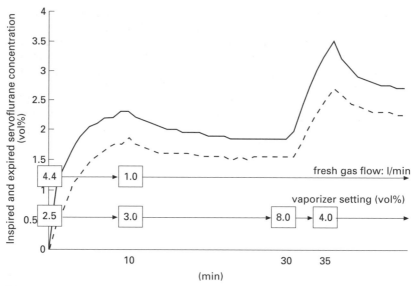

Figure 10.18   Inspired (——) and expired (– –) sevoflurane concentrations (mean values) during the course of low flow anaesthesia. Inspired and expired sevoflurane concentrations increase rapidly if use is made of the maximum output of the agent-specific vaporizer, although the fresh gas flow is maintained at the low rate of 1.0 l/min. (From Baum et al.[41])

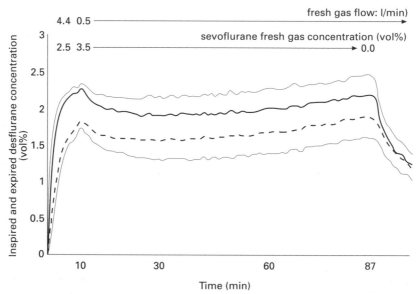

Figure 10.19   Inspired (——) and expired (– –) sevoflurane concentration (mean values) during the course of minimal flow anaesthesia. Inspired and expired sevoflurane concentrations decrease slightly directly after fresh gas flow rate reduction from 4.4 to 0.5 l/min, although the fresh gas concentration is increased from 2.5 to 3.5 vol%. After a short time the concentrations increase again, slowly but continuously. Enveloping curves: standard deviation. (From Baum et al.[41])

hydroxide lime is used, which does not degrade sevoflurane, neither in desiccated condition nor if containing the normal amount of water[43,44]. To date there have been no reports of clinically relevant permanent impairment of renal function, even after prolonged low flow anaesthesia. Sevoflurane, therefore, was approved in all the countries of the European Union to be used without any flow restriction. With respect to the ongoing scientific discussion on nephro- and neurotoxic effects of compound A, minimal flow anaesthesia with sevoflurane should not exceed a duration of 2–3 h, unless calcium hydroxide lime is used as absorbent. Low flow sevoflurane anaesthesia (1.0 l/min) can be assumed to be safe even in longer-lasting cases as the continuous discharge of excess gas guarantees a sufficient wash-out effect. To minimize the risk of compound A generation, it would be prudent at least to use potassium-free soda lime. The use of barium hydroxide lime should be given up completely[43].

The facts concerning low flow anaesthesia with sevoflurane can be summarized as follows[41]:

- Due to the low solubility of sevoflurane, the initial high flow phase can be shortened to 10 min. An expired sevoflurane concentration equalling $0.8 \times MAC$ will be achieved during that time if the vaporizer is set to 2.5 vol% at an initial flow of about 4.0 l/min. The risk of accidental gas volume imbalances limit further reduction of the duration of the initial phase.
- After flow reduction to 1.0 l/min, the sevoflurane concentration will decline only insignificantly if the dial of the vaporizer is set to 3.0 vol%. The quotient $Q_{i/f}$ amounts to about 0.7 in low flow anaesthesia. If minimal flow anaesthesia is performed at flow reduction the fresh gas concentration has to be increased to 3.5 vol% to maintain an expired concentration of about 1.7 vol%. The quotient $Q_{i/f}$ amounts to about 0.5–0.55.
- If use is made of the full range of the vaporizer, the sevoflurane concentration can be raised with sufficiently short time constants even in low flow techniques.
- For safety reasons, sevoflurane should not be used with flows lower than 1.0 l/min in cases lasting longer than 2–3 h, unless calcium hydroxide lime is used consistently.
- To minimize sevoflurane degradation, potassium-free soda lime should be used consistently.

10.4   Gas volume deficiency

Gas volume deficiency may always occur if the gas volume supplied into the system does not meet the gas volume lost by total gas uptake and leakages. Due to the high total gas uptake, the frequency of accidental gas volume deficiency is highest directly after flow reduction as, at that time, there is only a small amount of excess gas available for compensation. During the course of the anaesthetic procedure this risk declines significantly. If minimal flow anaesthesia is performed on a strong patient with correspondingly high oxygen and nitrous oxide uptake it may be wise after finishing the initial wash-in to reduce the flow rate to only 0.7 l/min (0.35 l/min O_2, 0.35 l/min N_2O) during the following period of 15 min.

By careful setting of the ventilator monitor alarm limits, any accidental gas volume deficiency will be recognized rapidly as this will instantly result in a corresponding decrease of the minute volume and the peak and plateau pressures.

When anaesthetic ventilators featuring active support of the bellows' expiratory expansion are used, the ventilatory patterns may even change from IPPV to APV. In some anaesthetic machines this problem will be announced by a clear text message at the alarm display, and one machine even features a special monitor, called 'Econometer', which provides continuous information about the gas volume circulating within the breathing system (Cicero EM, Dräger Medizintechnik, Lübeck, Germany).

In the event of accidental gas volume deficiency, the fresh gas flow rate must be increased over a period of at least 1–2 min to top up the anaesthetic gas volume. If this is accomplished the flow may then be reduced again. If this problem, however, occurs repeatedly, the flow first has to be increased to meet the additional gas loss and then the leak should be identified.

Assuming the anaesthetic machine proved to be sufficiently gas tight in the pre-use technical check, leaks are mostly due to insufficient gas tightness of the cuff, the connection between the endotracheal tube and the Y-piece, the bacterial filter, the HME, the flow sensors, or the ISO connectors of the hoses. The latter is a particularly common site for leaks as, following repeated thermodisinfection, the connection between the hoses and the connectors becomes so loose that the connector rotates within the tubing. Gas volume deficiency also may occur in minimal flow anaesthesia if the gas sample return tube is accidentally not connected to the machine. All compact breathing systems have to be fitted to their mountings carefully to avoid any leakage.

When conventional anaesthetic machines are used without any gas reservoir it is wise to switch from controlled to manual ventilation only during the inspiratory phase. Otherwise a considerable amount of gas may be trapped in the ventilator, resulting in insufficient filling of the manual ventilation bag. Similarly, the change from manual to controlled ventilation should only be made if the manual bag is compressed and the gas volume is delivered into the lung of the patient. The exhaled gas is then routed back to the ventilator, thus guaranteeing a sufficient filling of the bellows.

If the anaesthetic ventilator features a gas reservoir, however, gas volume deficiency can be balanced over a limited period of time by the emptying of the reserve volume into the breathing system. Gas volume deficiency will not become manifest unless the reservoir is emptied completely.

If the reservoir bag is serving as the gas reservoir, it should not be suspended from the loop fixed at its top, but should be placed freely on the chassis of the machine. Otherwise the gas volume contained in the reservoir may be emptied into the breathing system by the traction exerted by the weight of the connecting hose whenever the excess gas discharge valve opens. Gas volume deficiency will only become manifest in anaesthetic machines featuring floating bellows if the gas volume, filling the bellows during expiration, falls below the pre-set tidal volume.

10.5   Water condensation within the hosing

The considerably higher temperature and humidity of the anaesthetic gases in low flow anaesthesia, compared with high flow techniques, cause increased water condensation in the patient hose assembly, especially if the ambient temperature in the theatre is kept low by air conditioning.

The accumulation of condensed water at the lowest point of the hoses can generate bubbling sounds, with the airway pressure curve showing corresponding peaks and oscillations. In this case, the ventilator should be switched off and the hoses disconnected from the breathing system. The condensed water should then be emptied into the reservoir jar of the suction apparatus, the hoses reconnected to the circuit, and finally the ventilator switched on again. This very simple action is performed routinely every day in nearly all intensive care units, where heated humidifiers are used in controlled ventilation. The use of additional water traps may be considered but, in the author's experience, these devices are rarely positioned properly.

However, careful attention should always be paid to the fact that the hoses should form a siphon on their way from the Y-piece to the connector at the breathing system. These siphons serve as reservoirs which ensure that condensed water will not flow directly into the breathing system. This may be an essential safety measure as, where compact breathing systems are concerned, water entering the control tubes within the system may cause clinically relevant failure of the valves.

Further attention should be paid to giving the port used to connect the sample gas tube to the breathing system an upward direction and, thus, to prevent condensed water from entering the sample gas tube, which may disturb the function of the gas analyser in the event that the water trap is not performing properly.

After having passed the gas analyser the sample gas has, at least in minimal flow anaesthesia, to be returned into the breathing system. A small bacterial filter should be attached to the outlet of the analyser to avoid any bacterial contamination. If the sample gas contains much water vapour this filter may be liable to blocking by water condensation, causing a failure of the gas monitor. In this case the bacterial filter has to be changed.

Water condensation within the hosing can be reduced significantly by using heated hoses[45] which recently became commercially available, for instance for use with the Cicero EM anaesthetic machine (Dräger Medizintechnik, Lübeck, Germany). As these hoses are considerably more expensive than the conventional corrugated hoses their use can only be recommended under the provision that bacterial filters are consistently inserted between the Y-piece and the tube connector. If this is the case, the hosing need only be changed once a day, minimizing the number of hoses to be kept in stock.

10.6   Economy and efficiency

The low anaesthetic potency of desflurane requires the establishment and maintenance of a comparatively high alveolar concentration. Using this agent in high flow anaesthesia a huge amount of desflurane vapour will be discharged out of the system as one of the components of the excess gas during each expiratory phase. A correspondingly large amount of agent has to be supplied into the breathing system just to replenish the required alveolar partial pressure, despite the fact that the individual uptake of just this anaesthetic is extremely low. Depending on the duration of the anaesthetic, a disproportionately high amount of desflurane may be discharged as waste out of the system, although to meet the individual uptake only a very small amount of this agent would be needed.

The efficiency of an inhalation anaesthetic procedure can be clarified with the efficiency coefficient (see Section 6.2.1). It is calculated by dividing the amount of agent taken up by the patient by that being delivered into the system, the latter of course being the true consumption. Applying this formula, the efficiency of a high flow desflurane anaesthesia of 2-h duration with a fresh gas flow of 4.4 l/min and an inspired concentration of 6.0 vol% is only 0.07. No more than 7% of the amount of agent used is actually taken up by the patient, the remaining 93% is needlessly wasted. Only by performing low or minimal flow anaesthesia can the consumption of the agent and the corresponding costs be reduced adequately, increasing the efficiency to an acceptable range of 0.23 or 0.32, respectively (Figure 10.20). By applying low flow techniques, the efficiency of desflurane anaesthesia can be raised by a factor of 3.3, or even 4.6.

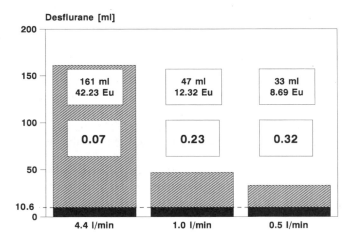

Figure 10.20   Comparison of anaesthetic agent consumption, costs (Eu = euro) and efficiency (depicted by the efficiency coefficient) in desflurane anaesthetics performed with different fresh gas flow rates: high flow anaesthesia (4.4 l/min), low flow anaesthesia (1.0 l/min) and minimal flow anaesthesia (0.5 l/min). Calculation base: duration of the anaesthetic procedure, 2 h; body weight of the patient, 75 kg; desired expired desflurane concentration, 6.0 vol%; cumulative uptake during 2 h, 10.6 ml fluid desflurane

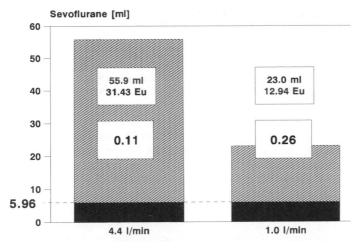

Figure 10.21   Comparison of anaesthetic agent consumption, costs (Eu = euro) and efficiency (depicted by the efficiency coefficient) in sevoflurane anaesthetics performed with different fresh gas flow rates: high flow anaesthesia (4.4 l/min) and low flow anaesthesia (1.0 l/min). Calculation base: duration of the anaesthetic procedure, 2 h; body weight of the patient, 75 kg; desired expired sevoflurane concentration, 1.7 vol%; cumulative uptake during 2 h, 5.96 ml fluid sevoflurane

This also holds for sevoflurane, as this agent is also characterized by comparatively low anaesthetic potency and low solubility. If high flow anaesthesia is compared with a low flow technique for an adult patient of normal weight, then an expired concentration of 1.7 vol%, and fresh gas flows of 4.4 or 1.0 l/min respectively assumed, the efficiency quotient increases from 0.11 to 0.26. Thus, by increasing the efficiency by a factor of 2.4, a significant reduction of sevoflurane consumption and a corresponding cost saving can be achieved (Figure 10.21).

To complete the picture, inhalation anaesthetics with isoflurane and enflurane using different fresh gas flows are also depicted (Figures 10.22 and 10.23). Comparing high and minimal flow anaesthesia, it becomes quite obvious that only by adequate flow reduction can the efficiency be increased by a factor of 3.1 or 2.6, respectively. The increase in efficiency is higher the lower the anaesthetic potency and the solubility of the respective inhalation anaesthetic.

From the aspect of economy and efficiency the use of the newer anaesthetic agents desflurane and sevoflurane can only be justified if low flow anaesthetic techniques are performed consistently. (Table 10.2)

10.7   The laryngeal mask airway

The laryngeal mask, introduced by Brain in 1983[46,47], is a unique concept of airway management. The device consists of a silicone mask, formed to fit the anatomy of the hypopharynx, attached to a silicone tube (Figure 10.24). The mask is available in six different sizes which makes it suitable

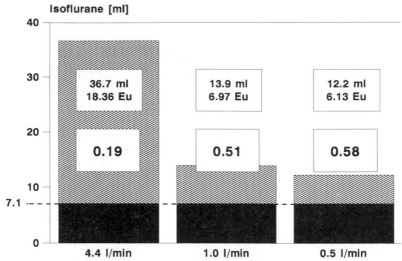

Figure 10.22 Comparison of anaesthetic agent consumption, costs (Eu = euro) and efficiency (depicted by the efficiency coefficient) in isoflurane anaesthetics performed with different fresh gas flow rates: high flow anaesthesia (4.4 l/min), low flow anaesthesia (1.0 l/min) and minimal flow anaesthesia (0.5 l/min). Calculation base: duration of the anaesthetic procedure 2 h; body weight of the patient, 75 kg; desired expired isoflurane concentration, 0.9 vol%; cumulative uptake during 2 h, 7.1 ml fluid isoflurane

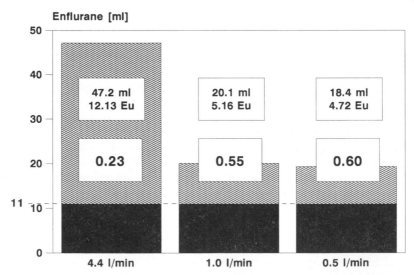

Figure 10.23 Comparison of anaesthetic agent consumption, costs (Eu = euro) and efficiency (depicted by the efficiency coefficient) in enflurane anaesthetics performed with different fresh gas flow rates: high flow anaesthesia (4.4 l/min), low flow anaesthesia (1.0 l/min) and minimal flow anaesthesia (0.5 l/min). Calculation base: duration of the anaesthetic procedure, 2 h; body weight of the patient, 75 kg; desired expired enflurane concentration, 0.9 vol%; cumulative uptake during 2 h, 11 ml fluid enflurane

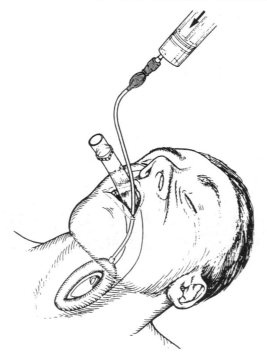

Figure 10.24   Laryngeal mask: correct position directly over the laryngeal orifice; the sealing cuff is inflated (from Brain[47], by permission)

for all age groups from the neonate to the large adult. The opening of the laryngeal mask is positioned over the laryngeal orifice. Once the sealing cuff is inflated, it provides an adequate seal to the airway. Computer tomographic investigations of the position revealed a perfect seal to the airways if the mask was inserted properly[49,50]. Handling of the device is simple and can be easily learnt, but it must be admitted that it requires some training to become familiar with its use.

The following are the advantages of this new airway, which is technically an intermediate between the face mask and the endotracheal tube[49,51]:

- Simple positioning without laryngoscopy, which means only minor circulatory responses upon insertion.
- Accidental oesophageal or bronchial malpositioning is impossible. Insertion is less traumatic than with endotracheal intubation, improving the postoperative comfort of the patient.
- Only minor irritation of the pharynx. After the initial phase, during which, however, anaesthesia has to be sufficiently deep, the device is tolerated virtually to complete recovery.
- Diminished occurrence of laryngospasm compared with endotracheal intubation.

Table 10.2   Standardized concept for performance of minimal flow anaesthesia

All the data given for gas flow and volatile anaesthetic control are clinically proven guidelines. However, they have to be carefully adapted in each single case according to the individual reactions of the patient and to surgical requirements.

Premedication
– In the usual way

Induction
– Preoxygenation
– Intravenous hypnotic
– Relaxation and intubation
– Or: insertion of a laryngeal mask
– Connecting the *patient on to* a circle absorber system

Initial phase
– Duration at least 10, in general 15–20 min (depending on the anaesthetic agent and the patient's constitution)
– 1.4 l/min oxygen
– 3.0 l/min nitrous oxide
  Vaporizer setting:
    halothane 1.0–1.3 vol%
    enflurane 2.0–2.5 vol%
    isoflurane 1.0–1 .5 vol%
    sevoflurane 2.0–2.5 vol%
    desflurane 4.0–6.0 vol%

Monitoring
– Inspired oxygen concentration: lower alarm limit 28–30 vol%
– Disconnect alarm: lower alarm limit 5 mbar below peak pressure
– MV monitoring: lower alarm limit 0.5 l/min below nominal value
– Inspired volatile anaesthetic concentration: upper alarm limit
    halothane, enflurane and isoflurane: 2.0–2.5 vol%
    sevoflurane: 3.0 vol%
    desflurane: 8.0 vol%

Fresh gas flow reduction
– 0.25–0.3 l/min oxygen
– 0.25–0.2 l/min nitrous oxide
  Vaporizer setting:
    halothane 2.5–3.0 vol%
    enflurane 3.0–3.5 vol%
    isoflurane 2.0–2.5 vol%
    sevoflurane 3.0–3.5 vol%
    desflurane +1.0–1.5 vol% (5.0–7.5 vol%)

In *longer lasting cases* (>2–3 h), unless calcium hydroxide lime is used, sevoflurane should be used with low flow technique: fresh gas flow 1.0 l/min (0.4–0.5 l/min O_2, 0.6–0.5 l/min N_2O), vaporizer setting 2.5–3.0 vol% sevoflurane. If calcium hydroxide lime, however, is used, the fresh gas flow rate – without any restriction – may be reduced to its outmost extent even in long cases.

Changes in fresh gas setting
Inspired oxygen concentration drops to lower limit
- Increase oxygen flow by 50 ml/min
- Decrease nitrous oxide flow by 50 ml/min

Increasing the anaesthetic depth with long time constant
- Maintain fresh gas flow at 0.5 l/min
- Increase vaporizer setting by 1–2 vol%
- When the desired depth of anaesthesia has been achieved, set vaporizer to a concentration about 0.5–1.0 vol% higher than desired nominal concentration

Decreasing anaesthetic depth with long time constant
- Maintain fresh gas flow at 0.5 l/min
- Decrease vaporizer setting by 1–3.5 vol%
- When the desired depth of anaesthesia has been achieved, set vaporizer to a concentration about 1.0–2.0 vol%

Rapidly increasing or decreasing anaesthetic depth with short time constant
- Set vaporizer to the aspired inspired concentration
- Increase fresh gas flow to 4.4 l/min (1.4 l/min O_2, 3.0 l/min N_2O)
- When the desired depth of anaesthesia is achieved, usually in about 5 min, re-*establish* again low fresh gas flow of 0.5 l/min (0.3 l/min O_2, 0.2 l/min N_2O)
- Set vaporizer to a value 0.5 vol% above, or 1.0–2.0 vol% below starting value respectively
- If sevoflurane or desflurane are used, due to their low solubility and the wide dialling range of the vaporizers, the anaesthetic concentration can be increased or decreased, even if low flow technique is maintained. Doing so, however, anaesthetic agent monitoring is indispensable
- Alternative option for increasing anaesthetic depth rapidly: intravenous injection of supplementary doses of hypnotics or opioids

Gas volume deficiency; peak pressure and minute volume decrease
- Replenishing the anaesthetic gas reservoir by short-term increase of the fresh gas flow
- Check for leaks
- If leakage persists: increase the fresh gas flow by 0.5 l/min and change over to low flow anaesthesia

Emergence and recovery
- Switch off the vaporizer 10–20 min prior to the end of the surgical procedure
- Maintain the fresh gas flow at 0.5 l/min
- Lead patient to spontaneous breathing by manual ventilation or SIMV
- Wash out anaesthetic gases with 5.0 l/min of pure oxygen 5–10 min prior to extubation
- Give patient postoperative care according to the generally used scheme

- Unhindered spontaneous breathing is guaranteed more reliably than via a conventional face mask. Provides safer protection from accidental aspiration than the face mask.
- Simplifies performance of anaesthesia, as the hands of the anaesthetist are kept free.

- Compared with the face mask, the laryngeal mask airway (LMA) considerably facilitates monitoring with the aid of capnometry or measurement of the expired gas volume.
- Transition from spontaneous breathing to ventilation and vice versa is rendered very easy.
- It is an alternative tool for airway management in cases of unexpectedly difficult endotracheal intubation.

On the other hand, it must be pointed out that aspiration cannot reliably be precluded in the case of regurgitation, since endoscopy has revealed that in 6% of the cases the seal of the inflated cuff toward the oesophagus was insufficient[49]. However, it can be assumed that protection against aspiration is more reliable than in anaesthesia using a conventional face mask. Controlled ventilation via the laryngeal mask is possible in most cases if the airway pressure does not exceed $17-20 \, cmH_2O$.

In comparison with the conventional face mask, the better gas seal of the connection to the patient's airway is an essential advantage of the laryngeal mask. This lessens the contamination of the operating room atmosphere with anaesthetic gases, thus helping to satisfy the requirements of increasingly stringent regulations on occupational safety and health (see Section 6.3.1).

Furthermore, the use of the laryngeal mask facilitates the performance of low flow anaesthesia techniques in short-term surgical interventions on spontaneously breathing patients. During controlled ventilation, older type conventional anaesthetic machines work without an anaesthetic gas reservoir. This operating mode needs precise adaptation of the fresh gas flow to that gas volume being lost by uptake and leaks (see Section 7.2.6.1.1) so as to prevent changes in ventilation. However, if these machines are used on spontaneously breathing patients, the manual bag, which is attached directly to the breathing system, assumes the function of a gas reservoir. In this way, performance of low flow anaesthesia is considerably simplified since adaptation of the fresh gas flow to the gas volume being lost is made much easier. Possible imbalances are compensated for by the changing degree of filling of the manual bag.

In the author's department, the laryngeal mask is used exclusively on patients with an empty stomach and for surgical interventions which, in principle, can be performed with spontaneous breathing. If, however, artificial ventilation can be carried out without problems, intermittent positive pressure ventilation (IPPV) or synchronized intermittent mandatory ventilation (SIMV) is used in order to prevent atelectasis. Initially, the sealing cuff is inflated with a volume according to the instructions for use.

In 1994–1996, nearly 20% of all cases undergoing inhalational anaesthesia were performed with the use of the laryngeal mask. The average duration of anaesthesia was about 55 min and minimal flow anaesthesia could be realized in about 90% of these cases, in spite of the fact that different modes of controlled ventilation (IPPV, SIMV) were applied on nearly 85% of the patients (Figure 10.25). In 1999, the laryngeal mask airway was used in 32% of all inhalation anaesthetics. Due to the fact, however, that this device was increasingly used also in very short-lasting procedures, the proportion of low flow techniques actually decreased to

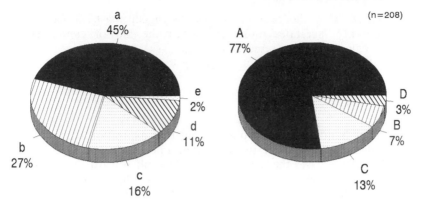

Figure 10.25 Minimal flow anaesthesia via the laryngeal mask. Left pie: percentage of different ventilation modes (a, IPPV; b, SIMV; c, ventilation possible only with muscle relaxation; d, spontaneous breathing). Right pie: performance of minimal flow anaesthesia (A, without any problem; B, 1–2 × refilling of the gas reservoir necessary; C, no attempt was made to reduce the flow rate; D, flow reduction impossible)

Table 10.3 Different techniques to perform inhalational anaesthesia (figures from the author's department, 1994)

	A	B	C	D
Anaesthesia with face mask	13.0%	14.8 min	4.1%	3.1%
Anaesthesia with endotracheal intubation	67.3%	68.4 min	85.7%	61.2%
Anaesthesia with laryngeal mask	19.7%	55.7min	87.5%	56.3%

A: Incidence of respective technique, in relation to the total number of inhalation anaesthetics; B: average duration; C: proportion of cases performed with minimal flow anaesthesia, related to the respective technique; D: proportion of time during which the flow was reduced to 0.5 l/min, related to the total time performed with the respective technique.

72%. Controlled ventilation is only possible without any problem if the body mass index (BMI) is less than $28 \, kg/m^2$ and the airway pressure does not exceed 18–20 mbar. The actual proportion of time during which a flow of 0.5 l/min was administered amounted to about 60%. Different methods of inhalational anaesthesia and the total proportion of time during which the flow was actually reduced to 0.5 l/min are listed in Table 10.3.

The present author agrees with the clinical experience of other authors that low flow anaesthetic techniques can be performed on most patients in whom the laryngeal mask airway is used[51–53]. A reduction in the use of face mask anaesthesia in favour of the laryngeal mask is recommended in order to reduce the workplace contamination by inhalational anaesthetics to an even greater extent.

The author's experiences can be summarized as follows. Barbiturates or propofol should be given in generous induction doses to achieve a deep initial anaesthetic level together with an appropriate inhibition of reflexes.

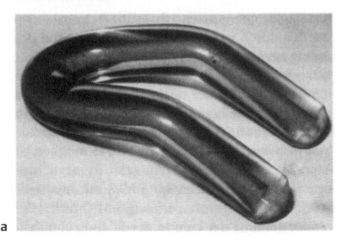

a

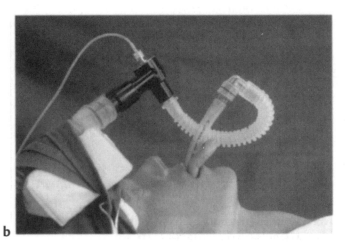

b

Figure 10.26 A simple gag which both protects against occlusion and ensures the correct position of the laryngeal mask airway (from Sachs and Baum[54]). Laryngeal mask airway and gag *in situ*. Smooth connection between the Y-piece and the tube connector via a short flexible silicon hose additionally ensures the correct position of the laryngeal mask (from Baum and Sachs[55]).

In most cases the laryngeal mask can be inserted without any problems. The correct position can easily be verified by checking whether sensitive manual ventilation can be carried out with only slight elastic resistance. Should insufflation be difficult and high pressures build up, the laryngeal mask has to be removed immediately and a new attempt made at insertion. After insertion of the laryngeal mask, the tube is protected by a gag. A special disinfectable device made of plastic has proven to be advantageous (Figure 10.26a and b), not only for bite protection but also for fixing the tube in the midline, thus providing an additional aid to proper positioning and sufficient sealing of the laryngeal mask[54,55]. This device is now commercially available at all the distributors of the laryngeal mask airway. Where elderly patients are concerned, it may happen in the individual case that the laryngeal mask dislocates spontaneously from its originally correct position into the oropharynx. This must be attributed to age-related atrophic alteration of the pharyngeal profile and reduced turgor of the tissues. In two patients we observed complications resulting from intentional reduction of the pressure within the sealing cuff of the laryngeal mask with the aid of a cuff pressure measurement device[56]. The pressure should not be less than 60 mbar. If the sealing cuff is not inflated sufficiently, the hard body of the laryngeal mask may exert pressure directly to the mucous membrane surrounding the entrance of the larynx, resulting in painful ulcers. The laryngeal mask is impressively well tolerated during emergence and may be kept in place until full awakening, which ensures optimum protection of unhindered spontaneous breathing.

In summary, the following statements seem to be justified:

- The gas tightness of a correctly positioned laryngeal mask in about 90% of all patients is sufficient for performing low flow techniques, even with a fresh gas flow rate as low as 0.5 l/min.
- In most of these cases (85%) controlled ventilation can be carried out.
- Limiting factors in the use of the laryngeal mask airway, at least with controlled ventilation, are old age, obesity $(BMI > 28 \, kg/m^2)$ and airway pressure exceeding 18–20 mbar.

The laryngeal mask is thus a valuable means of reduction of emission of inhalational anaesthetics. This new device facilitates low flow anaesthesia in short surgical interventions and also the performance of low flow techniques with conventional anaesthesia machines on spontaneously breathing patients. This tool, however, does not reliably prevent aspiration.

10.8 Paediatric anaesthesia

Every anaesthetist who has gained sufficient practical experiences in low flow techniques on adult patients should be able to perform this method even in paediatric anaesthesia without any deficit in safety. However, reviewing the literature, only a few articles deal with this topic[57,58]. An excellent overview on the different aspects of low flow anaesthesia in paediatric anaesthesia was published recently by G. H. Meakin[59]. The lack of interest in paediatric low flow anaesthesia may be due to traditional reservations, as even nowadays many colleagues are of the opinion that in paediatric anaesthesia preferentially or even obligatorily non-rebreathing systems should be used. We are, however, in a time of change: in 1985 Rügheimer still questioned the use of low flow techniques, even for adult patients[60], while in 1993 Altemeyer predicted low flow anaesthetic techniques would become acknowledged methods in the near future in paediatric anaesthesia[61].

As a rule, the techniques of low flow or minimal flow anaesthesia can be applied on all paediatric patients in whom use is made of a rebreathing

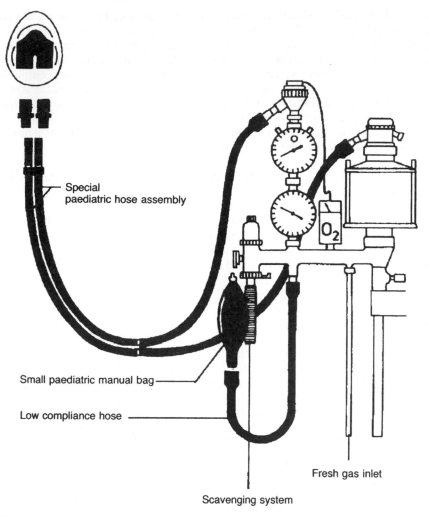

Special
paediatric hose assembly

Small paediatric manual bag

Low compliance hose

Fresh gas inlet

Scavenging system

Figure 10.27   Ulmer-Kreissystem (Dräger Medizintechnik, Lübeck, Germany): circle absorption system for use in paediatric anaesthesia. (From Striebel and Kretz[64], by permission)

system. An indispensable precondition must be, however, that the small tidal volumes and the high ventilatory stroke frequency required in paediatric anaesthesia are included in the technical features of the respective anaesthetic machine. Special paediatric circle absorber systems[62,63] such as the Ulmer Kreissystem (Dräger Medizintechnik, Lübeck, Germany) are available for this purpose (Figure 10.27). Such systems feature appropriately small ventilation bellows, an absorber canister with reduced volume, a specially scaled volumeter and a patient hose assembly with small diameter tubing characterized by very low compliance[64]. Meakin comes to the conclusion that if ventilation is controlled in neonates, and either controlled or assisted in infants, an adult circle system fitted with small bore tubing and a reduced capacity reservoir bag is suitable for paediatric patients of all ages[59]. Paediatric anaesthesia with low fresh gas flow can be performed even more easily without any age restriction with the newer generation of anaesthetic machines, such as the Cato and Cicero (Drägerwerk, Lübeck, Germany). The software controlling the ventilator operation permits setting of tidal volumes down to 20 ml and features compliance compensation[65]. This enables the anaesthetist to use rebreathing systems even on newborns and very small infants.

The following advantages result from the use of rebreathing systems if compared with the use of non-rebreathing systems:

- less pollution of the workplace atmosphere with inhalational anaesthetics;
- less emission of waste anaesthetic gases;
- exact monitoring of ventilation parameters such as expired volume and airway pressure is rendered possible;
- the unrestricted possibility of carbon dioxide monitoring;
- improved climatization of the anaesthetic gases;
- less loss of heat and humidity[57];
- the possibility of controlled mechanical ventilation;
- less liability to accidental carbon dioxide rebreathing; and
- considerable cost savings.

The equipping of modern anaesthetic machines with comprehensive gas monitoring and the introduction of the newer anaesthetic agents characterized by low solubility and decreased anaesthetic potency are further arguments in favour of paediatric low flow anaesthesia.

The terms low and minimal flow anaesthesia are traditionally defined by the fresh gas flow rate. If these techniques, using a flow of 1.0 or 0.5 l/min, respectively, are performed on adult patients, the rebreathing fraction can be assumed to be at least 50%. Thus, both methods, by definition, are low flow anaesthetic techniques. However, if the same flow is used in infants and small children, due to their significantly smaller uptake, this will result in a considerable increase of excess gas and a corresponding decrease of the rebreathing fraction. Furthermore, the gas-containing space, i.e. the volume of the lungs and, if special paediatric components are attached to the machine, the volume of the breathing system too, is comparatively small. Thus, the time constant is correspondingly short and changes in fresh gas composition take place in the paediatric breathing system within a relatively short period of time, even if low fresh gas flows are used. Low flow anaesthesia using a fresh gas flow of 1.0 l/min performed on an infant approximately resembles in its characteristics a high flow technique on an adult patient. The difference between the fresh gas composition and that of the respired anaesthetic gas is smaller, and the time constant shorter, than in adult low flow anaesthesia. In paediatric anaesthesia a fresh gas flow rate of 1.0–1.5 l/min in children up to an age of about 10–12 years is ample. Nevertheless, in the interest of an unambiguous terminology, the generally acknowledged terms should be used also in paediatric anaesthesia (see Chapter 4).

Table 10.4   MAC with respect to the patient's age

	0–6 months	3–5 years	20–30 years	≈40 years	≈50 years	≈65 years
Halothane	1.1	0.9	0.8	0.8	∅	∅
Enflurane	∅	2.4	∅	1.7	∅	∅
Isoflurane	1.9	1.6	1.3	1.2	∅	1.1
Sevoflurane	3.3	2.5	∅	2.1	1.7	∅
Desflurane	9.4	8.6	7.3	∅	6.0	5.2

(from: Conzen P, Hobbhahn J. Sevoflurane-Kompendium, Wissenschaftliche Verlagsabteilung, Abbott GmbH, Wiesbaden, 1996[69])

The special calculation of an individual fresh gas flow, as was suggested by Cuoto da Silva and Aldrete[66], is by no means helpful in any case, as gas flows as low as 56 ml/min oxygen or 84 ml/min nitrous oxide, which for instance are calculated for a 1-year-old child with a body weight of 10 kg, can not be set on most available anaesthesia machines. In daily clinical practice, even in paediatric anaesthesia, generally we have to be content with a flow of about 0.5 l/min, although with single machines the flow may even be reduced to 0.3 or even 0.2 l/min. Using extremely low flows, however, the sample gas used for side-stream analysis of the anaesthetic gas composition necessarily has to be delivered back into the breathing system. Since the excess gas proportion is comparatively high, which compensates for minor gas losses, low flow anaesthesia can also be performed with uncuffed endotracheal tubes if their size is selected appropriately. The same holds for the use of the laryngeal mask in low flow anaesthesia on children[59,67,68].

Generally, with respect to induction, maintenance and recovery, there is no difference between low flow anaesthesia on children or on adult patients. In paediatric anaesthesia the standardized settings, as recommended for use in low flow anaesthesia on adults, will result in significantly higher inspired and expired anaesthetic concentrations. This applies equally for enflurane, isoflurane and sevoflurane. The MAC values of these agents for children, however, are higher than for adults (Table 10.4), justifying the application of the standardized dosing schemes. Alterations of the fresh gas composition will become effective much faster, as the gas volume contained in the patient's lung and in the anaesthetic machine, as well as the individual uptake, are small. If anaesthetic machines with anaesthetic gas reservoirs are used, it is advisable to replace the special paediatric manual bag (0.5 litres), which is used during induction, with a large volume (2.0 litres) manual bag prior to flow reduction. Thus, after flow reduction, a large gas volume will be available to compensate for possible gas volume imbalances. The manual bag should be detached from its mount and left resting freely to prevent unwanted gas loss via the excess gas discharge valve (see section 10.4). Meakin, contrarily, recommends using a smaller reservoir bag (800–1000 ml), enabling better visual assessment of spontaneous ventilation possible in children aged more than 1 year[59].

In paediatric anaesthesia low flow anaesthetic techniques can always be performed if use is made of a rebreathing system. The smaller the child, the more the characteristic of the procedure resembles a high flow technique, as the excess gas volume increases whereas the rebreathing fraction decreases.

10.9   Low flow anaesthesia in cases of short duration (day-case surgery)

If an attempt is made to adopt low flow techniques in very short surgical interventions, such as are frequently performed in day-case surgery, the following points must be considered. An initial high fresh gas flow is needed to ensure adequate denitrogenation, achievement of the desired anaesthetic gas composition within the breathing system within the short time available and bridging of possible initial gas volume imbalances. For sufficient denitrogenation, a flow of 4–6 l/min has to be used over a period of at least 6–8 min. The desired anaesthetic concentration needed to permit the surgical intervention to start can only be achieved quickly by setting comparatively high fresh gas concentrations, so as to increase the alveolar–blood partial pressure difference, thus accelerating uptake of the respective volatile anaesthetic. Nevertheless, the problem of the initial high nitrous oxide uptake with the resulting possibility of gas volume imbalances remains unresolved if the flow is reduced to 0.5 l/min just after denitrogenation. Unfortunately, this holds also for the use of desflurane, although wash-in of a desired concentration of this agent, according to its favourable pharmacokinetic properties, is accomplished rapidly[39].

Stepwise reduction of the fresh gas flow may be an alternative method to adopt for low flow techniques, even in very short anaesthetics. In the first 5 min the flow is set to 4.4 l/min (1.4 l/min O_2, 3.0 l/min N_2O), over the following period of 10 min to 1.0 l/min (0.4 l/min O_2, 0.6 l/min N_2O) and then finally to 0.5 l/min (0.25 l/min O_2, 0.25 l/min N_2O). Applying this scheme of stepwise flow reduction, the vaporizer setting can be standardized at 3.0 vol% for isoflurane (Figure 10.28) and 4.0 vol% for enflurane.

But if this technique is judged honestly, no real advantage will be gained. During a 15-min anaesthetic performed with stepwise flow reduction, only 24 litres of nitrous oxide but no volatile anaesthetic can be saved in comparison with minimal flow anaesthesia maintaining a high flow 4.4 l/min over the whole initial period of 15 min. Due to shortening of the nitrogen wash-out, this gas will accumulate at a comparatively high level even after a short time. The technique is involved, as flow adjustments are required just at the time when the anaesthetist is occupied by setting of monitors, positioning of the patient and preparation for the surgical intervention. Accordingly, timely flow adjustments will often be omitted. And the better climatization of the anaesthetic gases, resulting from flow reduction, only become effective after a certain time delay.

However, compared with high flow anaesthesia (4.4 l/min), if minimal flow anaesthesia is applied according to the aforementioned standardized scheme during an anaesthetic lasting only 60 min, about 34% (9.86 US$)

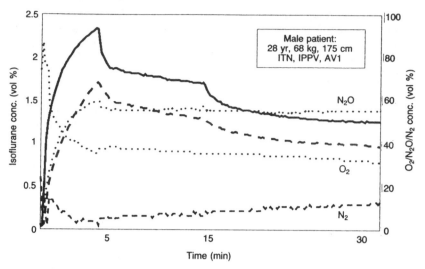

Figure 10.28   Course of anaesthetic gas composition during performance of short-term anaesthesia by stepwise control of the fresh gas flow (5 min: 4.4 l/min; 10 min: 1.0 l/min; then 0.5 l/min); vaporizer setting maintained at 3 vol% (male patient aged 28 years, weight 68 kg, height 1.75 m). Computer-based on-line record, gas analyser: Capnomac (Datex, Helsinki, Finland)

of the otherwise overall costs of about 29 US$ can be saved, in spite of the use of more expensive supplementary drugs like propofol, atracurium, alfentanil and the use of the laryngeal mask. Even in a 30-min anaesthetic, 15% (3.15 US$) of the total cost of 21 US$ can be saved just by the appropriate use of available rebreathing equipment. Thus, if short duration day-case surgical procedures are performed under general anaesthesia with inhalational anaesthetics, low flow anaesthetic techniques should be applied consistently whenever the surgical intervention lasts longer than 10–15 min.

10.10   References

1. Bergmann H. Das Narkosegerät in Gegenwart und Zukunft aus der Sicht des Klinikers. *Anaesthesist* 1986; **35**, 587–594.
2. Baum J. Contaminazione Batterica dei Sistemi Ventilatori. La Riduzione del Flusso Aumenta il Rischio? In Giunta F, ed., *Anesthesia a Bassi Flussi e a Circuito Chiuso*. Piccin Nuova Libraria, Padova, 1992, pp. 173–180.
3. Baum J, Enzenauer J, Krausse Th and Sachs G. Atemkalk – Nutzungsdauer, Verbrauch und Kosten in Abhängigkeit vom Frischgasfluß. *Anaesthesiol Reanim* 1993; **18**, 108–113.
4. Bengtson JP, Brandberg Å, Brinkhoff B, Sonander H and Stenqvist O. Low-flow anaesthesia does not increase the risk of microbial contamination through the circle absorber system. *Acta Anaesth Scand* 1989; **33**, 89–92.
5. Deutsche Gesellschaft für Anästhesiologie und Intensivmedizin. Hygienische Maßnahmen als Bestandteil der Anwendungssicherheit medizinisch-technischer Geräte. *Anästh Intensivmed* 1984; **24**, 79–82.

6. Stober HD, Lüder M, Bensow Ch, Jung G and Reinartz P. Experimentelle Untersuchungen über die mikrobielle Kontamination von Narkosegeräten und Zubehör und die Bedeutung für den infektiösen Hospitalismus. 2. Mitteilung: Zur Frage der aerogenen Keimverbreitung während der Inhalationsnarkose. *Anaesthesiol Reanimat* 1982; **7**, 85–93.
7. Stober HD, Lüder M, Markwardt J and Bensow Ch. Experimentelle Untersuchungen über die mikrobielle Kontamination von Narkosegeräten und Zubehör und die Bedeutung für den infektiösen Hospitalismus. 3. Mitteilung: Quantitative Kontaminationsmessungen an drei verschiedenen Narkose-Kreissytemen. *Anaesthesiol Reanimat* 1983; **8**, 53–61.
8. Mazze RI. Bacterial air filters. *Anesthesiology* 1981; **54**, 359–360.
9. Luttropp HH and Berntman L. Bacterial filters protect anaesthetic equipment in a low-flow system. *Anaesthesia* 1993; **48**, 520–523.
10. Kohler P, Rimek A, Albrecht M, Frankenberger H, Mertins W and van Ackern K. Sind Feuchtigkeitsfilter in der Inspirationsluft während der Narkose notwendig? *Anästhesiol Intensivmed Notfallmed Schmerzther* 1992; **27**, 149–155.
11. Gregorini P. Effect of low fresh gas flow rates on inspired gas composition in a circle absorber system. *J Clin Anaesth* 1992; **4**, 439–443.
12. Barton FJ and Nunn F. Totally closed circuit nitrous oxide/oxygen anaesthesia. *Br J Anaesth* 1975; **47**, 350–357.
13. Parbrook GD. The levels of nitrous oxide analgesia. *Br J Anaesth* 1967; **39**, 974–982.
14. Don H. Hypoxemia and hypercapnia during and after anesthesia. In Orkin FK and Cooperman LH, eds, *Complications in Anesthesiology*. Lippincott, Philadelphia, 1983, pp. 183–207.
15. Westenskow DR. How much oxygen? *Int J Clin Monitor Comput* 1986; **2**, 187–189.
16. Halsey MJ. A reassessment of the molecular structure – functional relationships of the inhaled general anaesthetics. *Br J Anaesth* 1984; **56** (Suppl. 1), 9S–25S.
17. Terrell RC. Physical and chemical properties of anaesthetic agents. *Br J Anaesth* 1984; **56** (Suppl. 1), 3S–7S.
18. Lowe HJ. Dose-regulated penthrane anesthesia. Abbott Laboratories, Chicago, 1972.
19. Nemes C, Niemer M and Noack G. Datenbuch Anästhesiologie. Fischer, Stuttgart, 1979.
20. Weiskopf RB. Inhalation anaesthetics: today and tomorrow. In Torri G and Damia G, eds, *Update on Modern Inhalation Anaesthetics*. Worldwide Medical Communications, New York, 1989, pp. 23–28.
21. Zbinden AM. *Inhalationsanästhetika: Aufnahme und Verteilung*. Wissenschaftliche Verlagsabteilung, Deutsche Abbott, Wiesbaden, 1987.
22. Eger II EI. New inhaled anesthetics. *Anesthesiology* 1994; **80**, 906–922.
23. Eger II EI. The pharmacology of isoflurane. *Br J Anaesth* 1984; **56** (Suppl. 1), 71S–99S.
24. Baum J. Minimal flow anaesthesia with isoflurane. In Lawin, P, van Aken H and Puchstein Ch, eds, *Isoflurane. Anaesthesiologie und Intensivmedizin*, Bd. 182. Springer, Berlin, 1986, pp. 325–331.
25. Schwilden H, Stoeckel H, Lauven PM and Schüttler J. Pharmakokinetik und MAC – Praktische Implikationen für die Dosierung volatiler Anästhetika. In Peter K, Brown BR, Martin E and Norlander O, eds, *Inhaltionsanaesthetika*. *Anaesthesiologie und Intensivmedizin*, Bd. 184. Springer, Berlin, 1986, pp. 18–26.
26. Torri G, Salvo P, Righi E, Calderini E and Bordoli W. Pharmacokinetic profile of Isoflurane in children. In Lawin P, van Aken H and Puchstein

Ch, eds, *Isoflurane. Anaesthesiologie und Intensivmedizin*, Bd. 182. Springer, Berlin 1986, pp. 24–28.

27. Hendrickx JFA, Soetens M, Van der Donck A, Meeuwis H, Smolders F and De Wolf AM. Uptake of desflurane and isoflurane during closed-circuit anesthesia with spontaneous and controlled mechanical ventilation. *Anesth Analg* 1997; **84**, 413–418.

28. Eger II EI Complexities overlooked: things may not be what they seem. *Anesth Analg* 1997; **84**, 239–240.

29. Robson JG, Gillies DM, Cullen WG and Griffith HR. Fluothane (halothane) in closed circuit anesthesia. *Anesthesiology* 1959; **20**, 251–260.

30. Zinganell K. Halothane im geschlossenen Kreislauf. *Anaesthesist* 1969; **18**, 88–94.

31. Bennets NB. Halothane and the liver – the problem revisited. Proceedings of a Symposium at Bristol University Medical School, 11th April 1986. Sir Humphry Davy Department of Anaesthesia, Bristol Royal Infirmary, 1986.

32. Brown BR Jr and Gandolfi AJ. Adverse effects of volatile anaesthetics. *Br J Anaesth* 1987; **59**, 14–23.

33. Hobbhahn J, Hansen E, Conzen P and Peter K. Der Einfluß von Inhalationsanästhetika auf die Leber. *Anästh Intensivmed 1991*; **32**, 215–220 and 250–256.

34. Scholz J and Tonner PH. Kritische Bewertung der neuen Inhalationsanästhetika Desfluran und Sevofluran. *Anaesthesiol Reanimat* 1997; **22**, 15–20.

35. Biebuyck JF. New inhaled anesthetics. *Anesthesiology* 1994; **80**, 906–922.

36. Eger II EI. Physicochemical properties and pharmacodynamics of desflurane. *Anaesthesia* 1995; **50** (Suppl.), 3–8.

37. Smith I, Nathanson M and White PF. Sevoflurane – a long-awaited volatile anaesthetic. *Br J Anaesth* 1996; 76, 435–445.

38. Baum J, Berghoff M, Stanke HG, Petermeyer M and Kalff G. Niedrigflußnarkosen mit Desfluran. *Anaesthesist* 1997; **46**, 287–293.

39. Lee DJH, Robinson DL and Soni N. Efficiency of a circle system for short surgical cases: comparison of desflurane with isoflurane. *Br J Anaesth* 1996; **76**, 780–782.

40. Hargasser S, Hipp R, Breinbauer B, Mielke L, Entholzner E and Rust M. A lower solubility recommends the use of desflurane more than isoflurane, halothane, and enflurane under low-flow conditions. *J Clin Anesth* 1995; **7**, 1–5.

41. Baum J and Stanke HG. Low Flow- und Minimal Flow Anästhesie mit Sevofluran. *Anaesthesist* 1998; **47** (Suppl.), S70–S76.

42. Kharasch ED. Putting the brakes on anesthetic breakdown. *Anesthesiology* 1999; **91**, 1192–1194.

43. Baum J and van Aken H. Calcium hydroxide lime – a new carbon dioxide absorbent. A rationale for judicious use of different absorbents. *Eur J Anaesth* 2000; **17**, 597–600.

44. Murray JM, Renfrew CW, Bedi A, McCrystal CB, Jones DS and Fee JPH. Amsorb: a new carbon dioxide absorbent for use in anaesthetic breathing systems. *Anesthesiology* 1999; **91**, 1342–1348.

45. Baum J, Züchner K, Hölscher U, Sievert B, Stanke HG, Gruchmann T and Rathgeber J. Klimatisierung von Narkosegasen bei Einsatz unterschiedlicher Patientenschlauchsystme. *Anaesthesist* 2000; **49**, 402–411.

46. Brain AIJ. The laryngeal mask – a new concept in airway management. *Br J Anaesth* 1983; **55**, 801–805.

47. Brain AIJ. The Intavent laryngeal mask. Instruction manual, Intavent, 1990.

48. Calder I, Ordman AJ, Jackowski A and Crockard HA. The Brain laryngeal mask airway. An alternative to emergency tracheal intubation. *Anaesthesia* 1990; **45**, 137–139.
49. Leach AB and Alexander CA. The laryngeal mask – an overview. *Eur J Anaesth* 1991; Suppl. 4, 19–31.
50. Silk JM, Hill HM and Calder I. Difficult intubation and the laryngeal mask. *Eur J Anaesth* 1991; Suppl. 4, 47–51.
51. Hönemann Ch. Die Sicherung der Atemwege bei Inhalationsnarkosen. Inaugural-Dissertation der Medizinischen Fakultät der Westfälischen Wilhelms-Universität, Münster, 1995.
52. Möllhoff T, Burgard G and Prien Th. Low-flow and minimal flow anaesthesia using the laryngeal mask airway. *Eur J Anaesth* 1996; **13**, 456–462.
53. Stacey MRW and Shambrook A. Laryngeal mask airway and low flow anaesthesia. *Anaesthesia* 1992; **47**, 1108.
54. Sachs G and Baum J. Ein einfacher Beißschutz für die Kehlkopfmaske. *Anästhesiol Intensivmed Notfallmed Schmerzther* 1994; **29**, 309–310.
55. Baum J and Sachs G. Comment on J. Brimacombe's statement 'The laryngeal mask airway – fixation, gags and stability'. *Anästhesiol Intensivmed Notfallmed Schmerzther* 1995; **30**, 130.
56. Burgard G, Möllhoff Th and Prien Th. Intraoperative Druckreduktion im Cuff der laryngealen Maske senkt die Inzidenz postoperativer Halsschmerzen. *Anaesthesist* 1993; **42** (Suppl. 1), S140.
57. Gebhardt R and Weiser UK. Die Niedrigflußnarkose bei Neugeborenen – Vorteile und Risiken. *Anaesthesiol Reanimat* 1999; **24**, 41–46.
58. Igarashi M, Watanabe H, Iwasaki H and Namiki A. Clinical evaluation of low-flow sevoflurane anesthesia for paediatric patients. *Acta Anaesthesiol Scand* 1999; **43**, 19–23.
59. Meakin GH. Low-flow anaesthesia in infants and children. *Br J Anaesth* 1999; **83**, 50–57.
60. Rügheimer E. Low-flow and closed circuit anaesthesia. In Dick W, ed., *Kombinationsanästhesie. Klinische Anästhesiologie und Intensivtherapie*, Bd. 29. Springer, Berlin, 1985, S116–S129.
61. Altemeyer KH. Narkosebeatmung – Prinzipien. In Fösel Th and Kraus GB, eds, *Beatmung von Kindern in Anästhesie und Intensivmedizin*. Springer, Berlin, 1993, S36–S49.
62. Altemeyer KH. Narkose- und Überwachungssysteme für die Kinderanästhesie. *Anästhesiologie und Intensivmedizin*, Bd. 170. Springer, Berlin, 1985.
63. Altemeyer KH, Fösel Th, Berg-Seiter S and Wick C. Besonderheiten der endotrachealen Intubation und der Narkosesysteme. In Dick W, ed., *Kinderanästhesie – Kombinationsnarkosen im Kindesalter*. Springer, Berlin, 1986, S33–S39.
64. Striebel HW and Kretz FJ. Narkosesysteme. In Kretz FJ and Striebel HW, eds, *Basisinformationen Kinderanästhesie*. Editiones Roche, Basel, 1991, pp. 78–82.
65. Peters JWB, Bezstarosti-van Eden J, Erdmann W, Meursing AEE. Safety and efficacy of semi-closed circle ventilation in small infants. *Paediatr Anaesth* 1998; **8**, 299–304.
66. Cuoto da Silva JM and Aldrete JA. A proposal for a new classification of anesthetic gas flows. *Acta Anaesth Belg* 1990; **41**, 253–258.
67. Fröhlich D, Schwall B, Funk W and Hobbhahn J. Laryngeal mask airway and uncuffed tracheal tubes are equally effective for low flow or closed system anaesthesia in children. *Br J Anaesth* 1997; **79**, 289–292.
68. Weiser UK. Praktische Erfahrungen mit Narkoseverfahren bei reduziertem Frischgasflow (Low-flow- und Minimal-flow-Anästhesie) im Säuglings- und

Kleinkindesalter. In Fösel Th and Kraus GB, eds, *Beatmung von Kindern in Anästhesie und Intensivmedizin*. Springer, Berlin, 1993, S50–S59.

69. Conzen P and Hobbhan I. *Sevofluran-Kompendium: Inhalationsanästhetikum*. Wissenschaftliche Verlagsabteilung, Abbott GmbH, Wiesbaden, 1966.

Low flow anaesthetic techniques without nitrous oxide

11.1 The routine use of nitrous oxide as carrier gas – pros and cons

Most anaesthetists still assume nitrous oxide to be a more or less inert anaesthetic gas which thus is used every day as a matter of course. Nitrous oxide has been used since the very first days of clinical general anaesthesia, even though the first clinical demonstration to alleviate pain in surgical interventions by Horace Wells (1815–1848) in January 1845 was a failure. Since about 1860 the development of anaesthetic machines and breathing systems has assumed the routine use of nitrous oxide in different anaesthetic techniques[1–3]. As early as 1800, in the first scientific monograph on this gas, Humphrey Davy (1778–1829) mentioned the analgesic potency of nitrous oxide and its potential for use during surgery: 'As nitrous oxide in its extensive operation appears capable of destroying physical pain, it may probably be used with advantage during surgical operations in which no great effusion of blood takes place'[4]. Davy, a true polymath, seemed to lose interest in nitrous oxide after his treatise was published and did not pass his exceptional idea on to any surgeon, neither did any physician recognize that this was already the concept of inhalational anaesthesia. Davy was a man too far ahead of his time – the world was simply not yet ready to exploit his idea.

Thus for many years a mixture of oxygen and nitrous oxide has been used as the carrier gas to deliver inhalational agents, with no thought given to its true value or disadvantages. Although with total intravenous anaesthesia the concurrent use of any gaseous anaesthetic should be unnecessary, this technique is frequently carried out with the additive use of nitrous oxide. For most anaesthetists the following arguments support the continuing use of nitrous oxide[5–9]. According to the concept of 'balanced anaesthesia', nitrous oxide is assumed to exert a quite powerful analgesic and, along with the other inhalation anaesthetics, a modest but significant hypnotic effect. Short but painful interventions can be performed without any additive narcotic[10]. By using nitrous oxide the doses of supplementary opioids and other anaesthetics can be considerably reduced. The rapid wash-out of this gas, together with its dose-reducing effect, favourably accelerates recovery from anaesthesia. During mask induction in paediatric anaesthesia the second gas effect accelerates the wash-in of inhalation anaesthetics, hence shortening the induction time. Its mild sympathetic effect counteracts the depressive effects of the volatile agents on the cardiovascular system. Nitrous oxide is widely assumed to be an essential factor in the prevention of intra-operative awareness and in suppressing spinal reflex movements caused by intense surgical stimulation.

The common opinion, however, that nitrous oxide is a near inert, albeit anaesthetic, gas which can be used without any problem is no longer sustainable in the light of current knowledge[5–7,9,11]. Generally accepted contraindications to the use of nitrous oxide include all situations where there is confinement of air in tissues or hollow spaces of the body such as ileus, pneumencephalon, pneumothorax or occlusion of the Eustachian tube. In abdominal operations of long duration the diffusion of nitrous oxide into gas-containing spaces will cause bowel distension with consequent impairment of operative conditions and delays in the recovery of bowel function[12]. Nitrous oxide causes increased cerebral blood flow and so is contraindicated in patients with head injuries and raised intracranial pressure[13]. In patients with compromised coronary perfusion the administration of nitrous oxide results in a significant decrease in myocardial contractility with a secondary increase in the left ventricular end-diastolic pressure[14–16]. For this reason nitrous oxide should be avoided in all patients with severe cardiac disease and latent myocardial insufficiency[7]. In patients suffering from chronic vitamin B_{12} deficiency the use of nitrous oxide may cause myeloneuropathy, characterized by progressive demyelination and axonal lesions of the peripheral nerves and cervicothoracic spinal cord[17,18]. Furthermore, in cases suffering from congenital neutropenia, nitrous oxide may cause agranulocytosis[19]. After long-term nitrous oxide use megaloblastic alterations of the bone marrow with anaemia, thrombopenia and leucopenia were observed[5–7,9,11]. Due to its proven harmful effect on DNA synthesis, nitrous oxide may be considered to be contraindicated in pregnant women during the first two trimesters, during preparations for *in vitro* fertilization, or in immunosuppressed patients with impaired function of lymphocytes and reduced neutrophil responsiveness[11]. Although the results of meta-analyses of scientific publications on this topic were somewhat ambiguous, nitrous oxide seems to play a role in postoperative vomiting and probably nausea also[20,21]. In all patients who have on previous occasions suffered from severe postoperative nausea and vomiting (PONV) the use of nitrous oxide should be avoided[5–7,9]. It remains a matter of scientific discussion whether chronic exposure to trace gas concentrations of nitrous oxide really endangers theatre personnel, although embryotoxic and teratogenic effects were found in animal experiments. Most countries stipulate a maximum workplace concentration for nitrous oxide. In Germany, the measurement of workplace contamination is a statutory requirement[22,23]. Nitrous oxide is also not inert in respect to ecology, as it is known to have a significant greenhouse gas effect and is a potent destroyer of the stratospheric ozone layer. Although the emission of anaesthetic nitrous oxide, comprising not more than about 1% of the total global output, seems to be negligible if compared with the vast amount generated by bacterial metabolism in fertilized soil, anaesthetists should be obliged to fully utilize currently available technology to minimize unnecessary wastage of this gas[24,25].

11.2 Inhalation anaesthesia without nitrous oxide – general considerations with special respect to low flow anaesthetic techniques

The ecologically and economically justified demand to avoid any unnecessary waste of anaesthetic gases can already be met by the consistent use of low flow anaesthetic techniques. Maximum use is made of the rebreathing technique, thus minimizing consumption and emission of anaesthetic gases[26]. During a 2-h anaesthetic, the nitrous oxide consumption is decreased from about 360 litres at 4.4 l/min fresh gas flow to 70 or 85 litres at a flow of 0.5 or 1.0 l/min. While the problems of workplace contamination and nitrous oxide emission into the atmosphere are both minimized by using low flow techniques[27,28], the exposure of patients to the gas and its possibly harmful consequences remain. The latter can only be resolved by consistently renouncing any use of nitrous oxide in inhalation anaesthesia, even if low flow techniques are performed.

The loss of analgesia resulting from omitting nitrous oxide has to be compensated for by an increased use of opioids and the loss of hypnotic effect by increasing the concentration of the volatile anaesthetic agent. According to the findings of Eger *et al.*[6] and Röpcke and Schwilden[29,30], the anaesthetic effect of a 60 vol% concentration of nitrous oxide can be adequately replaced by increasing the concentration of the chosen volatile agent by $0.2–0.25 \times MAC$. In line with the recommendations given in Sections 10.2–10.3, the following expired anaesthetic concentrations may be appropriate in the absence of nitrous oxide: isoflurane 1.2 vol%, sevoflurane 2.2 vol% and desflurane about 5.0 vol%[26,29,30]. As has already been explained comprehensively beforehand, when using nitrous oxide an initial high flow phase of about 4.0 l/min has to precede the flow reduction. During this phase denitrogenation is completed, the desired anaesthetic concentration established within the whole gas-containing space, a sufficient anaesthetic level gained, and the time of initial high nitrous oxide uptake also allowed for. If, however, nitrous oxide is not used at all, no nitrogen wash-out is required and it is axiomatic that nitrous oxide wash-in is not needed. Thus, the duration of the initial phase is determined only by the time needed to establish the agent concentration required to guarantee a sufficient anaesthetic depth. This time is determined by the pharmacokinetic properties of the respective agent and the technical features of the agent-specific vaporizer. Generally, the omission of nitrous oxide can be assumed to significantly shorten the time of the initial high flow phase. Furthermore, as only oxygen and the volatile agent are being taken up by the patient, the total gas uptake decreases and hence the amount of excess gas can be expected to increase considerably. This, for its part, will reduce the risk of accidental gas volume deficiency when using fresh gas flow rates as low as 1.0 or 0.5 l/min.

11.3   Low flow anaesthetic techniques without nitrous oxide – clinical practice

11.3.1   Minimal flow anaesthesia without nitrous oxide

Pre-medication and intravenous induction follow the routinely used scheme, there are no procedure-specific requirements. However, renouncing the use of nitrous oxide, it seems wise to routinely give a supplemental dose of 0.1–0.2 mg fentanyl or 0.5–1.0 mg alfentanil to enhance analgesia. Following endotracheal intubation or insertion of a laryngeal mask and connection of the patient to the circle system an initial fresh gas flow rate of 4.0 l/min (1.0 l/min O_2, 3.0 l/min air) is set. The fresh gas concentration can be standardized at 2.5 vol% for isoflurane, 3.5 vol% for sevoflurane, and 6.0 vol% for desflurane. In the following 10 min the inspired oxygen concentration will be about 40 vol% (Figure 11.1), the expired anaesthetic concentrations 1.2–1.4 vol% for isoflurane, 2.2–2.4 vol% for sevoflurane and 4.5–5.5 vol% for desflurane (Figure 11.2). After 10 min the fresh gas flow rate can be reduced to 0.5 l/min, at which time the oxygen concentration of the fresh gas should be increased to 67 vol% (0.3 l/min O_2, 0.2 l/min air). Only by increasing the fresh gas oxygen content so markedly is it possible to compensate for the oxygen-depleted expired gas exhaled back into the circuit and the increase of that gas volume being discharged out of the breathing system as waste. Compared with minimal flow anaesthesia using nitrous oxide, an even higher fresh gas oxygen content is needed in order to prevent the development of hypoxic gas mixtures. The continuous monitoring of inspired oxygen concentration remains indispensable during nitrous oxide-free minimal flow anaesthesia. With fresh gas flow reduction, the isoflurane concentration has to be increased to 5.0 vol%, the sevoflurane fresh gas

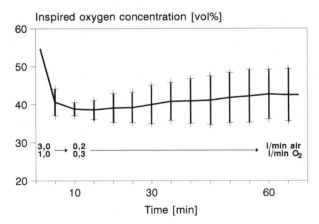

Figure 11.1   Inspired oxygen concentration during performance of minimal flow anaesthesia with an oxygen–nitrogen mixture as carrier gas. Mean values and standard deviations are shown. Details on fresh gas flow rate and its composition are given in the figure. Sample of patients: $n = 17$; mean body weight, 76.8 kg; mean body size, 169.5 cm; mean age, 48.8 years. (From Baum et al.[26])

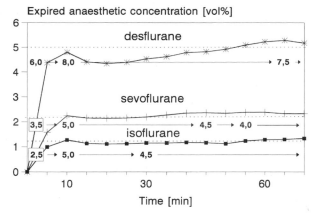

Figure 11.2   Expired anaesthetic agent concentration during performance of minimal flow anaesthesia with an oxygen–nitrogen mixture as carrier gas, mean values. Details on vaporizer settings given in the figure; broken lines: respective nominal values for expired agent concentration. Samples of patients – isoflurane: $n = 10$; mean body weight 69.3 kg, mean body size 162.2 cm, mean age 54.4 years; sevoflurane: $n = 10$, mean body weight 68.9 kg, mean body size 172 cm, mean age 33.8 years; desflurane: $n = 9$, mean body weight 86.5 kg, mean body size 172.4 cm, mean age 44.4 years. (From Baum et al.[26])

concentration to 5.0 vol%, or the desflurane concentration to 8.0 vol% to maintain the required expired agent concentration. Assuming that these fresh gas settings are used, the inspired oxygen concentration will be 35–45 vol% in most cases (Figure 11.1), whereas the expired anaesthetic concentration will be maintained at roughly the MAC value, about 1.2 vol% for isoflurane, about 2.0–2.2 vol% for sevoflurane, and about 4.5–5.0 vol% for desflurane (Figure 11.2). Further adaptations of the fresh gas concentration of the inhalational agent will have to be made according to the patient's individual response and to suit the surgical procedure.

The clinical experiences with consistent performance of minimal flow anaesthesia without nitrous oxide, gained by the author over 18 months, can be summarized as follows[26].

The initial high flow phase really can be finished after 10 min, and the fresh gas flow reduced to 0.5 l/min, as denitrogenation and wash-in of nitrous oxide are no longer considerations. Further shortening of the initial phase is unlikely to be possible, especially when isoflurane is used, as the desired end-tidal concentration of 1.2 vol% will not be established in that time and maintained after flow reduction, unless higher initial fresh gas flows were used, thus resulting in increasing waste of the anaesthetic agent.

The limited maximum output of conventional vaporizers outside the circuit is the main obstacle to increasing the amount of agent supplied to the patient. Desflurane and sevoflurane have the advantage that their vaporizers with their higher output allow for a significant increase in vapour delivery into the system, while their low solubility has the further advantage of reducing the amount of agent that needs to be taken up by the patient[31,32].

If the carrier gas does not contain any nitrous oxide, the patient only takes up oxygen and an adequate amount of volatile agent. Thus a higher volume of excess gas is available in nitrous oxide-free minimal flow anaesthesia, resulting in an improved gas filling of the breathing system and hence a significant decrease in the risk of accidental gas volume deficiency. This considerably facilitates the performance of minimal flow anaesthesia in routine clinical practice.

There is absolutely no contraindication to the use of a carrier gas containing only oxygen and nitrogen. The pressure within the cuffs of endotracheal tubes and laryngeal masks does not increase during the course of anaesthesia.

The hypnotic and analgesic effect exerted by 60 vol% of nitrous oxide in clinical practice proved to be remarkably less than generally assumed. Indeed, according to the author's own clinical experiences, an increase of not more than $0.2–0.25 \times$ MAC of the respective anaesthetic agent, together with only small supplemental doses of opioids, was adequate to replace the missing effects of nitrous oxide[6]. The additional consumption of fentanyl over 9 months in 1999 amounted to about 58.7%, and that of alfentanil 24.1%, compared with the same period in 1998.

In the case of strong surgical stimulation, for instance with repeated skin incisions during stripping of varicose veins, spinal motor reflex actions were observed on occasions, especially during the author's team's early experiences with nitrous oxide-free anaesthesia. These motor reactions were not problematic in any way, and were not accompanied by any sympathetic cardiovascular response.

Eger et al.[6] and von Tramer et al.[21] assumed that renouncing the use of nitrous oxide would increase the risk of intra-operative awareness. In the author's own clinical experience of more than 2700 inhalation anaesthetics performed without nitrous oxide, not a single case of intra-operative awareness was reported. Even the generally assumed cardiovascular suppression resulting from the higher concentration of volatile agents could not be verified, agreeing with the similar observations reported by Eger et al.[6]. On the contrary, the performance of inhalation anaesthesia without nitrous oxide proved to be so astonishingly simple and easy, that it became increasingly difficult to still define a convincing indication for the further use of nitrous oxide.

However, some anaesthetic machines, particularly older types, do not meet the technical preconditions to perform low flow anaesthetic techniques without nitrous oxide. The flowmeter tubes for air are not graduated in the low flow range, but only start with a minimum flow of 0.8–1.0 l/min; indeed some are not equipped with any system for the supplying and metering of air.

A highly significant advantage, which could result from the consistent renunciation of nitrous oxide, would be the fact that the technical infrastructure for nitrous oxide supply and the nitrous oxide logistics would become completely dispensable. The nitrous oxide manifold and central gas piping system for a major hospital costs about 7700–15 350 Euros, depending upon its dimension and design, while further equipment, comprising tubes, check valves, pressure regulators and wall outlets, costs about 1300 Euros per operating theatre. Additional costs result from routine technical maintenance and checks of the whole central gas piping system, and from the required regular measurement of workplace contamination by a certified company and also from the purchase and transportation of nitrous oxide. All in all, there is considerable potential for savings.

11.3.2   Non-quantitative closed system anaesthesia in clinical practice

The renunciation of nitrous oxide, resulting in significant improvement of the gas filling of the breathing system in minimal flow anaesthesia, even enables the performance of non-quantitative closed system anaesthesia with conventional anaesthetic machines in routine clinical practice[26]. When the initial high flow phase is finished and the desired gas concentrations established, the admixture of air can be stopped completely and the supply of oxygen into the system can be reduced to a flow equalling the oxygen uptake calculated by applying Brody's formula, i.e. about 250 ml/min in average adults. Thus, the amount of carrier gas delivered into the system meets approximately the respective total gas uptake of the patient, and no further excess gas is discharged. As the oxygen consumption can be assumed to be nearly stable, the oxygen flow can be maintained unchanged during the whole course of anaesthesia, unless increased gas loss due to leaks necessitates the replenishment of the gas volume. If sevoflurane is used, the vaporizer has to be set to 8.0 vol%, and with desflurane to 10 vol%. This will meet the need to maintain the desired expired anaesthetic concentration, even with such low fresh gas flows. With this fresh gas flow, however, the limits of conventional isoflurane vaporizers are exceeded. Even if the maximum output is set, an expired concentration of 1.2 vol% cannot be maintained (Figure 11.3). This requires either prolongation of the initial high flow phase, intermittent use of a higher flow of 0.5 l/min or the supplemental administration of opioids.

Again, it has to be strongly emphasized that the use of sevoflurane with such low fresh gas flows is only acceptable if the soda lime is maintained properly (see Sections 9.1.2.2.4 and 9.1.2.2.8). Potassium-free soda lime should always be used, and if low flow techniques of long duration are performed with this agent, the consistent use of calcium hydroxide lime (Amsorb™) should be mandatory.

Even the expert is likely to be surprised by the ease with which closed system anaesthesia can be realized in daily clinical practice with conventional anaesthetic machines, simply by abandoning the use of nitrous oxide. As, however, Brody's formula only allows rough calculation of the individual oxygen uptake, and the volatile agent, using VOC (vaporizer outside the circuit), can by no means be supplied quantitatively, this technique must be referred to as non-quantitative closed system anaesthesia (see Section 1.2.4).

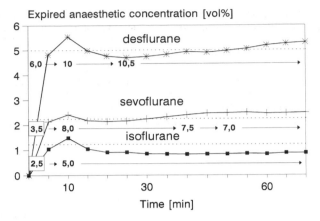

Figure 11.3 Expired anaesthetic agent concentration during performance of non-quantitative closed system anaesthesia with an oxygen–nitrogen mixture as carrier gas, mean values. Details on vaporizer settings given in the figure; broken lines: respective nominal values for expired agent concentration. Samples of patients – isoflurane: $n = 12$, mean body weight 72.6 kg, mean body size 166 cm, mean age 58 years; sevoflurane: $n = 11$, mean body weight 76.7 kg, mean body size 170 cm, mean age 36.4 years; desflurane: $n = 8$, mean body weight 80.4 kg, mean body size 172 cm, mean age 45.9 years. (From Baum et al.[26])

11.4   Economics of low flow anaesthetic techniques without nitrous oxide

If consistent use is made of the rebreathing technique by performing minimal flow anaesthesia, especially being facilitated by the renunciation of nitrous oxide, in a 2-h long anaesthetic the additional costs resulting from increased consumption of the anaesthetic agent amount to 1.50–2.60 Euros, compared with minimal flow anaesthesia using nitrous oxide (Tables 11.1–11.3). Furthermore, a somewhat increased consumption of opioids has to be expected – according to the author's own experiences, this will result in additional costs of 0.13–0.26 Euros per patient.

In 1998 the author's department performed 3640 inhalation anaesthetics. It was possible to precisely calculate the corresponding nitrous oxide consumption as being 320 000 litres gaseous nitrous oxide. As the gas cylinders of the major manifold, for safety reasons, have to be changed although still containing a residue of 20%, the nitrous oxide consumption was calculated to be 384 000 litres. In fact, however, in the year 1998 a total number of 32 gas cylinders containing 600 000 litres were consumed via the central gas piping system! Although one has to keep in mind that all cylinders have to be changed still containing a residue of 20%, about 100 000 litres of gaseous nitrous oxide were missing. This deficit can only be explained by gas loss via leaks from the central gas piping system and its terminal units. Thus, instead of the amount of nitrous oxide really used in anaesthetics equalling 18 gas cylinders, containing 37.5 kg liquefied

Table 11.1   Comparison of costs: high and minimal flow anaesthesia with – versus minimal flow anaesthesia without nitrous oxide, volatile anaesthetic: isoflurane

	1.4 l/min O$_2$ 2.0 l/min N$_2$O exp. Iso: 0.9%	0.3 l/min O$_2$ 0.2 l/min N$_2$O exp. Iso: 0.9%	0.3 l/min O$_2$ 0.2 l/min air exp. Iso: 1.2%
Vaporizer setting base for calculation	60 min: 1.5 vol% 60 min: 1.2 vol%	15 min: 1.5 vol% 105 min: 2.5 vol%	10 min: 2.5 vol% 30 min: 5.0 vol%
Oxygen consumption costs	1.68 l 0.09 Euro	52.5 l 0.03 Euro	43 l 0.02 Euro
N$_2$O or air consumption costs	360 l 2.93 Euro	66.1 l 0.54 Euro	52 l 0.01 Euro
Isoflurane consumption costs	37.3 ml 14.77 Euro	12.1 ml 4.81 Euro	16.4 ml 6.68 Euro
Total costs	17.79 Euro	5.38 Euro	6.71 Euro

Table 11.2   Comparison of costs: high and minimal flow anaesthesia with – versus minimal flow anaesthesia without nitrous oxide, volatile anaesthetic: sevoflurane

	1.4 l/min O$_2$ 3.0 l/min N$_2$O exp. Sev: 1.7%	0.3 l/min O$_2$ 0.2 l/min N$_2$O exp. Sev: 1.7%	0.3 l/min O$_2$ 0.2 l/min air exp. Sev: 2.2%
Vaporizer setting base for calculation	15 min: 2.2 vol% 105 min: 2.0 vol%	15 min: 2.5 vol% 105 min: 3.5 vol%	10 min: 3.5 vol% 110 min: 5.0 vol%
Oxygen consumption costs	1.68 l 0.09 Euro	52.5 l 0.03 Euro	43 l 0.02 Euro
N$_2$O or air consumption costs	360 l 2.93 Euro	66.1 l 0.54 Euro	52 l 0.01 Euro
Sevoflurane consumption costs	59.6 ml 46.43 Euro	19.7 ml 15.30 Euro	23.8 ml 18.49 Euro
Total costs	49.45 Euro	15.87 Euro	18.52 Euro

nitrous oxide each, 32 gas cylinders had to be bought at a purchase price of 4193 Euros. Thus, additional costs of 1.50–2.60 Euros per 2 hours of inhalation anaesthesia resulting from renunciation of nitrous oxide have to compare with 1.15 Euros per 1 hour of anaesthesia (1 hour being the mean duration of the 3640 inhalation anaesthetics in 1998) resulting from

Table 11.3 Comparison of costs: high and minimal flow anaesthesia with – versus minimal flow anaesthesia without nitrous oxide, volatile anaesthetic: desflurane

	1.4 l/min O_2 3.0 l/min N_2O exp. Des: 4.0%	0.3 l/min O_2 0.2 l/min N_2O exp. Des: 4.0%	0.3 l/min O_2 0.2 l/min air exp. Des: 4.0%
Vaporizer setting base for calculation	15 min: 5.0 vol% 105 min: 4.5 vol%	10 min: 5.0 vol% 105 min: 6.0 vol%	10 min: 6.0 vol% 110 min: 8.5 vol%
Oxygen			
consumption	168 l	47 l	43 l
costs	0.09 Euro	0.03 Euro	0.02 Euro
N_2O or air			
consumption	360 l	52 l	52 l
costs	2.93 Euro	0.42 Euro	0.01 Euro
Desflurane			
consumption	120.2 ml	27.9 ml	36.7 ml
costs	43.53 Euro	10.05 Euro	13.21 Euro
Total costs	46.55 Euro	10.50 Euro	13.24 Euro

Gas consumption and costs in high-and minimal flow anaesthetics with, versus without, nitrous oxide. Costs are calculated with the computer program CIA[33]. Actual German prices which were the base for calculation, state September 1999: 0.53 Euro/m^3, N_2O: 8.16 Euro/m^3, air: 0.04 Euro/m^3, isoflurane: 99.13 Euro/250 ml, sevoflurane: 1194.64 Euro/250 ml, desflurane: 86.49 Euro/240 ml. (from Baum *et al.*[26]).

nitrous oxide consumption. When considering these calculations, however, one has to keep in mind that, due to the consistent performance of minimal flow anaesthesia at our department, the nitrous oxide consumption *per se* was already extremely low in 1998. Additional savings, furthermore, will result from the cancellation of technical maintenance of the nitrous oxide gas pipeline system and the required measurement of workplace contamination.

11.5 Are there any specific indications for the use of nitrous oxide?

Concluding this chapter, four reviews on nitrous oxide shall be cited synoptically, as doubts seem to be justified in respect of the question of whether a legitimate indication can be defined for the use of nitrous oxide in modern inhalation anaesthesia. In his conclusions concerning the use of nitrous oxide Schirmer[9] states: 'Generally, nowadays general anaesthesia could be performed satisfactorily, although renouncing the use of nitrous oxide, with the available modern anaesthetics'. The following recommendations for the use of nitrous oxide, however, only list syndromes and surgical interventions in which favourably this gas should *not* be used; a clear indication is, missing. Similarly to James[7], Dale and Husum[5] conclude in their editorial: 'Nitrous oxide should not automatically be included as the basis of any anaesthetic but, like other anaesthetic agents, should be administered after careful consideration of the needs of the individual patient in relation to the planned surgical procedure'. Again this statement is followed by a list of contraindications whereas a clear definition of any indication for this gas is not given. Eger et al.[6], judging the results of their comprehensive clinical investigation, conclude: 'In summary, we found that the addition of N_2O to isoflurane for maintenance of anesthesia only subtly, if at all, altered the course of anesthesia and the development of untoward outcomes. The use of N_2O may have diminished the risk of remembrance and fear during anesthesia. In some patients, its use may have increased the incidence of vomiting and sore throat. Our findings do not indicate that the use of N_2O is dangerous in a typical patient having elective surgery'. Whether this résumé justifies the further use of nitrous oxide remains the question. Brodsky and Cohen[11], however, refer to an editorial in *Lancet* from 1978 entitled 'Nitrous oxide and the bone marrow' which stated 'In fact, N2O would probably not be released if it were a new drug being considered for introduction into clinical practice today'.

Because of the great number of arguments against the use of nitrous oxide, the lack of any justified indication for its use, and clinical experience that inhalation anaesthesia without nitrous oxide can be performed easily, economically and judiciously in respect to ecology, anaesthetists should consistently renounce the further use of this gas.

11.6 References

1. Baum JA. Who introduced the rebreathing system into clinical practice? In Schulte am Esch J. and M. Goerig, eds, *Proceedings of the Fourth International Symposium on the History of Anaesthesia*. Dräger, Lübeck, 1998, pp. 441–450.
2. Duncum B. Nitrous oxide. In Duncum B, *The Development of Inhalation Anaesthesia*. Royal Society of Medicine Press Ltd, London, 1994, pp. 273–310.
3. Smith WDA. Under the influence: a history of nitrous oxide and oxygen anaesthesia. The crucial experiment, its eclipse and its revival. The Wood Library–Museum of Anesthesiology, Park Ridge, IL, 1982, pp. 53–66.
4. Davy H. *Researches, Chemical and Philosophical; Chiefly Concerning Nitrous Oxide, or Dephlogisticated Nitrous Air, and its Respiration*. J. Johnson, London, 1800, p. 556.
5. Dale O and Husum B. Nitrous oxide: from frolics to a global concern in 150 years. *Acta Anaesth Scand* 1994; **38**, 749–750.
6. Eger EI, Lampe GH, Wauk LZ, Whitendale P, Cahalan MK and Donegan JH. Clinical pharmacology of nitrous oxide: an argument for its continued use. *Anesth Analg* 1990; **71**, 575–585.
7. James MFM. Nitrous oxide: still useful in the year 2000? *Curr Opin Anaesthesiol* 1999; **12**, 461–466.
8. Parbrook GD. The levels of nitrous oxide analgesia. *Br J Anaesth* 1967; **39**, 974–982.
9. Schirmer U. Lachgas – Entwicklung und heutiger Stellenwert. *Anaesthesist* 1998; **47**, 245–255.
10. Vic P, Laguette D, Blondin G, Blayo M, Thirion S, Queinnec C, Lew J, Mehu G and Broussine L. Use of 50% oxygen–nitrous oxide mixture in a general pediatric ward. *Archives de Pediatrie* 1999; **6**, 844–848.
11. Brodsky JB and Cohen EN. Adverse effects of nitrous oxide. *Med Toxicol* 1986; **1**, 362–374.
12. Scheinin B, Lindgren L and Scheinin TM. Perioperative nitrous oxide delays bowel function after colonic surgery. *Br J Anaesth* 1990; **64**, 154–158.

13. Watts A, Luney SR, Lee D and Gelb AW. Effect of nitrous oxide on cerebral blood flow velocity after induction of hypocapnia. *J Neurosurg Anaesthesiol* 1998; **10**, 142–145.
14. Eisele JH, Reitan JA, Massumi RA, Zelis RF and Miller RR. Myocardial performance and N_2O analgesia in coronary-artery disease. *Anesthesiology* 1976; **44**, 16–20.
15. Hohner P and Reiz S. Nitrous oxide and the cardiovascular system. *Acta Anaesthesiol Scand* 1994; **38**, 763–766.
16. Stowe DF, Monroe SM, Marijic J, Rooney RT, Bosnjak ZK and Kampine JF. Effects of nitrous oxide on contractile function and metabolism of the isolated heart. *Anesthesiology* 1990; **73**, 1220–1226.
17. Sesso RMCC, Iunes Y and Melo ACP. Myeloneuropathy following nitrous oxide anesthesia in a patient with macrocytic anaemia. *Neuroradiology* 1999; **41**, 588–590.
18. Takàcs J. N_2O-induzierte akute funikuläre Myelose bei latentem Vitamin-B_{12}-Mangel. *Anästhesiol Intensivmed Notfallmed Schmerzther* 1996; **31**, 525–528.
19. Fiege M, Wappler F and Pothmann W. Gefährdung von Patienten mit schwerer chronischer Neutropenie durch Lachgasexposition. *Anästh Intensivmed* 1998; **39**, 347–350.
20. Hartung J. Twenty-four of twenty-seven studies show a greater incidence of emesis associated with nitrous oxide than with alternative anesthetics. *Anesth Analg* 1996; **83**, 114–116.
21. von Tramer M, Moore A and McQuay H. Omitting nitrous oxide in general anaesthesia: meta-analysis of intraoperative awareness and postoperative emesis in randomized controlled trials. *Br J Anaesth* 1996; **76**, 186–193.
22. Marx T, Zwing M, Köble R, Fröba G, Klampp D and Georgieff M. Lachgas als Leitsubstanz zur Beurteilung der Arbeitsplatzbelastung mit Narkosegasen. *Anästhesiol Intensivmed Notfallmed Schmerzther* 1998; **33**, 27–31.
23. Schulte am Esch J. Gefahren der Narkosegasbelastung am Arbeitsplatz. *Anästh Intensivmed* 1998; **35**, 154–161.
24. Logan M and Farmer JG. Anaesthesia and the ozone layer. *Br J Anaesth* 1989; **53**, 645–646.
25. Radke J and Fabian P. Die Ozonschicht und ihre Beeinflussung durch N_2O und Inhalationsanästhetika. *Anaesthesist* 1991; **40**, 429–433.
26. Baum J, Sievert B, Stanke HG, Brauer K and Sachs G. Lachgasfreie Niedrigflußnarkosen. *Anaesthesiol Reanimat*, 2000; **25**, 60–67.
27. Imberti R, Preseglio I, Imbriani M, Ghittori S, Cimino F and Mapelli A. Low flow anaesthesia reduces occupational exposure to inhalation anaesthetics. *Acta Anaesthesiol Scand* 1995; **39**, 586–591.
28. Virtue RW. Low flow anesthesia: advantages in its clinical application, cost and ecology. In Aldrete JA, Lowe HJ and Virtue RW, eds, *Low Flow and Closed System Anesthesia*. Grune & Stratton, New York, 1979, pp. 103–108.
29. Röpcke H and Schwilden H. Interaction of isoflurane and nitrous oxide combinations similar for median electroencephalographic frequency and clinical anesthesia. *Anesthesiology* 1996; **84**, 782–788.
30. Röpcke H. Klinische Pharmakologie von Stickoxidul im Vergleich und im Zusammenwirken mit volatilen Anästhetika. Abstract DAK, 1999.
31. Baum J, Berghoff M Stanke HG, Petermeyer M and Kalff G. Niedrigflußnarkosen mit Desfluran. *Anaesthesist* 1997; **46**, 287–293.
32. Baum J and Stanke HG. Low Flow- und Minimal Flow-Anästhesie mit Sevofluran. *Anaesthesist* 1998; **47** (Suppl. 1), S70–S76.
33. Stanke HG and Baum J. Costs of inhalation anaesthesia (CIA), vers. 3.OE. Computer program for the calculation of costs resulting from anaesthetic gas consumption. Damme, 1999.

Future perspectives

12.1 Future technical developments

Currently available anaesthetic machines of the new generation, being equipped with adequate safety features and perfectly gas-tight compact breathing systems, are especially designed for the utilization of rebreathing by the use of even the lowest fresh gas flows. It may be assumed that in the future electronic flow control and metering systems will replace the conventional combination of fine needle valves, flowmeter tubes and plenum vaporizers, a technique which was realized for the first time in 1910 with Neu's nitrous oxide oxygen anaesthetic apparatus. New technical concepts will enable not only the fresh gas flow independent supply of volatile anaesthetics, but also the metering of anaesthetics by computer-controlled closed-loop feedback according to pre-selected nominal values. Such a technical concept is already realized in one commercially available anaesthetic machine, the PhysioFlex (Dräger Medizintechnik, Lübeck, Germany).

12.2 Environmental protection and occupational health and safety

The growing environmental awareness and increasingly stringent regulations on occupational safety and health make obligatory the judicious use of available anaesthetic equipment to reduce as far as possible the consumption of anaesthetic gases. The discussion on environmental pollution by inhalational anaesthetics will be even more accentuated in so far as, according to the London Protocol of 1990, the production of fully halogenated fluorochlorocarbons (CFCs) should have been stopped completely by the year 2000. This means that the proportion of volatile anaesthetics in the total yearly production and consumption of CFCs will increase, which in turn raises the question of environmental compatibility of uncontrolled and unnecessary emission of anaesthetic gases. Furthermore, the production of the partially halogenated CFCs, to which the inhalation anaesthetics halothane, enflurane and isoflurane belong, also has to cease completely by the year 2030[1]. Hydrocarbons which are exclusively fluorosubstituted, like sevoflurane and desflurane, are not included in these regulations, as they have significantly less ozone-depleting potential. However, they contribute considerably to the greenhouse effect, hence by no means can they be referred to as environmentally friendly. In view of these aspects, it can be expected that the future will bring even more stringent requirements for the most sparing use, and perhaps even recycling, of inhalational anaesthetics[2,3].

12.3   Future inhalational anaesthetics

A common tendency with respect to molecular structure can be observed in the development of new volatile anaesthetics[4]. The integration of halogen atoms ensures non-inflammability. The exclusively fluorosubstituted molecules feature great chemical stability, minimal metabolism and, according to present-day knowledge, a lower potential for ozone-layer destruction. An ether analogue structure of the molecules results in a lower incidence of cardiac dysrhythmias. However, the anaesthetic potency of volatile anaesthetics of such molecular structure tends to be low, they are less soluble in blood and of higher volatility. With high flow anaesthetic techniques, the use of such inhalational anaesthetics will be extremely uneconomical, favouring again the consistent use of low flow anaesthetic techniques.

12.3.1   Xenon*

Along with helium, neon, argon, krypton and radon, xenon is one of the noble gases, that is, it is an element whose outer shell is filled with electrons. While the two lowest molecular weight noble gases, helium and neon, have very small electron shells and no anaesthetic actions, the anaesthetic properties of xenon have been recognized for almost 50 years[5]. With its filled outer electron shell, xenon exists as a monatomic gas under normothermic and normobaric conditions. It is virtually inert and does not form covalent bonds with other elements, except under extreme conditions. The very large electron shell of xenon can be polarized and distorted by nearby molecules, creating an induced dipole. This distortion of the electron orbitals permits xenon to interact with and bind to proteins such as myoglobin[6] as well as to bilayer lipids, particularly in the region of the more polar headgroups[7]. Its oil–gas partition coefficient of 1.9 is the highest of all noble gases. The ability of xenon to interact with cell proteins and cell membrane constituents is presumably responsible for its anaesthetic potency. It has been shown to inhibit the plasma membrane Ca^{2+} pump[8]; an action similar to the volatile anaesthetics and that may be responsible for a rise in neuronal Ca^{2+} concentrations and altered excitability.

Xenon has an extremely low solubility in blood with a blood–gas partition coefficient of 0.115, and during the past decade it has begun to

---

* This paragraph is mainly based on the review article: Lynch C 3rd, Baum J, Tenbrick R, Xenon anaesthesia. *Anesthesiology* 2000; **92**, 865–868.

receive increasing study as an anaesthetic agent with many attractive properties. Based on reports from one of the most recent meetings of the the American Society of Anesthesiologists xenon has been shown to not alter voltage-gated ion channels in the myocardium, nor does it sensitize the myocardium to the dysrhythmogenic effects of epinephrine. Studies in patients and in cardiomyopathic dogs have demonstrated that xenon does not depress the myocardial contractility. Effects on the vasculature remain to be better defined, but xenon has no apparent effects on mesenteric vascular resistance. This apparent lack of effect on cardiovascular tissues may be responsible for its minimal effects on the cardiovascular system, and may make xenon particularly useful in situations where cardiovascular stability needs to be maintained. In addition to cardiovascular stability, a number of features make xenon a nearly ideal anaesthetic gas: rapid induction and emergence, a sufficient analgesic and hypnotic effect in a mixture with 30% oxygen, the absence of metabolism, undisturbed ventilation and pulmonary function and lack of triggering of malignant hyperthermia. With a human MAC value of 0.71[9] the gas is optimally suited to be used as an inhalation anaesthetic in a mixture with 30% oxygen. However, at concentrations greater than 60%, xenon increases the cerebral blood flow[10] and there can be retention of considerable amounts of the gas in the bowels and fatty tissues. Up to this point no data are available concerning the suitability of xenon in patients suffering from increased intracranial pressure or bowel obstruction. Nevertheless, the use of xenon as an anaesthetic agent is promising and it has been submitted for legal medical approval in Europe.

Xenon is the rarest noble gas, present in atmospheric air in a concentration of not more than 0.086 ppm. Thus, the air of a normal living room with a volume of $50 \, m^3$ contains only 4 ml of xenon. While the high molecular weight of xenon (131.2 Da) gives it a density over four times greater than air, xenon is recovered in the process of air liquefaction. After several separation processes, a purity of 99.995% can be obtained. The current annual world production of xenon is about 6 million litres. One million litres of xenon per year are already expended in medical uses, half of this amount being used for anaesthetic purposes. The yearly production is predicted to increase during the next three years to 9.5 million litres. Corresponding to its rarity, xenon is quite expensive. During the last 2 years the price has risen from about 5 US$ to about 10 US$ per litre, and further changes are unpredictable[11].

Due to the fact that xenon is extremely rare and expensive, the use of this gas as an anaesthetic agent can be justified only if its waste is reduced to the absolute minimum. It must be administered via rebreathing systems using the lowest gas flows. Even if xenon were administered with a minimal flow technique, using a fresh gas flow as low as 0.5 l/min or even lower during a 2-h anaesthetic procedure, the efficiency would not even reach 20%. That is, less than 20% of the xenon delivered into the breathing system would actually be taken up by the patient, leaving over 80% (about 34 litres) to be spilled out into the atmosphere as waste[12]. Closed system anaesthesia is the only economically acceptable technique for application of xenon for anaesthetic purposes and this is possible at present only by an electronically controlled anaesthesia delivery system, which monitors and controls the addition of gases to the circuit. The gas concentrations inside the breathing circuit are measured continuously (xenon concentration by thermal conductivity) and, with the aid of closed loop feedback control, xenon and oxygen are delivered into the system only in those amounts needed to keep the gas concentrations and the circulating gas volume constant[13]. Due to its high density, the presence of xenon may degrade the accuracy of certain respiratory flowmeters[14].

For practical clinical use, nitrogen must first be washed out upon induction by applying high flow pure oxygen over a period of at least 5 min, typically accompanied by administration of a combination such as fentanyl (3 µg/kg), propofol (2 mg/kg), and a muscle relaxant. After endotracheal intubation, the patient is connected to the ventilator of an appropriate anaesthetic delivery system. The desired xenon concentration of 65–70% is established with a high fresh gas flow of 5 l/min in a short initial period of about 2.5 min. A small supplementary dose of fentanyl may be given just before skin incision. Based on clinical experience to date, the uptake of xenon during the initial 15 min is about 1 litre xenon per 10 kg body weight. In the first hour xenon consumption amounts to 12–14 litres, and in each following hour about 4 litres of xenon have to be supplied into the system[15,16]. Luttropp gives somewhat lower figures: if xenon is administered via a closed rebreathing system after complete denitrogenation, 60–70% inspired xenon results in about 6 litres being taken up in the first hour in an average adult, with 9–15 litres being consumed over the first 2 h of the xenon administration[17]. Wash-out of the drug follows a similar time course. Because xenon is substantially less soluble than nitrous oxide, its equilibration and wash-out causes less diffusion hypoxia[18]. In addition, because of its low solubility it may also permit a faster emergence than with nitrous oxide[19].

If the total yearly production of about 6 million litres of xenon were available exclusively for anaesthetic purposes, no more than 400 000 anaesthetic procedures could be performed with this amount of gas. Recycling of the xenon contained in the gas escaping via the exhaust port rather than wasting it into the atmosphere is the one and only way to guarantee the availability of a sufficient amount of xenon for routine use as an anaesthetic gas in clinical practice. With currently available prototypes of recycling devices (Figure 12.1), about 70–90% of the xenon delivered into the system can be recovered, with a purity of about 90%. Oxygen and nitrogen make up the bulk of the impurities[20,21].

Due to its considerable expense and the fact that it cannot be synthesized, but rather must be extracted from the atmosphere, it is most unlikely that xenon will gain widespread use. However, should delivery systems (totally closed circuit) become available along with appropriate techniques for recycling the gas, xenon anaesthesia may become more readily available. It may be a highly useful alternative in very specially indicated patients, for instance those with limited cardiovascular reserve, or in plastic surgery if really rapid emergence is needed. Without any doubt, due its extremely limited availability, xenon can hardly ever become a generally used inhalation anaesthetic. The next few years,

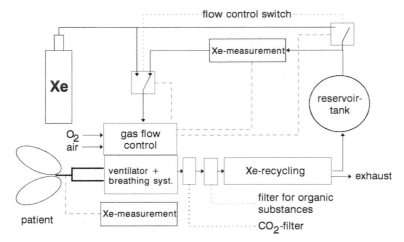

Figure 12.1 Technical concept of the combination of an anaesthetic machine with a device for recycling of xenon (with permission of R. Dittmann, Dräger Medizintechnik, Lübeck, Germany)

however, should reveal better definition of its pharmacological characteristics at the cellular level, as well as its effects in clinical trials.

12.3.2 Oxygen as carrier gas

Probably in the next years, due to the strong tendency to no longer routinely use nitrous oxide as a carrier gas, its consumption will decrease considerably, and after 150 years its use as an anaesthetic gas may even come to an end. Alternatively an oxygen–nitrogen (oxygen–air) mixture seems to be the carrier gas of choice, enabling the anaesthetist to freely choose an inspired oxygen concentration meeting the individual needs of the respective patient. Recently, a scientific discussion was launched on whether it would not be advantageous to apply nearly pure oxygen during anaesthetics. Significant reduction of wound infections[22] and of postoperative nausea and vomiting[23] are the arguments in favour for this alternative. Sessler and co-workers succeeded in demonstrating that pulmonary function was not impaired after 4 h of administering 80% inspired oxygen[24]. It seems generally accepted, in spite of its acknowledged possibly harmful effects, that the use of 100% oxygen over a period of 12 h is acceptable, as it will not significantly impair pulmonary function[25-27]. It remains a matter of discussion whether the application of a distinct inspired oxygen concentration of 80% is significantly less harmful than a somewhat higher concentration, as it is stressed by Sessler and co-workers[24].

To only use oxygen obviously would be another step towards facilitating the performance of low flow anaesthesia without nitrous oxide. Only the oxygen flow would have to be set at the controls of the gas flow control system. Furthermore, this would increase patient safety in respect of the possibility of development of hypoxic gas mixtures and hypoxaemia.

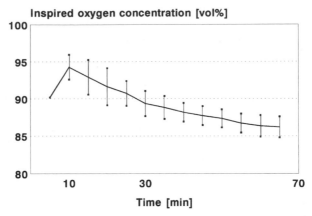

Figure 12.2 Inspired oxygen concentration (mean values and standard deviation) during clinical performance of non-quantitative closed system anaesthesia using pure oxygen as carrier gas

Nevertheless, patients suffering from chronic obstructive lung disease, prematurely born infants and pregnant women, for instance, should perhaps preferably not be exposed to pure oxygen.

During performance of non-quantitative closed system anaesthesia (see Section 11.3.2) in the initial 10 min, the oxygen flow can be set to 4.0 l/min and then reduced to the oxygen uptake of the patient, about 250–300 ml/ min in adults. Due to delayed wash-out of nitrogen from the tissues of the patient, after flow reduction the inspired oxygen concentration will slowly decrease to 90–85 vol% during the following 60 min (Figure 12.2). In this way the author has routinely performed inhalation anaesthetics for 6 months, and to date in not a single case were any harmful effects observed. However, until the developing scientific discussion on this topic comes to an acknowledged conclusion, the author cannot recommend this technique for general use in clinical practice.

Another aspect of using pure or nearly pure oxygen, however, shall be mentioned in connection to these considerations: if a sufficient supply with carbon dioxide absorbents could be guaranteed, low flow techniques then could be performed even under the most unfavourable conditions. Imagine oxygen supply by the aid of an oxygen concentrator and the availability of a syringe pump delivering a sufficient amount of anaesthetic agent into the breathing system independently of the fresh gas flow rate. Without further logistical requirements, only electric current would be needed to operate a suitable anaesthetic machine fitted with an electrically driven ventilator and an emergency air inlet valve allowing air to entrain the system in case of gas volume deficiency.

12.4   Improvements in patient care

Low flow anaesthesia results in a distinct improvement of the anaesthetic gas climate. This protects the function and the morphological integrity of the respiratory epithelium and reduces humidity and heat losses. The effect can be achieved simply by judicious use of available anaesthesia machines equipped with a rebreathing system. Although humidification is increased significantly by flow reduction alone, the loss of heat at the hosing with the corresponding decrease of inspired gas temperature remains a matter of concern. The use of heated hoses will solve the problem[28], thus making dispensable the additional use of heat and moisture exchangers, which, being disposable items, merely increase the problem of waste and expense.

Continuous measurement of oxygen uptake in quantitative closed system anaesthesia may pave the way for new dimensions in patient monitoring, permitting the early detection of subtle changes in haemodynamics and metabolism. The precise physiological data that can be obtained in quantitative closed system anaesthesia may in the future enable the exact measurement of the carbon dioxide production and the respiratory quotient. The control of artificial ventilation according to a pre-set nominal value of expired carbon dioxide concentration, or even continuous monitoring of the cardiac output, may be possible.

12.5 Conclusions

All the arguments put forward speak in favour of a judicious use of rebreathing systems by consistent reduction of the fresh gas flow. Technically advanced anaesthetic machines featuring appropriate safety facilities including the required monitoring are already available. Further development will facilitate quantitative closed system anaesthesia in routine clinical practice. Anaesthetists should not close their eyes to this development, but rather should study the theoretical background and practical management of low flow anaesthetic techniques to the benefit of their patients and the environment[29].

12.6 References

1. Marx Th. Umwelt- und Arbeitsplatzbelastung durch Anästhesie. *Anästhesiol Intensivmed Notfallmed Schmerzth* 1997; **32**, 44–46.
2. Marx Th, Gross-Alltag F, Ermisch J, Hähnel J, Weber L and Friesdorf W. Experimentelle Untersuchungen zur Rückgewinnung von Narkosegasen. *Anaesthesist* 1992; **41**, 99–102.
3. Waterson CK. Recovery of waste anaesthetic gases. In Brown Jr BR, Calkins JM and Saunders RJ, eds, *Future Anaesthesia Delivery Systems. Contemporary Anaesthesia Practice*. F. A. Davies, Philadelphia, 1984, pp. 109–124.
4. Weiskopf RB. Inhalation anaesthetics today and tomorrow. In Torri G and Damia G, eds, *Update on Modern Inhalation Anaesthetics*. Worldwide Medical Communications, New York, 1989, pp. 23–28.
5. Cullen SC and Gross EG. The anaesthetic properties of xenon in animals and human beings, with additional observations on krypton. *Science* 1951; **113**, 580–582.
6. Trudell JR, Koblin DD and Eger IE, II. A molecular description of how noble gases and nitrogen bind to a model site of anaesthetic action. *Anesth Analg* 1998; **87**, 411–418.

7. Xu Y, Tang P. Amphiphilic sites for general anaesthetic action? Evidence from 129Xe-[1H] intermolecular nuclear Overhauser effects. *Biochim Biophys Acta* 1997; **1323**, 154–162.

8. Franks JJ, Horn J-L, Janicki PK and Singh G. Halothane, isoflurane, xenon and nitrous oxide inhibit calcium ATPase pump activity in rat brain synaptic plasma membranes. *Anesthesiology* 1995; **82**, 108–117.

9. Cullen SC, Eger EI, II, Cullen BF and Gregory P. Observations on the anaesthetic effect of the combination of xenon and halothane. *Anesthesiology* 1969; **31**, 305–309.

10. Luttropp HH, Romner B, Perhag L, Eskilsson J, Fredriksen S and Werner O. Left ventricular performance and cerebral haemodynamics during xenon anaesthesia. A transesophageal echocardiography and transcranial Doppler sonography study. *Anaesthesia* 1993; **48**, 1045–1049.

11. Garrett ME. The production and availability of xenon. Abstract book of the Annual Meeting of the Association for Low Flow Anaesthesia. Gent, 18–19 September 1998.

12. Baum J. Niedrigflußnarkosen mit Xenon. *Anästhesiol Intensivmed Notfallmed Schmerzther* 1997; **32**, 51–54.

13. Teeling MThA. Xenon – technical solutions to administer xenon. Abstract book of the Annual Meeting of the Association for Low Flow Anaesthesia. Gent, 18–19 September 1998.

14. Goto T, Saito H, Nakata Y, Uezono S, Ichinose F, Uchiyama M and Morita S. Effects of xenon on performance of various respiratory flowmeters. *Anesthesiology* 1999; **90**, 555–563.

15. Tenbrinck R, Leendertse K and Erdmann W. Xenon in the Physioflex: the first clinical experience. Abstract book of the Annual Meeting of the Association for Low Flow Anaesthesia. Gent, 18–19 September 1998.

16. Marx T, Georgieff M and Fröba G. Xenon application. Abstract book of the Annual Meeting of the Association for Low Flow Anaesthesia. Gent, 18–19 September 1998.

17. Luttropp HH, Thomasson S, Dahm S, Persson J and Werner O. Clinical experience with minimal xenon anaesthesia. *Acta Anaesthesiol Scand* 1994; **38**, 121–125.

18. Calzia E, Stahl W, Handschuh T, Marx T, Fröba G, Georgieff M and Radermacher P. Continuous arterial PO_2 and PCO_2 measurements during nitrous oxide and xenon elimination: prevention of diffusion hypoxia. *Anesthesiology* 1999; **90**, 829–834.

19. Lachmann B, Armbruster S, Schairer W, Landstra M, Trouwborst A, van Daal G-J, Kusuma A and Erdmann W. Safety and efficacy of xenon in routine use as an inhalational anaesthetic. *Lancet* 1990; **335**, 1413–1415.

20. Bäder S and Brand T: Rückgewinnung volatiler und gasförmiger Anästhetika. *Anästhesiol Intensivmed Notfallmed Schmerzther* 1997; **32**, 46–48.

21. Boso LR. Recycling technique. In F. Giunta, ed., *Abstract book: Expert Meeting on Xenon Anaesthesia*, Pacini Editore, Pisa, 1997, 77.

22. Greif R, Akca O, Horn EP, Kurz A and Sessler DI. Supplemental perioperative oxygen to reduce the incidence of surgical wound infections. *N Engl J Med* 2000; **342**, 161–167.

23. Greif R, Laciny S, Rapf B, Hickle RS and Sessler DI. Supplemental perioperative oxygen reduces the incidence of postoperative nausea and vomiting. *Anesthesiology* 1999; **91**, 1246–1252.

24. Akca O, Podolsky A, Eisenhuber E, Panzer O, Hetz H, Lampl K, Lackner FX, Wittmann K, Grabenwoeger F, Kurz A, Schultz AM, Negishi C and Sessler DI. Comparable postoperative pulmonary at electasis in patients given 30% or 80% oxygen during and 2 hours after colon resection. *Anesthesiology* 1999; **91**, 991–998.

25. Benumof JL. Hyperoxia (oxygen toxicity). In Miller RD, ed., *Anaesthesia*, 5th edn. Churchill Livingstone, Philadelphia, 2000; pp. 612–613.
26. Capellier G, Maupoil V, Boussat S, Laurent E and Neidhart A. Oxygen toxicity and tolerance. *Minerva Anesthesiol* 1999; **65**, 388–392.
27. Kleen M and Messmer K. Toxicity of high PaO$_2$. *Minerva Anesthesiol* 1999; **65**, 393–396.
28. Baum J, Züchner K, Hölscher U, Sievert B, Stanke HG, Gruchmann T and Rathgeber J. Klimatisierung von Narkosegasen bei Einsatz unterschiedlicher Patientenschlauchsysteme. *Anaesthesist* 2000; **49**, 402–411.
29. Baum J. Sind 'Niedriger Fluß' und 'Geschlossenes System' die Techniken der Zukunft? In Laubenthal H, Puchstein Ch, Sirtl C, eds, *Inhalationsanästhesie – eine Standortbestimmung*. Wissenschaftliche Verlagsabteilung Abbott, Wiesbaden, 1991, pp. 30–43.

Index

Access anaesthetic machine,
  technical characteristics of, 168
  technical details of, 147
Acetone, accumulation of, 197
Acidosis, influence on oxygen
  consumption, 38
Aestiva 3000,
  technical characteristics of, 168
  technical details of, 141
AFYA anaesthesia machine, 20
Age, influence on oxygen consumption,
  39
Air-Shields ventilator, 133
Airway pressure, accidental increase of,
  193
Alcoholism as a contraindication for
  low flow anaesthesia, 213
Ambu–Paedi system, 3
Anaesthetic gases,
  pharmacokinetics of, 38–52
  see also individual gases by name
Argon, accumulation of, 203
AS/3 ADU, technical characteristics
  of, 168
AS/3 ADU Plus Anaesthesia Delivery
  Unit, technical requirements
  of, 142, 145
Aspiration, protection against by
  laryngeal mask, 256
Ayre's T-piece, 3, 4
development of, 21
recommended fresh gas flows for, 6

Bacteria, growth of within equipment
  and use of low flow rates,
  222–225
Bag-in-bottle ventilators, technical
  details of, 134
Bain system, 3, 4
  development of, 21

recommended fresh gas flows for, 6
Barium lime, use in carbon dioxide
  absorption, 9
Bellows-in-box ventilators and floating
  bellows, technical details of,
  133
Boyle–Davis gag, 3
Breathing systems,
  advantages of, 15–16
  carbon dioxide absorption methods,
    126–128
  Cicero anaesthetic workstation, 138
  classification of, 1
    by functional criteria, 11–12
    by technical aspects, 12–14
  compact, 136, 137
  control of anaesthesia in, 75
  disadvantages of, 15–16
  fresh gas flow rates in, 14
  fresh gas utilization by, 125, 126
  function of, 1
  gas tightness of, 123–125
    leakage tolerances, 123
  historical aspects of development, 18
  hybrid, 10
  inertia of system and fresh gas flow
    rate, 80
  monitoring of volatile anaesthetics in
    cf. in fresh gas flow, 180
  non-rebreathing systems,
    flow-controlled, 2–7
    valve-controlled, 7
  specified range of operation for, 125
  technical aspects, 1–16
  technical details, system volumes,
    161
  technical details of, 123, 123,
    141–162
  utilization period, 126
    use of absorbers in tandem
      arrangement, 127

292　Index

Breathing systems (*cont.*)
  ventilators in, 128
  with ventilators, 133–135
  without anaesthetic gas reservoir, 2
  without gas reservoir, classification
      of, 14
  without ventilators, 128–132

Calcium hydroxide lime, cf. soda lime,
      96
Carbon dioxide,
  accumulation of, risk of with
      reduced fresh gas flow, 193
  effect of minute volume on partial
      pressure of, 139
  evaluation of production, 21
  monitoring of, 183–187
    artefacts in capnogram, 183–185
    implications for anaesthetic
        practice, 187
    soda lime exhaustion and, 186
Carbon dioxide absorption,
  capacity of absorbents, 94, 95
  consumption of absorbents in low
      flow anaesthesia, 94
  costs of absorbents, 96
  early absorbers used, 25, 26
  implications for anaesthetic practice,
      127
  indicator dyes used in absorbers, 10
  soda lime exhaustion simulation, 186
  technical requirements on absorbers,
      126
  types of absorber used, 9–10
  use of absorbers in tandem arrange-
      ment in closed system, 127
  utilization time for absorbents, 96,
      126
Carbon monoxide accumulation,
      198–203
Cardiac output, effect on gas uptake,
      80
Cato workstation,
  technical characteristics of, 168
  technical details of, 143, 145
  Children, paediatric anaesthesia,
      259–263
Chloroform, 18
  Simpson's technique for application
      of, 19
Chronic obstructive lung disease as a
      problem in anaesthesia, 130
Cicero EM workstation,
  technical characteristics of, 168

technical details of, 143, 146
Circle absorption systems, 3
  development of semi-closed, 32
  leakage tolerances for, 123
  of Sword, 31
  types of, 8
Classification of breathing systems,
  by functional criteria, 11–12
  by technical aspects, 12–14
Cleaning,
  of equipment in clinical practice, 220
  reduced fresh gas flow and possible
      increased bacterial contami-
      nation of equipment, 222
Closed breathing systems, classification
      of, 11
Closed circle system, Jackson's circle
      absorption system, 25
Closed system anaesthesia,
  characteristics of, 61
  definition, 56
  denitrogenation in, 62
  gas concentrations during, 69
  implications for use of, 166
  in clinical practice, 220–264
  leakage tolerances for, 124
  non-quantitative, 68–70
    cf. quantitative, 56
  problems with, 63
  procedure for performance of, 62
  quantitative, 70
  technical requirements for, 67, 115
  transition to, problems of early, 62
  use of vaporizers in, 64
  without nitrous oxide, 275
Coleman's economising apparatus, 24
Computer simulation programs,
  clinical relevance of, 74
  Gas Man, 73
  NARKUP, 73
  of induction phase, 75
Condensation within hosing, 249
Contraindications,
  for low flow anaesthesia,
    absolute, 214
    relative, 213
Control of anaesthesia, 73–87
  as a function of fresh gas flow, 85
  climatization of breathing gases, 100
  Conway's formula, 86
  emergence phase, 84
  environmental pollution with gases,
      98–100
  humidity of breathing gas during,
      103–105

improved gas climate, 100–107
induction phase, 75
maintenance of anaesthesia,
    adapting fresh gas flow to
    uptake, 79
process of, 75
rules for, 86
simulation programs, 73
    clinical relevance of, 74
technical requirements for, 111–169
temperature of breathing gas during,
    101–103
with desflurane, 86
with sevoflurane, 86
Conway's formula, 86
Costs,
    annual consumption of volatile
        anaesthetics, 90
    assumption of reduced costs in low
        flow cf. high flow anaesthesia,
        89
    desflurane, 250
    economy and efficiency of low flow
        anaesthesia, 250–251
    of 120-min anaesthetic, 90
    of anaesthetic gases as a function of
        fresh gas flow, 92
    of low flow anaesthesia without
        nitrous oxide, 276–278
    rebreathing cf. non-rebreathing
        systems, 92
    reduction of in low flow anaesthesia,
        cf. increase in soda lime con-
        sumption, 94–96
        through reduced anaesthetic gas
            use, 89–94
        savings as a function of flow
            reduction, 91
        savings as a function of procedure
            duration, 91
    sevoflurane, 251
Crystal oscillometry, effects of
    humidity on, 179
Cyclopropane, role in development of
    closed systems, 32

Datex multi-gas analysers, 176
Day-case surgery, 263
Denitrogenation, in closed system
    anaesthesia, 62
Depth of anaesthesia, judgement of, 76
Desflurane,
    economy and efficiency of, 250

expired concentrations in minimal
    flow anaesthesia without
    nitrous oxide, 273
in clinical practice, 241–245
induction phase levels, 78
uptake of, 50
uptake pharmacokinetics of, 93
use in paediatric anaesthesia, 262
vaporizers for, 120
Diabetes, as a contraindication for low
    flow anaesthesia, 213
Dieffenbach's modification of Morton
    Ether Inhalator, 19
Dogma anaesthetic machine,
    technical characteristics of, 168
    technical details of, 147
Dräger circle absorber system, 29
Dräger gas mixer, 115
Dräger gas monitors, 177
Dräger Lachgas-Narkose apparatus
    model A, 30
Dräger Narcylen apparatus, 28

EAS 9010,
    technical characteristics of, 168
    technical details of, 149
Econometer, 147
Efficiency,
    cost–benefit ratio, 93
    of flow-controlled non-rebreathing
        systems, 7
    of low flow anaesthesia, 250–251
    role in cost reduction, 93
ELSA,
    technical characteristics of, 168
    technical details of, 149
Emergence phase, 84
    in clinical practice, 239–241
    in minimal flow anaesthesia, 255
Enflurane,
    atmospheric pollution with, 99
    metering of during low flow
        anaesthesia, 235
    time-course of uptake, 49
    use in paediatric anaesthesia, 262
    vaporizers for, 120
    workplace concentration limits of,
        97
Environmental pollution,
    atmospheric, 98–100
    protection in the future, 281
    workplace exposure to anaesthetic
        gases, 96–98

Equipment,
  bacterial contamination of, 222
  causes of incidents with, 212
  for carbon dioxide concentration
      monitoring, 183–187
  for gas blending, 115
  for nitrous oxide concentration
      monitoring, 182–183
  for oxygen concentration
      monitoring, 178–179
  for volatile anaesthetic concentration
      monitoring, 179–182
  future developments, 281
  gags, 258
  gas flow control systems, 112
  gas supply systems, 111
  laryngeal mask, 251–259
  mainstream gas analysers, 174–177
  maintenance of, 113, 220–225
    importance of when using low
        fresh gas flows, 207
  multi-gas analysers, 187–188
  safety features required in, 211
  side-stream gas analysers, 174–177
  technical regulations for safety of
      inhalational anaesthesia
      machines, 174
  technical requirements for in reduced
      fresh gas flow, 111
  Ulmer-Kreissystem circle absorption
      system for use in paediatric
      anaesthesia, 260
Ethanol, accumulation of, 198
Ether, first use, 18
Excel SE,
  technical characteristics of, 168
  technical details of, 155
Excess gases,
  dangers of discharge, 33
  role of cyclopropane in reduction of,
      32
Exhaled gases,
  elimination of in flow-controlled
      non-rebreathing systems, 5
  evaluation of carbon dioxide bpro-
      duction, 21
  factors governing washout of, 6
  fresh gas flow and proportion of gas
      reaching absorber, 55
  techniques for discharge of, 4

Fabius anaesthetic machine, 136, 137
  technical characteristics of, 168
  technical details of, 151

Flow-controlled non-rebreathing
      systems,
  classification of by technical aspects,
      13
  development of, 20
  fresh gas flow rates in, 14
Flowmeter tubes,
  calibration of, 115
  importance of accuracy in, 113
  in minimal flow anaesthesia, 112
  inaccuracies in, 112
  special low flow tubes, 114
Foreign gases,
  accumulation of, 196–207
    acetone, 197
    argon, 203
    carbon monoxide, 198–203
    ethanol, 198
    haloalkenes, 204
    hydrogen, 204
    implications, 206
    methane, 203
    nitrogen, 196
  monitoring of, 176–177
Fresh gas decoupling valve, technical
      details of, 139
Fresh gas flow,
  adaptation of to uptake in mainte-
      nance of anaesthesia, 79
  airway pressure and ventilation and,
      130
  calculation of, 138
  changes in halothane concentration
      and, 34
  compensation techniques, technical
      details of, 135
  cost of gases as a function of, 92
  decoupling valves, 134
  definition of anaesthetic technique
      by rate of, 55, 56
  discontinuous and ventilator
      performance, 141
  effect of changes in on isoflurane
      levels, 76, 77, 78
  effect on nitrous oxide concentration
      in inspired gas, 42
  effect on oxygen concentration of
      inspired gas in rebreathing
      systems, 40, 41
  effect on vaporizer, 120
  effect on vaporizers in closed system
      anaesthesia, 64, 65
  electronic control of, 140
  excess gas discharge and, 32

function of breathing systems in
relation to, 14
gas tightness for, 123
importance of equipment
maintenance when using low
rates of, 207
importance of monitoring of oxygen
concentration when using low
rates of, 179
improvement of breathing gas
climatization by reduction of,
105
in different breathing systems, 14
in ventilators, 132
inertia of system and rate of, 80
management of anaesthesia as a
function of, 85
methods using reduced, 54–70
rate-specific artefacts in capnograms,
183–185
recommended rates for
flow-controlled non-
rebreathing systems, 6
reduction of, in minimal flow
anaesthesia, 254
relationship with minute volume, 54
risks specific to reduced rate of,
accidental airway pressure
increase, 193
accidental anaesthetic overdose,
194
carbon dioxide accumulation, 193
hypoventilation, 192
hypoxia, 191
role in cost reduction and efficiency,
93
role in function of rebreathing cf.
non-rebreathing systems, 16
safety of changing from low to high
rates, 180
technical requirements of equipment
for use with reduced, 111
use of excessive, 32, 34
use of fresh gas in, 125
Future developments, 281–287

Gags, 258
Gambro–Engstrom anaesthetic
delivery system, 118, 119
Gas analysers,
mainstream, 174–177
multi-, 187–188
side-stream, 174–177
Gas blending, equipment for, 115

Gas flow control systems, 112–116
technical requirements for, 112
Gas Man, 73
Gas reservoir,
anaesthetic machines with, 133–135
anaesthetic machines without,
128–133
Gas supply systems, 111
technical requirements for, 111
gas tightness of breathing systems,
123–125
leakage tolerances for, 123
points predisposed to leaks, 124
testing for, 221
gas volume deficiency,
during low flow anaesthesia, 247–249
during minimal flow anaesthesia, 255
Goldman vaporizer, 121
greenhouse effect, 98–100

Hale's closed rebreathing system, 23
Haloalkenes, accumulation of, 204–206
Halothane,
actual values cf. Lowe uptake model,
49
atmospheric pollution with, 99
changes in concentration with
changed fresh gas flows,
cumulative dose calculation
for, 48
metering of during low flow
anaesthesia, 235–238
role in development of closed
systems, 32
use in paediatric anaesthesia, 262
vaporizers for, 120
workplace concentration limits of,
97
Historical aspects of development of
breathing systems, 18
Hose systems,
for control of breathing gas
humidity during anaesthesia,
103–105
for control of breathing gas
temperature during anaesthesia, 101–103
Humidity,
effects on monitoring of volatile
anaesthetic concentrations by
crystal oscillometry, 179
of breathing gas during anaesthesia,
103–105

Humidity (*cont.*)
  range for gas climate during
    anaesthesia, 100
  reduced fresh gas flow and possible
    increased bacterial contami-
    nation of equipment, 222
  see also condensation
Humphrey ADE system,
  function of, 7
  recommended fresh gas flows for, 6
Hybrid breathing systems, 10
Hydrogen, accumulation of, 204
Hyperthermia (malignant) as a
    contraindication of low flow
    anaesthesia, 214
Hypoventilation, risk of with reduced
    fresh gas flow, 192
Hypoxaemia, prevention of, 40
Hypoxia,
  risk of with reduced fresh gas flow,
    191
  unsuitability of some equipment for
    prevention of, 113

Induction phase,
  control of anaesthesia during, 75
  desflurane levels in, 78
  in low flow anaesthesia, 225
  in minimal flow anaesthesia without
    nitrous oxide, 272
  isoflurane levels in, 76, 77
  sevoflurane levels in, 78
Infrared absorption, use in monitoring
    of volatile anaesthetic
    concentration, 179
Initial phase in minimal flow
    anaesthesia, 254
Isoflurane,
  atmospheric pollution with, 99
  concentration as a function of
    uptake, 81
  effect of vaporizer on concentration
    in closed system anaesthesia,
    66–67
  expired concentrations in minimal
    flow anaesthesia without
    nitrous oxide, 273
  induction phase levels, 76
  levels during closed system
    anaesthesia, 69
  levels during emergence phase, 85
  metering of during low flow anaes-
    thesia, 231–235
  setting alarm limits with, 181

uptake of, 50
use in paediatric anaesthesia, 262
vaporizers for, 120
workplace concentration limits of,
    97

Jackson Rees system, 3, 5
  recommended fresh gas flows for, 6
Jackson's circle absorption system, 25
Jackson's rebreathing circle system, 8
Jackson's to-and-fro absorption
    system, 26
Julian anaesthetic machine, 115
  technical characteristics of, 168
  technical details of, 151

Komesaroff vaporizer, 64, 121
Kuhn system, 3, 5
  development of, 21

Lack system, 2, 3
  development of, 21
  recommended fresh gas flows for, 6
Laryngeal mask, 251–259
Leaks, *see* gas tightness Lin uptake
    model, 48
Litigation,
  costs of absorbents and, 96
  role in choice of depth of
    anaesthesia, 33
Low flow anaesthesia,
  accumulation of foreign gases
    during, 196–205
  advantages of, 59
  annual consumption of volatile
    anaesthetics in, 90
  causes of incidents in, 212
  change from high to low flow, 226
  characteristics of, 57, 58
  choice of vaporizers for, 117
  consumption in 120-min anaesthetic,
    90
  contraindications for,
    absolute, 214
    relative, 213
  control of anaesthetics during, 238
  cost reduction as a function of flow
    reduction, 91
  definition, 55
  detection of soda lime exhaustion in,
    186–188
  economy and efficiency of, 250–251
  emergence phase, 239–241
  gas composition in, 227–239

gas volume deficiency during,
    247–249
implications for use of, 167
in clinical practice, 220–264
in day-case surgery, 263
induction techniques in, 225
initial phase of, 225
inspired oxygen concentration
    during, 227–231
length of time constant in as a safety
    factor, 208
metering of anaesthetics during,
    231–238
monitoring of oxygen concentration
    during, 178
nitrous oxide flow calculation in, 58
oxygen concentration changes in, 58
oxygen flow calculation in, 58
pre-medication techniques in, 225
procedure for performance of, 59
reduced costs in, 89
reduction of gas consumption in cf.
    high flow, 88
return of sampling gas to system in
    side-stream gas analysers, 176
safety aspects of, 191–214
special low flow tubes for use with,
    114
training in, 212
use in children, 259–263
use of desflurane in, 241–245
use of laryngeal mask during,
    251–259
use of sevoflurane in, 241, 245–247
water condensation within hosing
    during, 249
without nitrous oxide, 269–279
    clinical practice of, 272
    contraindications, 278
    costs of, 277
    economics of, 276
    reasons for its use, 269
    specific considerations in, 271
workplace exposure to anaesthetic
    gases and, 98
zero calibration in, 186–188
Lowe uptake model, 46

Magill system, 2, 3
    development of, 21
    recommended fresh gas flows for, 6
Mainstream gas analyser,
    cf. side-stream, 174–176
    zero calibration of, 185

Maintenance,
    cleaning, 220
        effects of reduced fresh gas flow
            on need for, 222
    importance of, 34
        when using low fresh gas flows,
            207
    of equipment, 113
        in clinical practice, 220–225
    testing for leaks, 221, 222
Mapleson non-rebreathing systems, 2,
    3
Mapleson systems, recommended fresh
    gas flows for, 6
Megamed 700,
    technical characteristics of, 168
    technical details of, 153, 154
Mentell's hybrid breathing system, 10
Methane, accumulation of, 203
Minimal flow anaesthesia,
    accumulation of foreign gases
        during, 177
    change from high to low flow, 226
    characteristics of, 57, 60
    choice of vaporizers for, 117
    definition, 55
    gas tightness for, 123
    implications for use of, 166
    in clinical practice, 220–264
    isoflurane concentration in cf. high
        flow, 81
    monitoring of nitrous oxide
        concentration during, 183
    oxygen consumption calculation in,
        60
    procedure for performance of, 60
    standardized procedure for, 254–255
    time constants cf. high flow, 82
    without nitrous oxide, 272–275
    workplace exposure to anaesthetic
        gases and, 98
Mivolan,
    technical characteristics of, 168
    technical details of, 153
Modulus SE,
    technical characteristics of, 168
    technical details of, 155
Monitoring, 174–188
    accumulation of foreign gases during
        minimal flow anaesthesia, 177
    artefacts in capnogram, 183–185
    importance of a second device for
        safety, 180
    in fresh gas cf. breathing system, 180
    in minimal flow anaesthesia, 254

Monitoring (*cont.*)
  mainstream gas analysers, 174–177
  multi-gas analysers, 187–188
  of anaesthetic gases,
      enflurane, 235
      halothane, 235–238
      isoflurane, 231–235
  of carbon dioxide concentration,
      183–187
  of equipment function, 175
  of nitrogen concentration, 176
  of nitrous oxide concentration,
      182–183
  of oxygen concentration, 176,
      178–179
  of physiological parameters, 175
  of volatile anaesthetic concentration,
      179–182
  positioning of sensors for gas
      concentration measurements,
      175
  return of sampling gas to closed
      systems to maintain volume,
      176
  setting alarm limits with isoflurane
      and position of monitoring
      system, 181
  side-stream gas analysers, 174–177
  technical regulations for safety of
      inhalational anaesthesia
      machines and, 174
Morton Ether Inhalator, 19
Multi-gas analysers, 187–188

Narcylen, first use of, 27
Narkomat,
  technical characteristics of, 168
  technical details of, 147
Narkomed 4,
  technical characteristics of, 168
  technical details of, 156
NARKUP, 73
Neff's circulator, 8
Nitrogen,
  accumulation of, 196
  levels of during closed system
      anaesthesia, 69
  monitoring of concentration, 176
Nitrous oxide,
  atmospheric levels of, 98
  consumption, in rebreathing cf.
      non-rebreathing systems, 88
  first use, 20

flow
  calculation in low flow
      banaesthesia, 58
  in closed system anaesthesia, 62
  implications for anaesthetic practice
      in, 42
  indications for its use, 278
  low flow anaesthesia without,
      269–279
  monitoring of concentration,
      182–183
  uptake, 41
  calculation of, 42
  changes during anaesthesia, 43
  use as a carrier gas, 269–270
  use in dentistry, 23
  wash-in phase, 43
  workplace concentration limits of,
      97
Non-quantitative closed system
      anaesthesia, 68–70
  characteristics of, 57
  definition, 56
Non-rebreathing systems,
  advantages of, 15
  concentration maintenance of
      volatile anaesthetics in, 45
  disadvantages of, 15
  elimination of exhaled gases in, 5
  excessive rebreathing in, 6
  flow-controlled, 2–7
      classification of by technical
          aspects, 13
      development of, 20
  gas consumption in cf. rebreathing
      systems, 88
  recommended fresh gas flows for, 6
  valve-controlled, 7
      classification of by technical
          aspects, 13
      development of, 19

Obesity,
  effect on gas uptake, 80
  influence on oxygen consumption, 39
Occupational health in the future, 281
Ohio vaporizer, 117
Open breathing systems,
  classification of, 11
  development of, 18
Overdose, accidental with volatile
      anaesthetics, risk of with
      reduced fresh gas flow, 194

Oxford Vaporizer, 20
Oxygen,
  pure as a future carrier gas, 285–286
  concentration in minimal flow
      anaesthesia without nitrous
      oxide, 272
  consumption, 38
    calculation of, 38
    in closed system anaesthesia, 62
    influencing factors, 38
  flow in low flow anaesthesia, 58
  flow in minimal flow anaesthesia, 60
  implications for anaesthetic practice
      in, 39
  inspired concentration of during low
      flow anaesthesia, 227–231
  levels of during closed system
      anaesthesia, 69
  maintenance of adequate supply in
      minimal flow anaesthesia, 61
  monitoring of concentration, 176,
      178–179
  uptake, 38
    calculation of, 38
    cf. nitrous oxide uptake, 40
Oxygen ratio controller, 113, 116
Ozone,
  effect of nitrous oxide on, 99
  effect of volatile anaesthetics on,
      99–100

Paediatric anaesthesia, 259–263
Patient care, future improvements in,
      286
Patient monitoring, improvements in,
      107
Penlon coaxial system, 3, 4
Penlon PPV Sigma vaporizer, 117
Pharmacokinetics of anaesthetic gases,
      38–52
Photoacoustic spectrometry, use in
      monitoring of volatile
      anaesthetic concentration,
      179
PhysioFlex system, 8, 70
  technical characteristics of, 168
  technical details of, 164, 165
  vaporization in, 121
Pollution,
  atmospheric levels of inhalation
      anaesthetics, 98–100
  environmental protection in the
      future, 281

workplace concentration limits of
    inhalation anaesthetics, 97
workplace exposure to anaesthetic
    gases, 96–98
Potassium hydroxide, use in carbon
    dioxide absorption, 9
Pre-medication,
  in minimal flow anaesthesia, 254
  in minimal flow anaesthesia without
      nitrous oxide, 272
  techniques in low flow anaesthesia,
      225
prEN ISO, 4135 1

Quantitative closed system anaesthesia,
    70
  characteristics of, 57
  definition, 56

Rebreathing, excessive, 6
Rebreathing systems,
  absorbers used, 7
  advantages of, 30, 15, 88–107
    reduction of gas consumption, 88
    circle absorption system, 3, 8
  classification of, 12
  design of, 54
  development of, 18-35
  disadvantages of, 31, 15
  early Kuhn system, 24
  effect of fresh gas flow on oxygen
      concentration in inspired gas
      in, 40, 41
  fresh gas flow rate and fraction
      rebreathed, 54
  fresh gas flow rates in, 14
  role of fresh gas flow in action of, 32
  to-and-fro absorption system, 3, 8
Recovery, after minimal flow anaes-
    thesia, 255
Regulations, technical, 111
Revell's circulator, 8
Risks,
  attributable to inadequate technical
      equipment,
    accidental airway pressure
        increase, 193
    accidental anaesthetic overdose, 194
    carbon dioxide accumulation, 193
    hypoventilation, 192
    hypoxia, 191
  attributable to reduction of fresh gas
      flow,

Risks (*cont.*)
   accumulation of foreign gases,
      196–207
   long time constant, 195
causes of incidents, 212
reduction of, 212

SA 2,
   technical characteristics of, 168
   technical details of, 156, 157
Safety, 191–214
   absorbant exhaustion and, 96
   artefacts in capnogram when
      monitoring carbon dioxide,
      183–185
   causes of incidents, 212
   contraindications for low flow
      anaesthesia, 213–214
   cost and, 94
   facilities on equipment, 175
   features of modern machines, 35
   features required in inhalation
      anaesthesia machines, 211
   importance of a second monitoring
      device for, 180
   improved knowledge of theory and
      practice, 210
   intermittent manual injection of
      volatile anaesthetics and, 120
   length of time constant in low flow
      anaesthesia as a factor, 208
   misdosage, 181–182
   monitoring of equipment function,
      175
   monitoring of physiological param-
      eters, 175
   monitoring of volatile anaesthetics in
      breathing systems cf. in fresh
      gas flow, 180
   occupational health in the future,
      281
   of changing from low fresh gas flow
      to high flow rates, 180
   reduced fresh gas flow risks,
      accidental airway pressure
         increase, 193
      accidental anaesthetic overdose,
         194
      accumulation of foreign gases,
         196–207
      acetone, 197
      argon, 203
      carbon monoxide, 198–203
      ethanol, 198

      haloalkenes, 204
      hydrogen, 204
      implications of, 206
      methane, 203
      nitrogen, 196
   carbon dioxide accumulation, 193
   hypoventilation, 192
   hypoxia, 191
   long time constant, 195
setting alarm limits with isoflurane
   and position of monitoring
   system, 181
technical regulations for inhalational
   anaesthesia machines, 174
use of multi-gas analysers, 187–188
Schimmelbusch mask, 3
Semi-closed breathing systems,
   classification of, 11
Semi-closed rebreathing systems,
   development of use, 32
schematic flow diagram of, 33
Semi-open breathing systems,
   classification of, 11
Septicaemia as a contraindication for
   low flow anaesthesia, 214
Servo Anaesthesia System, 118
   technical details of, 158, 159
Servo-ventilator, technical
   characteristics of, 168
Sevoflurane,
   economy and efficiency of, 251
   expired concentrations in minimal
      flow anaesthesia without
      nitrous oxide, 273
   in clinical practice, 241, 245–247
   induction phase levels, 78
   reduced costs in paediatric
      anaesthesia with, 89
   uptake pharmacokinetics of, 93
   use in paediatric anaesthesia, 262
   vaporizers for, 120
Side-stream gas analyser,
   cf. mainstream, 174–176
   zero calibration of, 185
Siemens Anaesthesia system 711,
   technical details of, 158, 160
Siemens vaporizer, 119
Simpson's technique for application of
   chloroform, 19
Smoking, as a contraindication for low
   flow anaesthesia, 214
Snow's closed system, 22
Snow's ether inhaler, 22
Soda lime,
   capacity of, 94, 95

consumption in low flow anaesthesia offsetting savings in gas use, 94

costs of, 95

exhaustion and zero calibration, 186

use in carbon dioxide absorption, 9

utilization time, 96

Sodium thiopental, role in use of cyclopropane, 32

Standardization of breathing system classification, 1

Standards, common European standard for leakage tolerances, 124

Starvation, as a contraindication for low flow anaesthesia, 213

Sulla 800/808, technical characteristics of, 168

Sulla 808 V, flow diagram for, 129

Sulla 909,
technical characteristics of, 168
technical details of, 160, 161

Sword circle absorber system, 31

TEC 4 vaporizer, 117

TEC 5 vaporizer, 117

TEC 6 desflurane vaporizer,
characteristics of, 122
safety features of, 122

TEC 6 vaporizer, 117

Technical developments, 281

Technical regulations, safety features required in inhalation anaesthesia machines, 211

Technical regulations and standards, 111

Technical requirements,
characterisitics of anaesthesia machines, 168
for electronically controlled gas delivery systems, 162
of Access system, 147
of Aestiva, 3000 141
of anaesthetic machines with gas reservoirs, 133
of anaesthetic machines without gas reservoirs, 128
of AS/3 ADU Plus Anaesthesia Delivery Unit, 142, 145
of breathing systems, 123
of carbon dioxide absorbers, 126
of Cato workstation, 143, 145
of Cicero EM workstation, 143, 146

of Dogma system, 147
of EAS, 9010 149
of electronic control of fresh gas flow, 140
of electronic control of ventilator performance, 140
of ELSA, 149
of Excel SE, 155
of Fabius, 151
of fresh gas decoupling valve, 139
of gas flow control systems, 112
of Julian system, 151
of Megamed, 700 153, 154
of Mivolan, 153
of Modulus SE, 155
of Narkomat, 147
of Narkomed, 4 156
of PhysioFlex, 164, 165
of SA, 2 156, 157
of Servo Anaesthesia system, 158, 159
of Siemens Anaesthesia system, 711 158, 160
of specific anaesthetic machines, 141–162
of Sulla, 909 160, 909 161
of system volumes, 161
of vaporizers, 116
of ventilators, 128
of ventilators without fresh gas flow compensation, 135

regulations and safety facilities, 174

Temperature,
influence on oxygen consumption, 38
of body during anaesthesia, 105
in closed cf. semi-closed system, 106
of breathing gas during anaesthesia, 101–103

Terminology,
classification by fresh gas flow rate cf. by degree of rebreathing, 54
standardization of, 1

Time constant, 80-84
calculation of, 83
in minimal flow cf. high flow anaesthesia, 82
reduction of fresh gas flow and increased, 195
role in wash-in and wash-out processes, 83
safety implications of increased length when using low flow rates, 208

To-and-fro absorption system, 3
To-and-fro rebreathing system,
    development of, 21
    Jackson's, 26
    leakage tolerances for, 123
    Water's, 27
Total gas uptake, 51–52
Training, 212

Ulmer-Kreissystem circle absorption
    system for use in paediatric
    anaesthesia, 260

Valve-controlled non-rebreathing
    systems, classification of by
    technical aspects, 13
    development of, 19
    fresh gas flow rates in, 14
Vaporizers, 116–123
    discussion of requirement for, 121
    early, 32
    effect on isoflurane concentration,
        66–67
    evaporation cf. vaporization, 116
    limitations on output of, 120-121
    maximum output of, 64
    precision of, 117-119
    problems with use of, 65
    'pumping' effect of, 118
    requirements for, 118
    specified range of operation of, 121
    technical requirements of, 116
    types of, 64
    use in closed system anaesthesia, 64
Ventilation,
    changes in patterns of, risk of with
        reduced fresh gas flow, 192
    reduced and airway pressure, 130
    reduced and ventilation, 130
Ventilator 711, technical characteristics
    of, 168
Ventilators,
    Air-Shields ventilator, 133
    AV-E system, 131
    bag-in-bottle type, 134
    bellows-in-box design, 128
    bellows-in-box type, 133
    differentiation of, 128
    electronic control of performance,
        140
    fresh gas decoupling valve, 140
    gas reservoir,

    anaesthetic machines with,
        133–135
    anaesthetic machines without,
        128–132
    pressure and fresh gas flow, 132
    Sulla 808 V anaesthetic machine, 129
    technical details of, 128
    with fresh gas decoupling valve, 134
    without fresh gas flow
        compensation, 135
Ventilog anaesthetic ventilator, 135
Virtue scheme for control of
    anaesthesia, 80
Volatile anaesthetics,
    accidental overdose with, risk of
        with reduced fresh gas flow,
        194
    annual consumption of, 90
    atmospheric pollution with, 98–100
    Brody formula, 46
    computer simulation programs of
        uptake and distribution, 74
    control of concentration during low
        flow anaesthesia, 238
    cost of gases as a function of fresh
        gas flow, 92
    cumulative dose, 47
    future developments in, 282–286
        oxygen, 285
        xenon, 282–285
    implications for anaesthetic practice,
        50
    improving gas climate for, 100–107
    injection of in closed system
        anaesthesia, 63
    intermittent manual injection of and
        safety, 120
    Lin uptake model, 48
    Lowe uptake model, 46
    measurement techniques, 179
    metering of during low flow
        anaesthesia, 231–238
    monitoring of concentration,
        179–182
        in fresh gas cf. in breathing
            system, 180
        techniques for, 179
    pharmacokinetics of, 44
    positioning of sensors for gas
        concentration measurements,
        175
    priming dose, 47
    reduced consumption of in high flow
        cf. minimal flow anaesthesia,
        89

techniques for changing
        concentration of, 120
time-course of uptake, 49
transport of in body, 44
unit dose, 47
uptake of, 44–50
wastage rate, 94
Westenkow uptake model, 48
workplace concentration limits of, 97

Wash-in phase, 43
Wash-in process and time constant, 83

Wash-out process and time constant,
        83
Water condensation within hosing, 249
Westenkow uptake model, 48

Xenon, as a future anaesthetic,
        282–285

Zero calibration, 185
Zuntz equation, 45